"Catherine Taylor's voice is strong and su[...] subject shines through. Not only is her w[...] the discussion of how to best and most [...] but it is compelling and moving, beautifully wrought with her own story fluidly integrated. I trust her as a guide through this miraculous terrain and so, I'm sure, will mothers, potential mothers, and anyone interested in women's health."

—Peggy Orenstein, author of *Flux: Women on Sex, Work, Love, Kids, and Life in a Half-Changed World*

"*Giving Birth* is one of the most important books on childbirth. It should be read by aspiring and experienced midwives, hospital administrators, and every parent considering midwifery care. Catherine Taylor exposes the two faces of modern midwifery, taking readers on a colorful, anecdotal, and research-supported journey from both the mothers' and midwives' perspectives. *Giving Birth* serves us in the present, and will become a classic in midwifery-medical history for future generations."

—Pam England, nurse-midwife and author of *Birthing from Within: An Extra-Ordinary Guide to Childbirth Preparation*

"This is a really good read, written from a radical perspective. Catherine Taylor tackles some of the urgent questions about birth in our technocratic culture, bravely, and no-holds-barred."

—Sheila Kitzinger, author of *Rediscovering Birth*

"Combining both style and substance, Taylor deftly weaves together interviews, observation, the medical research, and her own evolution during her second pregnancy. This superb, inside look at the forces controlling U.S. maternity care is a 'must-read' for any woman who wants a safe and satisfying pregnancy and birth experience, and who wants to know why she is unlikely to get it without careful thought and planning."

—Henci Goer, author of *The Thinking Woman's Guide to a Better Birth*

Giving Birth

A Journey into the World of
Mothers and Midwives

Catherine Taylor

A Perigee Book

All names have been changed except for the midwives at the
Northern New Mexico Women's Health and Birth Center.

A Perigee Book
Published by The Berkley Publishing Group
A division of Penguin Putnam Inc.
375 Hudson Street
New York, New York 10014

Copyright © 2002 by Catherine Taylor
Text design by Tiffany Kukec
Cover design and art by Kiley Thompson

First edition: August 2002

Visit our website at www.penguinputnam.com

Library of Congress Cataloging-in-Publication Data
Taylor, Catherine, 1947–
Giving birth : a journey into the world of mothers
and midwives / by Catherine Taylor.
Includes index.
ISBN 0-399-52788-5
1. Midwives. 2. Midwives—Miscellanea. I. Title.
RG950 .T39 2002
618.2'0233—dc21
2001055157

Printed in the United States of America
10 9 8 7 6 5 4 3 2 1

For my midwife
and for my children, Maxwell and Emrys

CONTENTS

Acknowledgments   ix

Introduction: Beginnings   1

PART ONE
Prenatal/Conception

1. Shifting Ground: Midwives in the Hospital   19

2. In the Clinic   39

3. The Managed Midwife   69

PART TWO
First Trimester

4. Medical Midwives   95

5. Balancing Acts   129

6. Doula School:
   How Birth Attendants Soften the Blow   143

7. Home Birth   172

8. Choosing   185

PART THREE
Second Trimester

9. Challenges   205

10. "With Women"   221

PART FOUR
Third Trimester

11. Reaching the Summit:
    A Birth Center Fights for Families   239

12. Childbirth 101   270

13. An Earth Day Birthday   282

    Conclusions   292
    Notes   301
    Resources   311
    Index   315

ACKNOWLEDGMENTS

THIS book would not exist without the many generous women who allowed me into their lives: midwives, doulas, and mothers. Although I cannot name them all, I am particularly grateful to the midwives who went out of their way to include me in their work and to introduce me to their clients in such a way that made us all feel comfortable throughout the intimacy of birth. I am especially indebted to Susan Moore Daniels, an extraordinary individual, who reminded me not to lose sight of the magic in midwifery.

Looking back to the beginnings of this book, I would like to thank Celeste Frasier for her ardent, unapologetic feminism; her zest for life; and for first introducing me to midwifery through her passionately shared pregnancy. The midwives at the Durham Women's Clinic opened a door into a previously unknown world and made my first pregnancy especially sweet. Thanks as well to the Women's Studies Program at Duke University for their benevolent support of students and alumna.

Many thanks to Professor Leah Albers, whose rigorous research grounds the profession of midwifery, whose passionate commitment to the health of birthing women is inspirational, and whose critical eye helped keep my medical descriptions precise—although she is, of course, not responsible for any errors.

Thanks also to Jennifer Norden for her careful reading of my manuscript. Of the many researchers whose endeavors inform this book, I benefited greatly from Judith Pence Rooks's masterful work *Midwifery and Childbirth in America* and Pam England's insightful book *Birthing from Within: An Extra-Ordinary Guide to Childbirth Preparation*.

I am grateful to my agent, Heide Lange, whose enthusiasm for the subject and for my book made all the difference, to her assistant, Esther Sung, for her gracious facilitation of the process, and to my editor, Sheila Curry Oakes, and her assistant, Terri Hennessy.

Crucial to my efforts were my friends Eva-Lynn Jagoe, David Thomson, and Alden Bumstead, whose keen intellects, steadfast support, and constant love kept me going. Elaine Valby and Michael Hudock gave all of that as well as teaching me much about life, art, and commitment. An extra-special thanks to Peggy Orenstein for her encouragement, her friendship, and the example of her life and work.

I am indebted to my children's teachers and baby-sitters, who cared for them so well, especially Dana McCabe and the teachers and staff of Escuela del Sol Montessori, Kenna Josephene, and Vicky Ayala.

Finally, my gratitude and love to my family: to my parents, who taught me about the power of words and provided a room with a view; to Richard Milner, for standing by me, believing in me, and caring so well for me and for our children; and to my children, Max and Emrys, who suffered through my absences while I was writing and whose births are at the heart of this book and my life.

Beginnings

From behind a door, somewhere down the hall, comes a tiny but penetrating noise. A high-pitched mewling, a small animal sound, it is unmistakably the repeated rhythmic cry of a newborn baby. At once demanding and tender, it carries little identifiable emotional content. It is not quite the sound of despair, or rage, or anguish, or sorrow. It is a declaration song of existence and need. I am surprised by the mix of feelings it elicits. I'm thrilled by the sudden announcement of a new soul in our midst and relieved that the cry is received, here in the hospital, with a calm that signals all is well. I also feel a surge of jealousy and desire. This new baby is not mine, but I want one. I knew that I wanted a baby long before I heard this muffled wail; the sudden sharpness of my response merely confirms my yearning to be pregnant.

I do have a child—Max. He is beautiful, difficult, funny, challenging, and a source of incredible love. When he turned three, his babyhood started to seem like a thing of the past. I was thrilled to have conversations with him, glad to be able to reason with him, and fascinated to learn about the world through his eyes. But I found myself missing some of the joys of his early days. I missed the cuddles, the nursing, the warm, soft lump of baby. I began to wonder if he would be the only baby I would ever have. I started to dream of another one.

My life conspired against my desire. I was trying to finish my Ph.D., teach part-time, and raise a sparkling three-year-old. I had no time for a baby. Still, I yearned. I daydreamed about my next child. A boy or a girl? What would he look like? What lullabies would she want to hear—over and over? I had to stop myself from dreaming. I had finally started to write again, even if it was only my dissertation. Wouldn't a baby put an end to my degree and my dreams of writing? Besides, our family life as a threesome was already so full. And travel, already difficult, would become much harder and more expensive. I should be content.

When Max was almost four and I had finally finished my doctoral degree, I thought I would take some time to enjoy life beyond graduate school and not worry about whether or not to have another baby. But in the same week that I defended my dissertation, I found a lump in my left breast. It was like a tiny pebble or a dried pea.

I couldn't believe it. It hadn't been there the day before, had it? I spent all day rolling it under my fingers, willing it to disappear. When the sick feeling in the pit of my stomach and the evidence under my fingers didn't go away, I called the doctor. She scheduled a mammogram and sonogram appointment for the next day. The results weren't good. The doctors recommended an immediate biopsy. I called my friend Addie who had had breast cancer in her mid-thirties, and cried. She calmed me down and soothed my ragged nerves by telling me of all the friends she knew who had lumps that were not cancerous, and by reading to me from Susan Love's *Breast Book* about what to expect with a core biopsy.

After the biopsy, awaiting the results, I cried and cried, thinking that if I have cancer, my son might be raised without me. He probably won't even remember me. He needs to have his mother around for a lot longer, I sobbed. And then, the thought that I might never have another child jolted through me. Faced with this possibility, I found I desperately wanted a baby.

I wanted those moments of incredible tenderness that an infant brings. I wanted more of the love that having a baby brought into my life—mine for my child, my child's for me, and the love that the entire family shares. I also wanted Max to have a sibling. I wanted him to have the companionship I have with my own brother, the sense that, at least biologically, I am not alone in the world. I wanted to be special again in the way that pregnant women are special, taking up space in the world, my power written on my body, people smiling at my belly, holding doors, and offering seats (even as I want to reject the stereotype of the weak female). And despite the pain and fear of my first labor and childbirth, I wanted to have the primal power of birth thrust upon me again. Perhaps I wanted this because, unlike most of life's endeavors, there is no question of the importance, the significance, and the profundity of birth. Mostly, I just had a deep, powerful, and unreasoned yearning for a baby. I was a little surprised by the power and surety I felt. Suddenly my ambivalence about upsetting the carefully orchestrated pattern of my life disappeared. Sitting in the surgeon's office, I knew that if I didn't have cancer, I only wanted one thing—not to live each day as if it were my last—but to have another child as soon as possible. When I told my surgeon this, she shook her head and told me to wait until I knew the test results.

Finally, after two days of anguished waiting, the results came back. The lump was benign. No cancer. I could try to get pregnant. I was flooded with relief—and a newfound purpose in life.

After only a few months, I began consulting the calendar incessantly. Not the calendar that told me it was June in the southwest. I felt the windy dust storms of spring tapering off. I saw the cottonwood leaves turning from light, silvery green to a darker emerald shade, just in time for the hot, dry blast of summer. No, I focused instead on my internal almanac. Excited by ovulation, depressed by the first drop of blood, I wondered if I had waited too long. At thirty-four, was I too old? I knew this was ridiculous, but my desire for another child escalated fiercely and become entangled with a host of ready anxieties. I consoled myself by remembering that should I get pregnant, I would also get tired, and cranky, and volatile, and that should I have a baby, I would not be as mobile. This was a good time to work.

I decided to write about childbirth and midwifery, and I was determined to do so while I still had the time and energy. I had my first child with a midwife, and it was an experience that enriched my understanding of birth and opened a window into a world of traditional women's work redefining itself in modern society. Midwives offer a wealth of stories that are personal, political, life-affirming, and even death-defying. But more than anything else, my experience with midwives revealed to me that childbirth in the United States is shockingly behind the rest of the western world when it comes to both the physical and emotional health of mothers and babies. I wanted to find out more about midwifery for both personal and professional reasons. I wanted to get a glimpse into the world of these dedicated women and give others a portrait of their working lives. I wanted to know if they can provide the birth experience I sought for myself, should I get pregnant. And I wanted to know how are they changing the landscape and challenging the status quo of birth in America.

⌒

I had my first baby with a certified nurse-midwife (CNM) in a hospital in North Carolina. I had always assumed I would have an obstetrician, because that was all I had ever really heard of. But then a fellow graduate student and friend of mine—young, single, energetic, feminist, and very hip—became pregnant and had her baby with a midwife. She raved about their women-centered attitude, the length of time they spent with her at prenatal exams, and their stand against unnecessary interventions such as performing episiotomies to aid delivery (midwives are, in fact, four times less likely to cut an episiotomy than doctors, and episiotomies have never been shown to either improve the health of babies or decrease genital trauma in mothers).[1] My friend's experience sounded rewarding, so when I became pregnant a year later, at the age of thirty, I gave her midwives a call. The nine months I spent with the midwives in that practice proved to be not only an introduction to a remarkable group of women and their timeless profession, but also an experience that profoundly changed my ideas about childbirth. This book began with that experience.

The particular midwives I went to were a group of certified nurse-midwives who worked with an ob-gyn practice. The practice was affiliated with a local hospital, and you could have your prenatal exams and your delivery with a midwife as long as you had no complications. If anything unusual should occur, one of the obstetricians in the practice would take over your case. I figured a certified nurse-midwife in a hospital was the best-case scenario. I would receive all the expertise and equipment of a hospital if anything went wrong, but I would also benefit from the loving, constant care of a midwife during labor—someone who wouldn't arrive ten minutes before the baby was born, as I had heard was common with obstetricians. I learned, however, that I couldn't choose which midwife would attend my delivery, but I would get whoever was on call, and this bothered me a little. I decided to schedule prenatal appointments with all of the five or six midwives in the practice so at least I wouldn't be attended by a complete stranger.

At the time, I knew nothing about direct-entry midwives, sometimes called lay midwives, or how they differ from certified nurse-midwives. Simply put, certified nurse-midwives have a formal education with a nursing background, and direct-entry midwives usually come to the profession through a series of apprenticeships. With few exceptions, only nurse-midwives can practice in hospitals, and 95 percent of all midwife-attended births in the United States are by certified nurse-midwives. Some states have a licensing process for direct-entry midwives; some do not; and in some states this form of midwifery is illegal. Home birth was unlawful (although available as many women actively sought it out) in North Carolina at the time of my pregnancy, but it never occurred to me to have a home birth. It was already a big step for me not to have an obstetrician.

My decision to choose a midwife over an obstetrician was not a rejection of modern western medicine. I have had a number of positive experiences with modern medicine, including some fairly high-tech lung surgery which might have saved my life and definitely improved my quality of life. I was also working on a doctoral degree at a prestigious institution where science and technology, if not worshipped as gods, are certainly the most trusted realm of faith. And I am a physician's daughter. Although my father passed on a healthy dose of skepticism concerning the status of doctors, the medical profession itself was never seriously questioned. I opted for this alternative because I thought it would fulfill my long-held ideas about childbirth as a time for a particularly compassionate form of health care as well as an opportunity for empowerment.

I came of age when natural childbirth was having a resurgence and when feminism was demanding more from women's health care, including the care of birthing women. *Our Bodies, Ourselves* was one of the first books I purchased by myself as a young adult. I was too young to be a participant in the women's movement of the sixties and seventies, but I was an heir to their work. So when I arrived at my own childbearing years, I didn't assume that I would or should have children, but I did have a sense of entitlement to a birth experience that would include the highest-quality medical care, respect for myself as an individual, and at least the potential for a transformative, spiritual experience. I had high expectations.

My prenatal exams with the midwives were a comforting mix of information, attention, affection, and anticipation. Each month I looked forward to the next visit when I would spend thirty minutes chatting with one of the midwives about anything to do with my pregnancy, upcoming labor and delivery, or baby care. I loved arriving at their clinic with the oh-so-southern rocking chairs on the front porch, and I loved being part of the club of pregnant moms gathered there. I loved being connected to this age-old tradition. (One historian has proposed that the practice of midwifery is three or four million years old, dating back to when we humans switched to an upright posture.[2] Certainly it has been around since biblical times and before.) I confess that I also loved being part of something I saw as alternative. I relished announcing to the receptionist, "I'm a *midwife* patient." I became so comfortable with the idea of midwifery that I was surprised whenever people asked me, "Who's your doctor?" and I needed to explain midwifery to them.

My husband and I drove to a neighboring town to go to an alternative childbirth class, instead of simply taking the one the hospital offered. I practiced my breathing, my visualizations, and my mantras. But I had no idea how much labor would hurt. So when I found myself well into the merciless pain of labor, endlessly repeating one of the phrases we had learned in class ("The wave always hits the shore. The wave always hits the shore. The wave . . .") with a desperation I had never before experienced, I panicked. I felt as if I was drowning under those waves, and entering some dangerous mental zone from which I might never return. I stuffed myself into the small bathtub that the hospital had advertised as a soothing Jacuzzi. (They didn't mention that the water level in the tub wouldn't cover a large, pregnant belly, and, being so shallow, certainly wouldn't provide any buoyancy or much pain relief.) Then I threw up.

Feeling miserable, I cried. "They've got to help me! I need something!" I begged my husband to get some help. "Okay, okay," he muttered, looking around the prettily wallpapered hospital room. Where was our midwife? Where was the woman I was sure was going to be right there with me the whole time, focused on me and my pain, helping me through it, urging me on, encouraging me to stick it out a little longer, telling me I could do it? She was nowhere to be seen.

Other women were giving birth in that hospital that night, too, and our midwife, the only one on call, was alternately checking on them and then sitting at the nurses' station, writing up her notes, until one of us called for her. So when I first called out for help, she was too busy to come to me, then she was on a meal break, and when she finally did arrive, her first response to my pleas was to set up an intravenous drip, or IV, full of pain medicine. She had already inserted a "hep lock," an IV needle with a little cartridge ready to take the IV tubing, when I first arrived, "just in case." I had had to be careful whenever I moved, because bumping it hurt like crazy and threatened to knock it out. "Plus," she said now, "since your cervix has been at six centimeters for two hours and you've been in labor for five hours, let's give you some Pitocin to make your contractions stronger." At the time, I was in no mood to argue, and it did seem like I had been in pain forever, but now I know that two hours without a change in cervical dilation hardly constitutes being "stuck," and five hours is actually quite fast to have reached six centimeters for a first-time mom. What I didn't fully realize then is that I was "on the clock," as they say in labor and delivery wards; I had become subject to the standardized, time-based protocols of the hospital.

My water had broken the day before, and even though I was in active labor (spurred on by the downing of a "castor-oil cocktail," a natural labor-inducer often used by midwives, which the local pharmacist dispensed at his soda fountain, saying in a southern drawl, "Now, don't sip it like a fine wine"), the hospital's policy of giving intravenous antibiotics eighteen hours after one's water has broken was upon us. Because they were getting ready to give me an IV anyway, adding a pain killer and some Pitocin was easy to do. Also, it was past the supper-hour, and because my midwife was responsible for several other birthing women, she may well have been trying to ward off a difficult middle of the night for herself by speeding my labor along. This was not an entirely unreasonable move for her, given that she needed to be fresh enough to help with a number of deliveries.

As for me, I just wanted to be rescued from the bottom of the deep well of pain and fear I seemed to have fallen into. I wanted it all to be over, so I said, "Yes, okay, yes, let's do the Pitocin and the drugs." Promptly, a nurse appeared, bustled me over to the bed, and insisted I take off the loose, cotton dress I was wearing. "But this is what I want to wear," I protested. "Oh, no. It will just get all bloody," she said. "I know. That's why I chose it," I replied, gesturing toward its dark, purple and red swirls. "Its okay with me. Really," I managed to say, as another contraction began its unbearable pull. The nurse shook her head and said, "Just take it off." Defeated, I put on the thin, ugly, institutional, gray and blue hospital gown she held out to me. Then, as she reached to put the IV into my arm, I remembered to say, "You do know that I'm allergic to Demerol, right? It's in my chart." With a quick yank, she jerked the IV away. Frowning, she looked at my chart and then disappeared to find a different drug. "Oh God," I moaned, as the next contraction bore down on me.

The drugs didn't touch the pain. They only made me feel semi-conscious, disconnected, and lost between contractions. And yet there were positive moments. Our midwife reminded us to play the music we had brought with us, and listening to the warble of the dashboard-melted tape we had played on our honeymoon six years earlier was nice. Also, at one point when I was feeling especially miserable, the midwife looked me in the eyes and said, "You can do this," with such force that I believed her and regained a certain equilibrium, if not control.

Eventually, the drugs I had been given seemed to wear off, and around the same time my midwife said my cervix was almost completely dilated so I could try a push if I liked. I did, and it hurt like hell, but I was glad to have something to do and glad to be close to the end. At least now I felt more alert and active, even though I was yelling "It hurts! It hurts!" to anyone who would listen. I pushed for forty minutes with the nursing staff and the midwife yelling the whole time, "Push! Push! Hold your breath, tuck down, and push!! Puuush!!!" It seemed so loud, and violent, and urgent, as if the baby was in trouble. But the baby's heartbeat was fine, I hadn't had a long labor, and the length of my pushing phase was well within the range of normal.[3]

Occasionally, I would remember my child-birth class and the teacher's advice to "think of opening like a flower and breathing the baby out," and then I would cheat. Instead of holding my breath, I would let it escape noiselessly while happily picturing my baby's head crowning through a pink rose like some sweet flower-fairy. I felt guilty about this for years, wondering if I could have gotten him out faster if only I'd followed directions. Now I know that research shows that holding your breath excessively, in what is called "Valsalva pushing," can actually deny necessary oxygen to the baby (holding it just for a few seconds is preferable), and slow pushing in an unhurried atmosphere is more likely to prevent tearing.[4] Nonetheless, practitioners—doctors, nurses, childbirth educators, and even some midwives—don't always base their practice on current research. Often, they rely on their own education and the traditions of the hospital, which may be outdated. So I'm glad I "cheated" when pushing.

Finally, there was the burning agony of my baby's head crowning; seconds that seemed to last forever. Then, suddenly, the head was out, and all the pain began to subside. One last push and my baby's body slithered out—wet and gooey and covered with creamy white vernix, making him look like a deep-sea creature or a pale clown with ruby red lips. Apparently, my one dose of drugs four hours earlier had had little effect on him, because he was wide awake, eyes open and alert. As he was passed up to me, I pulled off the hospital gown and held him to my bare chest, both of us crying softly. He was so beautiful and so amazing, I couldn't stop smiling. A boy. My beautiful baby boy.

It was a wonderful moment, but soon it was time for the midwife to sew me up where I had torn. While she stitched, I remember telling my husband quite clearly, "We are never doing this again." Then it was time for our baby to be cleaned, weighed, and hustled off to the nursery. We had asked for "rooming in," where the baby would stay with us all the time, but were told now, for the first time, that the hospital could not allow him to be with us while we slept. Somebody would have to be awake at all times in order for him to stay with us, and as it was after midnight, it was clear that wasn't going to happen. So away he went, a first separation that opened a hole in my heart, and who knows what dark fears in my tiny newborn. The hospital had also told us that my husband could stay the night with me, but now it turned out that there were no rooms with extra beds or pull-out couches available. If he wanted to stay, he'd have to sleep on the floor. I begged the nurse to find us something. Finally, an hour and a half later, she turned up with a reclining chair to use as a make-shift bed. Exhausted, we slept.

⌒

By most standards, my birthing experience was a good one. My labor took a very typical twelve hours, there were no complications, I had minimal use of pain-killers and no emergency caesarean, I was an active participant in the process, and my baby was born healthy and whole. So why did I feel so disappointed? Why did I feel shattered by the pain? In the weeks following his birth, why did I find myself resenting my baby for putting me through such hell? How could I be so unreasonable?

In part, I think the answer lies in the fact that there is no preparation for the pain of childbirth. Years later I read Maren Hansen's insightful book, *Mother Mysteries,* and felt a lovely shock of recognition when she said, "No woman, personally or in the dozens of books I had read, adequately conveyed the terror, excruciating pain, and trauma of childbirth. They called it nice names like, 'hard work.'" Hansen adds, "women are disgustingly, pathologically nice and cheerful, not to mention liars." In part, I think my experience of disappointment also grew out of unfulfilled expectations. Because my prenatal visits were so satisfying—unhurried, comprehensive examinations of my body, my emotional life, and my ideas about parenting—I thought I would get the same kind of thorough attention at the birth. I expected my midwife to be with me throughout my labor, not just some of the time. And while I know that she was with me more than most doctors would have been, she gave me far less attention than I had anticipated. I do realize that even if she had been there, ultimately, I still had to give birth on my own. Nobody could do it for me. But the truth is that research has shown that the mere presence of a supportive, well-trained individual dramatically shortens labor, decreases the caesarean rate by 50 percent, decreases the need for forceps, and generally improves delivery outcomes for both mothers and babies.[5] Without such a person, I felt abandoned and vulnerable.

During my pregnancy, I was happy to tell people what a midwife is and what she does. After I gave birth, I realized that I didn't really know. I went to the library and found a number of wonderful books on historical midwifery, traditional granny midwives, midwives who serve the Amish, and resplendently spiritual, hippie midwives, but I found nothing that spoke to my experience and nothing that gave a broader picture of contemporary working midwives. So I began the research for this book. What I found was an extraordinarily diverse group of practitioners, most of whom share certain common goals: to respect birthing women, to treat pregnancy and birth as normal and natural situations (as opposed to the medical model's assumption of pregnancy and birth as pathological, i.e., as times of sickness and potential danger), to promote family-centered care, to treat the whole woman (not just her uterus), and—in differing degrees from one situation to the next—to avoid unnecessary medical interventions. I also found that the environment in which midwives work—hospitals, birth centers, government-run health clinics, or their clients' homes—all have tremendous power to influence the role of the midwife.

The dozens of midwives I interviewed and observed during my year of research were an eclectic and fascinating group. Whether they lived in the city and worked at a high-tech hospital or lived out in the mountains serving rural populations, they were never easy to categorize. Each woman's personality profoundly influenced the way she practiced, and each one approached the serious social and political obstacles facing midwives' reentry into the mainstream of birthing care with a different attitude and strategy. They all seemed to be both throwbacks to the past and modern pioneers in women's health care—competent professionals who are trained to provide compassionate, individualized care, and women embroiled in bitter political battles over the rights of birthing women to decent and caring medical services.

For more than a year, I followed a number of these midwives, trained as a birth assistant (or doula), and attended dozens of births, becoming a part of a community of birthing women and their attendants. I also read a great deal about childbirth, including the relevant medical literature. What I discovered was that, after spending several years thinking I could have avoided disappointment in my own birthing experience by expecting less, I should have, in fact, expected more—and so should all birthing women in America.

The United States currently ranks twenty-second in the world in maternal and infant mortality and morbidity rates.[6] This means that mothers and their infants are safer at birth nearly anywhere else in the industrialized world than they are in the United States, in spite of the fact that we spend more per capita on birthing women than any other nation. In western European countries, where infant mortality rates are lower than in the United States, midwives attend 75 percent of births; in America, midwives attend only 7 percent of births (although in some states, as many as 20 percent of births are attended by midwives).[7] The countries with the best statistics on maternal and infant well-being are those that have national health-care systems that allow universal access to care and rely heavily on midwifery care.

Great Britain has approximately thirty-five thousand midwives and only a few thousand obstetricians, with more than 75 percent of births attended by midwives; the United States has approximately six thousand nurse-midwives and about thirty-three thousand obstetricians.[8] Probably the most frequently cited example of a country with an excellent record of successful birth outcomes and a high proportion of midwives is the Netherlands. The Dutch have the lowest percentage of babies and mothers who die or are injured during childbirth. They also have the lowest rate of medical intervention during deliveries. Seventy percent of their births are attended by midwives, and one in three take place at home.[9]

International comparisons are notoriously difficult, with so many socio-cultural differences to account for. Some people argue that our poor international standing is because the United States is more like a third world in its ethnic and immigrant populations than these other countries. But this is still no excuse for one of the richest countries in the world to have such low standards of care for birthing women and their infants. Shockingly, the National Center for Health Statistics reports that the maternal death rate per 100,000 births for black women in New York is now 28.7, as compared with a still disappointing national average of 8.4 (Canadian rates are around 5.4, and Dutch rates are even lower).[10] It should be noted that of the countries that have better outcomes for their mothers and children than the United States, 100 percent provide universal prenatal care, while a number of Americans receive little or no prenatal care.[11]

A recent study showed that, after controlling for social and medical risk factors, "the risk of experiencing an infant death was 19 percent lower for certified nurse-midwife attended births than for physician attended birth, the risk of neonatal mortality [infant death in the first twenty-eight days of life] was 33 percent lower, and the risk of delivering a low birth weight infant 31 percent lower." Low birth weight is significant because it is a major predictor of infant mortality, disease, and developmental disabilities.[12] With statistics this favorable for midwifery, apart from the minority of women who truly need a doctor's medical expertise because of some unusual condition, why are so few American births attended by midwives?

One of the main reasons for the scarcity of midwives in this country is that the twentieth century saw a well-documented, systematic attack on the profession by doctors. For thousands of years, midwives, almost always women, were the primary care givers at birth. Doctors, until recently almost always men, began to dominate the scene only at the end of the nineteenth century. They soon used their institutional power, their power as men in a male-dominated society, and their promise to revolutionize childbirth with the progress they had brought to modern medicine to push midwives to the fringes. But unlike advances in other fields of medicine, advances in childbirth technologies were not of widespread benefit. As midwifery historian Judith Pence Rooks has found, wherever midwives were forced out of practice and doctors took over, more mothers and babies died. In the United States as a whole, as midwifery declined, deaths of babies from birth injuries rose by 44 percent between 1918 and 1925.[13]

Midwives survived the middle part of the century by attending impoverished and indigent women whom most doctors did not want to serve. In fact, attending under-served populations remains an important role of contemporary midwifery. It wasn't until the late 1960s when the natural birth movement and the feminist movement gained momentum and encouraged women to "take back their births" that midwifery began its comeback. One midwife writes, "A mere hundred years ago the midwife was still an important institution everywhere in the world. Today we are renegades, battling for our birthright—to help each other bring forth our babies."[14] With the rise of managed care in the 1980s, midwives' excellent outcomes combined with cost-effectiveness increased their availability and popularity.

In today's climate of medical cost-cutting, you might think that money alone would be a motivating factor in switching over to midwifery care. And in fact, in some places it is. One of the locations I observed was an HMO-run hospital where 95 percent of the vaginal deliveries are now attended by certified nurse-midwives due to the combined appeal of cost-effectiveness and customer satisfaction. Nationwide, midwife-attended births have actually increased tremendously in the last thirty years and have doubled in the last ten years alone.[15] Women appreciate the increased care and attention midwives offer compared to obstetricians, and many mothers who are having uncomplicated pregnancies want the less-invasive birth practices midwives offer.

Even women who want to have drugs for pain-relief available can choose to birth with a midwife. Most midwives working in this country are certified nurse-midwives working in hospitals where epidurals are available to their patients. When people hear I'm working on a book about midwives, they often ask me if I'm anti-epidural, and no, I'm not anti-epidural. I'm no martyr who thinks pain is good for you and that avoiding pain is for wimps. I'm glad to know they're available should I need one. After the agony of my first labor, I was ready to order an epidural then and there for any future labors I might have. I know there are many times when it can significantly aid a woman's labor. But I do wonder if women are being given the whole picture on pain control. What nonpharmaceutical options are available? What is the effect of a well-timed labor massage? How can women use meditation, hypnosis, or other mind-body approaches to prepare themselves in such a way that labor pain might be lessened? Certainly, women are all too rarely offered an epidural's best alternative: continuous, loving support from an experienced childbirth attendant.

I wonder, for myself, what do I trade away spiritually if I trade away pain? What about the way the experience of pain is integrated, or not, after the fact? Can't something hurt like hell and then either continue to wound you or disappear—or even become a source of strength? What is the difference between pain and suffering? What do midwives, women committed to serving birthing mothers, believe about these issues? And what about the whole question of technology at birth? Certainly, technology has a place at some births, but when, and why, and with what risks? Also, if home birth is as safe as studies show it is, why do so few people do it? What if something did go wrong? Is choosing home birth a way of placing the mother's experience over the safety of the baby? Is safety only to be found in the hospital and a positive experience only to be found at home? Or is that a false dichotomy? My list of questions blossomed profusely. This book traces my journey to find answers to these questions as I followed a diverse group of midwives and the path of my own pregnancy.

PART ONE

Prenatal/Conception

Shifting Ground:
Midwives in the Hospital

SKYLINE Hospital sits on the edge of a large southwestern city, wedged between a freeway, a dilapidated strip mall, and a neighborhood spotted with pale brown stucco houses. Surrounding the large, sprawling hospital is a swath of parking lots. During the day, the lots are generally packed. Today, there are even cars filling the area marked "Warning, Not Responsible for Landing Helicopter Damage." Inside, the hospital is cool, quiet, clean, newly carpeted, and surprisingly pleasant. There are framed art posters on the walls and, at least on the first floor, no foul hospital smells.

I am buzzed into Labor and Delivery, or as they call it here, the "Family Birthing Center." It is even more luxurious than the rest of the hospital. An interior designer has been here and left a trail of soothing dark blue, sea green, deep purple, and mauve décor. The hallways have noise-muffling carpet, and the rooms have hardwood floors—no ugly gray institutional vinyl here. The rooms look like hotel suites with their blonde wood furniture, armoires that conceal large televisions, floral sleeper-sofas for overnighting partners, and bathrooms with tubs that can be used to take the edge off labor pains. But on one side of the room is an electronic hospital bed, an IV pole tangled in plastic tubing, and a set of machines and monitors with metal dials, precision graphs, and twitching lights, which remind one that this is still a hospital. Back in the hallway, the lighting is subtle, with only the nurses station glowing in bright, white fluorescent light. So far, everything resembles a typical, newer hospital.

However, at Skyline, 80 percent of all deliveries and 90 percent of vaginal deliveries—more than two thousand yearly—are now attended by midwives. In the 1980s, Skyline decided to add certified nurse-midwives to the staff, a decision based on research that showed midwives provided greater customer satisfaction, lower caesarean rates, lower costs, and better overall outcomes for mothers and babies. The midwives are required to have graduated from an accredited program, be state-licensed as both a registered nurse (RN) and a midwife, and be certified nationally through the American College of Nurse Midwives (ACNM). After making the switch, the staff at Skyline quickly grew from a single midwife to the seventeen midwives employed today, because the department found that they really did live up to their reputation of providing safe, satisfying, and more cost-effective births.

So once I reach the nurses' station, I find an end to the similarities between Skyline and most of its counterparts, for the staff is not the typical mix of doctors and nurses. Instead, with only one doctor on call per shift—and that doctor not always present—nurses and midwives dominate the scene.

⌒

Today I am following nurse-midwife Sarah Walker-Adams. Sarah is in her late thirties, tall, and pretty, with long dark brown hair and apple cheeks that almost hide her sparkly brown eyes when she smiles. She is calm and confident and has a deliberately mellow way of speaking with her voice pitched low. Her hair is pulled back in a braided leather headband. She wears a white lab coat over faded blue jeans, a long-sleeve T-shirt with a Native American design on it, pine green wool clogs with cork soles, and oval wire-rim glasses.

Sarah did her training at the prestigious Yale University midwifery program, but she doesn't let her Ivy League education get in the way of bringing up mystical subjects like fairies, as she does now at the nurses' station. She matter-of-factly tells a story about something she and her daughter saw on a wooded mountaintop. She says it was a watery, nearly transparent shimmer that was "Maybe not a fairy, but definitely something not real." I look around to see how her listeners are taking this, expecting some skeptically raised eyebrows. Nobody bats an eye. Everyone, even the most seasoned nurse, is listening carefully. I suspect they like her. Without missing a beat, she deftly changes the subject and begins to tell me about the women in labor that day, carefully detailing their backgrounds and current medical situations.

Sarah leads me down a teal-colored corridor to check on a woman in early labor, a Hispanic teenager named Leticia. Lettie, as she calls herself, is sixteen years old and is here with her boyfriend and both her parents. Every two or three minutes, as her contractions come, she closes her eyes and breathes slowly and heavily. Sarah chats with Lettie briefly, then checks her cervix. She is three centimeters dilated and 90 percent effaced, meaning her cervix is nearly all the way thinned. Sarah asks if she's taken childbirth classes. Lettie has and says she wants to do natural childbirth, "Even though it hurts."

As another contraction catches Lettie, Sarah tells her, "This is some of the hardest physical work your body will ever do, but your body is made to do it." She then offers some options that might help Lettie—a walk on the hospital's walking track or maybe a warm bath. Having women up and active during labor is something midwives like to do because it keeps labor moving along and helps bring the baby down simply by using the force of gravity. Sarah's offer of a warm bath is a common way midwives provide drug-free pain reduction in labor.

Lettie shifts in the bed, but before she can respond to Sarah's suggestions, another contraction comes. She grabs the bed rail and moans softly. Sarah puts her hands on Lettie's shoulder and says gently, "Try not to tense up your shoulders." Immediately, Lettie visibly relaxes her body.

"Very nice. Good work," says Sarah.

Lettie closes her eyes and breathes hard.

"So, Lettie, what sounds good to you? Do you want to walk?"

"Yeah, and then the bath."

"Okay. I'll come check on you in a little bit," Sarah says. But as we leave the room, Lettie's mother follows us into the hall and catches Sarah by the arm. She looks worried, and asks if, because of her daughter's age, Lettie might be too small for the baby to fit through the birth canal. Sarah smiles and reassures her that this is unlikely to be a problem.

Lettie joins us in the hall and heads slowly toward the walking track. That the hospital offers a walking track, a private bath, and a single room for Lettie's labor, delivery, and recovery is a sign of the improvements many hospitals have made over the past twenty years.

Skyline is not alone in having converted from the usual layout of days gone by when at the eleventh hour (or more accurately, the tenth centimeter) birthing mothers had to be transferred from their labor rooms to sterile and surgical-looking delivery rooms and then to recovery rooms. The 1980s witnessed a definite trend toward providing parents with a more attractive birthing environment, including the genuine improvement of the single labor-delivery-recovery (LDR) room.

In fact, although many hospitals have yet to catch up with this trend, the seventies and eighties saw huge improvements in labor and delivery practices nationwide: in allowing fathers and other family members to attend births, in increased contact between parents and infants, and in more humane forms of anesthesia than the once common "twilight sleep" of morphine and scopolamine. Many of these advances grew out of the prepared childbirth movement (spearheaded by Lamaze followers) and out of the natural childbirth movement that arose in opposition to the, at times, brutal birth practices of the fifties and sixties when women often labored alone, frequently gave birth heavily sedated, birthed without their partners present, and were separated from their babies at birth.

Lettie will benefit from the improvements of the last few decades, but her birth will not be without challenges. As she shambles off, I check my watch. It is early evening, and I've promised my four-year-old that I will come tuck him in, so I leave for home.

⌒

A *few* hours later that night, having tucked my little boy into bed, just before I drift off to sleep, I decide to call the hospital to see what's happening. I pick up the phone, but there is no dial tone, so I hang up, and immediately the phone rings in my hand. It is Sarah, saying she just tried to call me. We laugh at our timing, and she tells me, "Young Lettie has progressed quite fast. It looks like we may have a baby soon. I thought maybe you'd like to come."

I'm on the road in a flash, leaving my child in my husband's care. Back at the hospital, I get buzzed into the Family Birthing Center hallway, and right away I can hear Lettie screaming. I feel my stomach plunge. As I rush into her room, I see her writhing on the bed yelling, "No! No more pain! I can't!" My stomach is instantaneously knotted, and I am overwhelmed by the desire to make her pain go away. I've been observing women here and in one other hospital for a few weeks, and now, suddenly, I understand why I so often hear nurses say, "Are you ready for your epidural yet?" when the woman hasn't even asked for pain medication. It is extremely hard to watch someone hurting.

Lettie's long wavy black hair is tied back in a thick loose braid that makes her look even younger than she is. Curls and wisps escape by the side of her face. She is flushed and, despite her pain, looks extraordinarily beautiful. Her boyfriend, Carlos, a thin young man—a boy really—with a shaved head, is standing between her naked legs while her mother and father each hold a hand. Another contraction hits, and for about ten seconds she tries some "hee hee hoo" patterned breathing she must have learned in her childbirth class. Then she stops and screams "I can't!"

"Ticha!" her mother says sharply, using her pet name. "Ticha! Push!"

She pushes, and everyone in the room says "Good . . . good," urging her on.

As this contraction passes, her mother and Carlos put an arch-shaped, steel railing, known as a "squat bar," into its slots in the hospital bed. Lettie pulls up to a kneeling position, then gets all the way up and stands on the bed, her head near the ceiling. As she leans back down over the bar, her mother goes right up to her ear and says, "You're doing great, sweetie pie. You've got to breathe deep, but you're doing great." Lettie nods and her mother passes her a drink of water. Lettie does not have an IV, often common practice in hospitals. The midwives take special care to make sure that their mothers keep drinking during labor to prevent dehydration, thus allowing them to avoid the discomfort and restriction of an IV's needle, tubing, bag, and pole.

As Lettie drinks, her mother glances over to the corner where Sarah has been squatting silently this whole time. Sarah nods back and smiles encouragingly, and the mother goes back to stroking her daughter's arm. Sarah is not exactly coaching, but is gently guiding Lettie and her family. She is, literally, on the fringes of this scene, and yet her presence is plainly reassuring. It is clear that her occasional comments not only help Lettie, but also give Lettie's family a model of how to best offer support.

Lettie has calmed down significantly in the past few minutes. Now she looks up for a moment and announces, "I just want to go. I'm hot and I'm tired, and I want to go home."

"In a couple of days, sweetie," says her mom.

"No, now," Lettie insists, completely serious.

Everyone smiles, and as the next wave hits Lettie, Sarah says, "A good, big, long, steady push now. That's it. Ah, your bottom was bulging with that last one." Lettie puts one thin but muscular leg up on the bar, revealing a rose tattoo on her ankle. She balances the way you do when you reach over to tie a raised shoe, and Sarah says, "Okay. That works." Midwives like to encourage a variety of labor and birth positions. They especially like to get women up off their backs, the medically termed "lithotomy position." Lying down is one of the worst positions to labor and birth in for several reasons. It causes compression of the major blood vessels, thus suppressing oxygen for the placenta; it makes it more difficult to push than in positions where gravity assists; and it increases the risk of perineal tears. It can also create a psychological loss of control as women become immobilized patients on whom the delivery is performed.[1] So, midwives often prefer more upright positions, but Lettie's position now, standing up on the bed with one leg raised like a ballerina at the barre, is pretty unusual, even for a midwife's client.

"Nice push," says Sarah. "Not too much longer and we're going to see the top of the head. Talk to your baby."

Lettie blurts out, "Come down, NOW!"

Everyone laughs and she adds, "Please."

Ginger, the nurse who just came on call says, "Push just like it's a poop. Good! Good!" Ginger taught Lettie's childbirth class, and she is clearly very happy to be here, smiling and actively encouraging her with every contraction. Now, Ginger brings a large, tilting mirror and asks, "Can you see that dark spot that gets bigger when you push? That's the baby's head."

Lettie looks, notices, and gives a good long push. She is now quite calm and seems far more focused.

Sarah puts on a long blue paper gown and a pair of latex gloves. Lettie's father says, "She wouldn't put her gloves on if you weren't going to have a baby." But Lettie seems disbelieving. She frowns, looks at Sarah, and says, "Pushing can take hours, right?"

"Yes," says Sarah, "But you're not going to have to push for hours." She smiles as the baby's head begins to show.

"Oh!" says Lettie. "It feels like I'm pushing him back in!"

"Yes, that's okay," Sarah reassures her, explaining, "Between contractions, the head does slip back in, but at a certain point, it will stay."

Through all this, Lettie's boyfriend has been very quiet. Now, he takes Lettie's hand and silently mouths to her, "I love you." She mouths back, "I love you, too!"

Lettie sits back down on the bed, pushing her feet against the squat bar. "Okay," says Sarah, approaching her, "I'm going to put my finger in. Can you feel my finger? Push here. Yes, very good." The baby's head bulges out, a dark oval shadow.

"Ohhh!" Lettie cries, "I can't! It burns! Take it out! It's not opening!"

"Yes it is!" calls out the nurse, pointing in the mirror. "See how you're stretching?" Around the wet, black fuzz of the baby's head, Lettie's skin is pulled taught, sleek, and pale.

Lettie looks and screams.

Loudly and forcefully, Sarah says, "LETTIE. Reach inside and find your strength." Lettie stops screaming, looks Sarah in the eye, pauses, and then focuses on pushing again.

As Sarah runs a finger under her labia, Lettie's mother calls out, "Here comes your baby, *mi hita!* My daughter! That's it, Lettie. That's it, baby!"

"Do they have to cut me open?" Lettie cries.

Both her mother and Sarah say, "No," firmly and at once. Sarah says she's stretching nicely and tells her to "Ease the baby out, a little more. Just like that, nice and slow." In fact, Lettie's contractions have slowed down a bit now, as they usually do at the end of the pushing stage. Ginger is at her ear, whispering, "Gentle pushes, baby pushes, gentle pushes."

Sarah comments, "Mothers call this 'The Ring of Fire.' Easy now, Lettie, easy, little push," and then, suddenly, "the head is out. Here come the shoulders." Lettie is looking in the mirror, and her face takes on a look of sheer amazement. The baby slides all the way out, a stretch of moist, plum-colored skin, and Sarah passes it up to Lettie in one smooth motion. Lettie pulls the baby up onto her chest. The room is silent for a moment. Then, "It's a girl!" her mother cries out, and she and Lettie's father start to laugh and to cry.

Lettie is smiling widely, the agony of the moment before gone.

"Hi, baby girl," she says, stroking her gently with the tips of her fingers. Then, still smiling, she turns and kisses her boyfriend. "Look, she has my nose. And, oh Carlos, she has your eyes." She cuddles her face down onto the baby's, looks up, and announces, "Her name is Jasmine."

As Jasmine lies on Lettie's chest, a nurse briefly suctions the mucus from the baby's nose. Lettie turns to her boyfriend again, and he starts to cry. Sarah asks him, "Carlos, do you want to cut the cord?" He nods and wipes his eyes, cutting and crying at the same time. I am crying now, too. The room is full of emotion. It feels electric, as if we have all been charged by some invisible current. And, in a way, we have. While Lettie births her placenta, her mother dabs her eyes and says, "Isn't this wonderful? What a miracle, *mi hita!* What a miracle."

Lettie looks surprised and proud, and, for a minute, it is silent again. She gazes around the room and says, "I did it! I really did it!"

"Yes," says Sarah, "You have a lot to be proud of."

Lettie nods and says, "Yes. Yes." Another moment passes and she declares, "I'm going to breast-feed." She tries to put the baby on, laughs, and says, "I may need a little help."

Sarah goes over to her, checks her position, and says, "Oh, you're doing a fine job. She's just learning. She may just want to look around a little bit. She's very content right there in your arms."

Lettie looks down at Jasmine and coos, "What's wrong, little one? Don't you want to eat?" Jasmine turns to look up at her.

"Ah. See. She knows your voice," says Sarah.

Lettie smiles broadly, and in the middle of this euphoric scene, Sarah quietly leaves the room.

I am a bit surprised by how far in the background Sarah manages to stay, despite the fact that I've heard a number of midwives explain that they believe it is important not to solicit thanks for their work or to take credit for the birth because it both undercuts the recognition that the mother and her family deserve and wrongly grants the power of birth to an authority outside the mother and her family. Two other Skyline midwives brought up this subject in interviews. One put it this way, "I have a Zen statement on midwives. She's there for the woman, and at the end, she slips out of the way. Let the mother have her experience. I love being at births because of the energy. I feed off that. I still shed tears sometimes, even though you're not supposed to. But I don't require thank-yous. If a person forgets your name, then you've done a good job—then truly the process was most important."

Another midwife elaborated, "We get the family to do the coaching, to do the work, because that's who the woman is going to have around with her the rest of her life. If someone thanks me just to be kind, that's nice, but I actually have a sense that if somebody is thanking me because they felt a dependence on me, I say 'Oh no.' I really love it when they say, 'You know, it was nice you were here, you're a nice person, but we could have done it by ourselves.' Then they've got the confidence that says, 'We grew a baby, we delivered a baby, we can be great parents.' We take that away from them as soon as we get them dependent on us."

As Sarah and I leave Lettie's room, Ginger, the nurse, follows us out and enthuses, "Oh! She did wonderfully! Once she got over her panic." She sees me scribbling in my notebook and pulls me aside, "What an amazing birth, *that* is why I work here. The midwives are so wonderful." I turn to talk with Sarah about Lettie's birth, but someone is asking her to bring a blanket to a cold person in the waiting room, and someone else is asking her to check a newly admitted woman. Apparently, no one can reach this woman's cervix. Sarah moves off down the hall, on to her next task.

As I stand outside Lettie's door, I think about how much support she had from her midwife. I saw how her family used their midwife's gentle coaching in what to say and how to act around Lettie while she was in pain. While some labor and delivery nurses can also offer this service, many are overworked and undertrained in the art of effective, loving labor support. And most obstetricians, who show up only in the final stages of labor, are unable to provide such continuous care. I am still overwhelmed by the powerful storm of Lettie's labor, with its squalls and calms, by the competence of her many attendants, and by the stunning arrival of a completely new being. Ginger pokes her head out of Lettie's room again, all smiles, and reports that the baby is nursing nicely. Then she, too, heads down the hall, back to work.

⌒

The next time I visit the hospital, Liz Donahue is one of two midwives on call. She is slim and attractive. Her pale brown hair is worn up in a loose chignon with long bangs. She is in her late thirties or perhaps early forties. She is poised and articulate and, despite a certain cool reserve, seems welcoming as well as knowledgeable. She is wearing blue surgical scrubs, making her indistinguishable from either the nurses or the few doctors around.

Liz has agreed to let me tag along with whatever clients give permission, and now she introduces me to the other midwife on call, Joanne White. Joanne is also in her early forties, and, like Liz, is slim and willowy with long hair, but hers is wavy, reddish-brown with streaks of gray throughout, and where Liz is poised and contained, Joanne is exuberant and relaxed. She is funny and animated and gestures with her whole body when she speaks. She has a slightly goofy energy and a lot of it.

At the nurses' station, Liz writes up some notes, in what soon seems to me like an endless river of paperwork. A baby is wheeled past in a clear, plastic bassinet, and one of the nurses says, "That baby's mother is a teenage slug. She's just been lying in bed all day, talking on the phone." I'm taken aback by her comment. Don't most mothers who have just given birth lie around for a while? Joanne has overheard this comment, and she waves her hand and shrugs as if to say, "Don't listen to her." She tells me the only thing she has to do right now is discharge somebody. "Booooring," she moans, "but you can come if you want." We head off down the hall and into a room where a young couple are sitting on the couch in their street clothes with their new baby, Harmony. Joanne coos over the baby and then asks the mother if she'll be breast-feeding or bottle-feeding. The mom replies, "Breast, but I only breast-fed my first one a little while since I had some difficulties."

"Those first two weeks are critical," says Joanne. "If you can get through that you're usually okay." She goes on to give her the number of a lactation consultant, providing just the kind of support for breast-feeding one might expect from a midwife. Joanne starts to ask the mom whether she is still sore from the birth when her pager suddenly goes off. Stopping mid-sentence, Joanne looks at the pager, looks back at the mom, and says, "Gotta go!" The next thing I know, we are jogging quickly down the hallway. As we approach the nurses' station someone calls out a room number and, without slowing, we veer into that room.

Liz comes over, smiling, and says, "She's feeling pushy." It turns out she had paged us so I could see a birth and doesn't need Joanne, which is just as well since the little room is packed. In addition to Liz and myself, the room holds the birthing mother, Denise, her husband, Frank, a nurse, and four adult women relatives as well as the usual furniture and equipment. Denise looks tense and scared. She says, "I feel pressure," and grabs her husband's hand. Her arm is shaking.

Denise is lying down in bed, her head slightly up. Liz says she wants to see what position the baby is in to prompt Denise into a good delivery position. She checks her and then gets her to sit up more and bend her knees, asking two female family members to hold Denise's feet, saying "You be stirrups." At first, I'm a little surprised, because midwives have famously opposed the obstetrical use of stirrups in delivery, preferring to move women into birthing positions that have been proven to be more effective, such as side-lying, squatting, kneeling, or on all fours.[2] In fact, the most commonly chosen birth positions worldwide are kneeling and squatting.[3] But Denise has had an epidural, and this is one of the few positions possible for someone who can't get out of bed and can't easily move herself around, so Liz's hands are a bit tied regarding birth positions.

The fact that this midwife is working with someone using

epidural anesthesia also stops me for a moment, even though I knew it was available, because I had always associated midwives with natural and low-intervention childbirth. Later, Liz tells me that at Skyline only about one third of their clients have natural childbirth, one third use analgesic pain relief like Fentanyl or Demerol, and one third opt for epidural anesthesia. While I am surprised that only one third of the midwives' deliveries are with mothers choosing natural childbirth, their epidural rate is actually quite low. Nationally, approximately two thirds of women now get epidurals,[4] and some private hospitals reportedly have epidural rates of more than 90 percent.[5]

When I ask Liz if, as a midwife, having only one third of her clients do natural childbirth feels odd to her, she says, "There are midwives who will look at a setting like Skyline and say, 'Well, what you're doing is not *real* midwifery.' But I would passionately argue that that's not true. A woman gets something from my being there to do her delivery that she wouldn't otherwise have gotten. I instill in her a sense that she's been successful, that she's brought a healthy baby into the world, and that she's capable of parenting this baby. That's a midwifery issue. That's not something that most doctors will bring into the room. And it doesn't really matter to me if she has an epidural or if she does it naturally. That's not my call. That's her call. She needs to have the birthing experience that she feels comfortable with."

As Denise enters the second stage of labor, her epidural is decreased so she can feel enough to push, and she is beginning to regain some sensation. "I feel something here," she says, pointing down.

"That's the baby," says Liz. "I can feel her head right in your vagina."

Denise has a contraction and moans and grunts.

"Push," Liz urges. "Push like you're having a bowel movement." To the nurse she says, "Put the back of the bed down," explaining to Denise, "it will help the baby's head go under the pubic bone." The nurse lies Denise down and then puts the monitor back on so Liz can see when she's contracting. Because of her epidural, Denise is not fully aware of the beginning and the end of each contraction, and Liz wants her to push throughout the length of each one. Her contractions are printed out on a strip of a paper, and the swooshing sound of the baby's heartbeat fills the room. Liz sees another contraction coming on the monitor and calls out again, "Push. Go ahead. Now is the time. Tuck your chin, that's good. Put your legs wide, wide open. Hard, hard, hard!"

Denise's husband, Frank, joins in now, saying, "Push, baby, push. Push, baby, push!"

Denise groans.

A new nurse comes in and the departing nurse updates her on the situation. I only catch the tail end of their exchange, but I hear the nurse who is leaving say, "It's the midwives," and she rolls her eyes. I'm not sure exactly what she was objecting to, but over the course of my observations, it becomes clear that the nurses are split on their opinions of the midwives. Some love the midwives and say they make working here a pleasure. Some even aspire to becoming midwives themselves. Others disapprove of the midwives' methods, particularly of natural approaches to labor management that can be more time-consuming and less convenient for the nursing staff.

Denise moans through another contraction, and Liz again urges her to push. Then, in the next lull, Liz leaves the room to check on another patient. Although I know this is standard procedure in the hospital, and no doubt the other patient needs checking, I am surprised. I didn't think that a midwife would leave a mother in the middle of pushing, even if this stage can take hours.

The new nurse steps up to Denise and puts her finger inside her vagina, taking over where Liz left off, saying, "Push down, down, down. A little more if you can. That's it. I can see the top of the head. Try to hold it real long and strong."

"Ay!" Denise cries. "I wish this baby would hurry up and come out!"

"She's stubborn like you," says her mother-in-law, who moves in closer to Denise and says, "Come on. Its time to get this baby out. Just like you're having a big bowel movement." I half expect this encouragement to work immediately, but Denise continues to push with no sign of the baby. The minutes stretch on, with Denise's lingering epidural making it hard for her to push effectively and impossible for her to get into a position that would get the force of gravity working for her.

Liz returns, bringing with her a squat bar she had asked the nurse to fetch twenty minutes before. A moment later the nurse ducks back in and says, "Oops, I forgot the squat bar," sees it's there, and then disappears again. As Liz attaches the bar to the bed, she tells Denise, "It takes two hours to push the baby out the first time." This seems like an oddly definite statement, so I assume she means it can take *up to* two hours, because, of course, it can take less and it can take more. Up to four hours is still within the range of "normal." While more time is considered long, it is not necessarily dangerous. Even so, hospitals sometimes limit pushing to two hours based on their calculation of what is safe for the mother and baby and what is prudent for the administration, given the litigious nature of our society. No doubt this protects the hospital, but it doesn't always protect the needs of the birthing woman.

Liz's midwifery training comes to the fore a few minute later, when she says, "Let's try a couple of squats and see if that helps. We'll try all the different positions until we get this baby out." Denise's epidural has finally worn out enough for her to move some. She struggles to pull herself upright by grabbing the squat bar. The nurse raises the bed up high and Denise ends up sitting with bent legs braced against the base of the arched bar, a little like someone driving a go-cart with their knees flopped outward. Liz looks, purses her lips, and nods, "The lotus pushing position. I like it."

With the next contraction, Liz urges her to push again, this time saying, "Push down as hard as you can. Good push. Beautiful, right into your bottom. The hardest part is getting it under the pubic bone, and that's what the head's doing right now."

Throughout, Liz is patient and supportive, urging, but not rushing Denise through her pushing. She is tirelessly encouraging. "Ready? Got another one coming? Good push, keep it coming. I can see the top of the baby's head. Good, Denise. Excellent. You did really good. Want to try it again? You're doing such a good job."

Several minutes go by. Several contractions, more pushing.

Finally, Liz says, "Okay. Let's try a couple of pushes on your side and see if that helps the baby turn. I want you to push my fingers out."

Denise rolls onto her side. Her leg is shaking. Frank gives her a kiss.

"Give yourself a little breather now," says Liz gently, and then, "Feel another coming? You can do it. It's almost close enough that I can grab the ears and pull."

Everybody laughs weakly.

"I hope she comes out," Denise moans.

"She will. We're not going to send you home with it still inside you," Liz says.

"I mean NOW," Denise insists amid general laughter.

"Well," says Liz, "Let's do one more and then I'll lay you down and check to see if I can help you with the soft suction cup."

"Ay! Ay! It hurts," Denise cries.

Liz lowers the bed, puts her fingers inside Denise, and says, "Oh yeah, let's have a baby. You did good." She puts on a blue paper gown and slides a blue paper and plastic pad under Denise's buttocks. "I need a little gel please," she says to the nurse.

Suddenly, Denise yells, "Ay! Ayyyy!"

"The head's right there," reports Liz. And sure enough, I can see a dark patch of hair appear begin to appear between Denise's legs. Everyone is gathered close around the bed now.

"It's got a lot of hair," Frank says.

"It hurts. I can't. Can you help? I can't do it," Denise pleads.

Liz says, "Yes, you can," but then in the same breath she turns to the nurse and says, "Okay, a little help," at which the nurse calls into the intercom, "I need a Mighty Vac and a baby nurse."

Meanwhile, the head is peeking out, a silent, slowly approaching tuft of black hair.

"I can't," Denise moans again.

Everybody in the room says, "Yes, you can." Just then, the baby nurse arrives and she and the other nurse rush to get the vacuum ready, even as Denise is giving birth. A few seconds later they pop the vacuum's suction cup on the baby's head.

"It burns. It hurts so much!" Denise yells.

Liz leans over and holds the head in both hands. The head comes out, slowly at first, then the whole body slides out with an audible gush. It is deep purple and dappled with blood. As the baby emerges, my eyes fill with tears. I wonder when midwives stop crying at births. For me, it is still so overwhelming. In this one moment, another being has joined us in the room; a new person has emerged into the world. It is a girl.

Liz suctions the baby and passes her up to Denise, at the same time asking the nurse to "get the baby crying to clear it out." The nurse rubs the baby's back, and we hear her cry. Frank, now a father, is also crying. He cuts the cord. Except for the midwife and the nurses, everyone is weeping quietly, blowing their noses and wiping their eyes. I remember reading birth researchers Marshall Klaus and John Kennell's comments that just after a birth, many observers will take on a look of ecstasy similar to that of the mother's. It is certainly true right now, for a stunned elation shines on every face.

The nurse takes the baby over to the warming table and checks her out. It seems too soon to be taking this baby from her mother, and I find myself bothered by the hospital protocol which doesn't allow the baby to be checked on her mother's breast and then taken to be cleaned up later. Meanwhile, Liz puts equipment away and tells Denise, "Now we have to watch for the placenta."

Denise asks, "Do I have to push?"

"Yes, but there are no bones. You're going to have more contractions to push the placenta out." The bluish-red bulk of placenta oozes out and Denise cries "Ow!" as her uterus contracts painfully.

Liz places the placenta in a stainless-steel tray. It looks like a large slab of meat. Poet George Ella Lyon described it more elegantly as "that valentine we all arrive with, / that red pad of which you were the lily / with the cord lying bleached across it / like a root pulled from the water / like a heartroot torn free."[6] Liz checks Denise's placenta to see if it is complete, to make sure there are no abnormalities, and to confirm that there are three vessels in the umbilical cord. She squishes it around and pronounces it okay. Then she checks on Denise and tells her, "You have one tiny little tear. I'm going to put in one stitch. Easy. This is going to poke. It is going to be tender for a moment. Use your breathing for a moment."

"Ay! Ay! Ay!" Denise cries out as Liz pierces her skin with the needle.

"You'll see a tiny purple thread. It will dissolve and drop out."

Now the nurse rubs Denise's belly, giving her a fundal massage intended to help stop the bleeding and get the uterus to contract and, thus, begin to return to its normal size. It clearly hurts, as Denise yells, "Ow! No!"

"We have to do this until you stop bleeding," the nurse tells her matter of factly and without much compassion.

"Is she boggy?" Liz asks. "No, she feels firm," the nurse reports, then says to Denise, "This is not so much fun now." I think to myself, *Fun? Was it fun earlier? I don't think so.*

As the nurse changes the bloody sheets for clean ones, a swarm of relatives, who have been waiting down the hall, surge in. Liz peeks at the baby and beams. "Oh, she's precious. Look at her smile." Then she washes her hands, and turning to the gathered family says, "We're going to leave the baby here for about a half hour, then she'll go to the nursery with Daddy. We're going to leave the IV in until you've been up and been to the bathroom. I'll check back with you guys later on this afternoon." Someone says thank you. Liz smiles, checks her pager, and leaves.

In the hallway, Joanne White is waiting to have lunch with Liz, who stretches and checks her watch. Joanne has a large, hinged hair clip in her hand; she smiles, holds it up, and, using a silly, squeaky voice, makes it talk like a puppet. It says, "Quesadilla." Liz laughs and nods, but a loud beep interrupts them. They both look at their pagers. It's Joanne's. She shrugs about the delayed meal and trots away down the hall.

As I drive away from the hospital, with the nearby mountains a blue beacon of calm just beyond the urban scene of red lights and backed-up traffic, I think about how Denise's birth was not exactly what I had expected. Her anesthesia, her relative immobility, and the use of the Mighty Vac all contributed to a much more medicalized scene than I anticipated with a midwife-attended birth. Yet, Denise's request for pain relief was attended to without judgment, the epidural was managed so as to allow for some movement and some pushing in the second stage, her midwife spoke to her in a way that was reassuring, and both mother and family were treated with a great deal of support and respect.

A doctor might have done all that, too, but I hear many stories about doctors who don't show their patients enough respect or patience with the sometimes slow process of birth. One midwife described a doctor-attended birth she saw, recalling, "It was a woman having her first baby, a normal pregnancy, normal course of labor, baby doing great. She had an epidural, and when she was completely dilated, this doctor let her push twice. When the baby wasn't born in two pushes, he cut an episiotomy, put on the forceps, and she got a fourth-degree tear. End of story. Unbelievable. There are doctors like that out there, but," she adds, "it's true that a doctor in our practice wouldn't dream of doing that." I use her words to remind myself that there is clearly a wide range of birth practices for both doctors and midwives.

After the birth, Denise was allowed to hold her baby right away, but only for a few precious minutes before it was whisked away to be cleaned and measured. Then she held her little girl again for only a short while before the baby was carried off to the nursery for more observation. This, too, was not exactly what I expected, or perhaps more accurately, it was not what I wanted to see.

I don't understand the hospital's need to separate mother and child; I don't understand their need to immediately quantify everything about the baby. Can't that wait an hour? And couldn't any observations that need to be done to asses the newborn's health be done with the baby lying with or on the mother if she wants it there? Perhaps my problem is with the way the hospital "allows" the mother certain things that then become "privileges," such as how much time she may spend with her baby. The mother does not make this decision, not even in collaboration with her midwife. If there were a legitimate health concern about the infant that would merit separation, that would make sense to me.

Of course, I realize that I am looking for a birth scene that might be mine some day, and I don't want to hold my baby for only five minutes if he or she is doing fine. I want to cradle and suckle my new baby, my own offspring that I nurtured, brought forth, and will nurture again for years to come, for as long as I need to. Even if I don't have the strength to hold my infant, I want it near me, the way infants have stayed near their mothers for millennia. Mother and child. Why break that chain, that dyad, that physical bond? Seas of separation might lie ahead, but here, at the beginning, the comfort of closeness is not a luxury. It is life itself. I realize again how much I want a baby.

In the Clinic

Aᴏᴛᴇʀ several months of trying, I am still not pregnant. I have joined the ranks of baby-wanting women who track the most fertile times of their cycles by charting their bodies' basal temperature. Each morning, I sense my fellow sisters-in-waiting, a tribe full of longing, thermometers poised. Today, my temperature rose, making a breath-catching peak on the gynecologist-provided graph paper. Ovulation. The most likely time to conceive. I don't want to miss this window. I remember reading somewhere that the opportunity for fertilization can be as short as six hours. I can't quite believe this, but I catch myself thinking, *great, I've probably missed my chance this month*. I know this is insane, but I want a baby, and I want it now.

With little but procreative sex on my mind, I drive all morning to reach my husband, who has already made the weekend journey to my parents' second home, a cabin in a desolate, but strikingly beautiful, valley. I arrive, get out of my truck, stretch my cramped legs, and gaze out at thousands of acres of hard, dusty, defeated land. After weeks of drought, the earth is the color of pale oatmeal. Light patches of stubborn grass persist, barely green, and clumps of gray-green sagebrush dot the scene. In the distance, a line of gray, sandy hills—badlands—rise in a jagged ridge—a dragon's spine tracing the edge of the valley over to the

Continental Divide five miles away. The wind is blowing hard, kicking up a series of animated dust clouds. The wind's insistent, impersonal groan is the only sound I can hear.

The sky, usually a high cup of blue punctuated with lofty cumulus tufts, is gray today from rim to rim. From as far as the distant rocky peaks a hundred miles to the north, all the way south to the blue-green bulge of a nearby range of hills, the sky is heavy with clouds. Finally, a dull, gray blanket promising rain. Already, in the far end of the valley a veil of white vapor—what meteorologists call "virga" and locals call "walking rain"—has descended and is gently ambling this way. It is a wet wash of hope in this otherwise barren scene.

I sit down on the porch steps and notice that a neighbor, who lives several miles up the valley, has parked his backhoe at our place today and on it sit two dozen yellow-headed blackbirds. They are small birds; the females are a humble black or dark dun color. But roughly half are males with vibrant egg-yolk hoods, coal-black capes, and black beaks. Colored like a flock of road signs, they neatly match the deep yellow of the backhoe. My Peterson's bird guide says they have a call that "suggests rusty hinges," but I can't hear them over the whine of the wind.

Inside, our four-year-old son is constructing miniature LEGO worlds. Today, he says he is building the ancient Mexican city of Tenochtitlan, and the rising jumble of multicolored plastic blocks is a surprisingly convincing rendition of Aztec glory. I am pretty sure this project will occupy him for some time. So, with a future sibling in mind, I tell him, somewhat insincerely, that Mommy and Daddy need to take a nap.

We duck into the only bedroom, a cool, white plastered addition from the 1940s, one wall striped with the dark and massive logs that once formed the exterior of the main cabin. This house was a one-room schoolhouse in the 1920s. I imagine a scraggly group of rural children, fighting and laughing as they crossed the threshold from high desert to enclosure. There is no transition zone here, no yard, no protective grove of trees, only wide open space. I imagine the sounds of those children and imagine that

they can call forth my next child. I close my eyes as the rain finally begins to ping hesitantly on the tin roof. The smell of water
meeting dust and the pungency of wet sage drifts into the room.
The drops increase steadily into the impassioned relief of a down-
pour.

In a few days, this rain will transform the barren scene around
me. Dormant seeds will germinate, and a green sea of grass will
spread across the landscape. It is a brief time of fertility in the
high desert. But to our eyes, even a transient lushness is delicious
and soothing. The drought will be broken, the land will bear life.
And so will I.

On Monday morning I'm back in the city, observing midwife
Sarah Walker-Adams at her prenatal and postpartum clinic visits
at one of Skyline's satellite medical buildings, a nondescript con-
crete and glass box of a building. Sheila, a client of Sarah's who is
twelve weeks pregnant, is lying on an examining table with her
denim shirt pushed up over her slightly rounded belly. The clinic
room is like any doctor's office with its blue-gray formica surfaces
and off-white walls. It is bland, sterile, and unmemorable. Sheila
has brought her daughter, Danielle, and her Aunt Betty to her
second prenatal check-up. Aunt Betty, an older woman, has come
to hear the heartbeat. Shaking her gray head, she says, "That's
new since I did this."

Sarah explains to the four of us squeezed into the tiny room
that she may not be able to find the heartbeat. Even if she does,
Sarah warns us, we'll probably hear static first, followed by an
echo of Sheila's heartbeat before "I finally zero in on the baby."
She places the small electronic wand of a handheld ultrasound
device, known as a Doppler, on Sheila's belly and right away a
rhythmic thumping fills the room. "Oh! That's the baby right
away," Sarah says, surprised and smiling. Sheila says softly, "Oh
my God." Aunt Betty beams, wide-eyed and a little teary. She
chuckles and says, "Sounds like a choo-choo train!"

We all listen to the heartbeat for a minute or so. Nobody

speaks. Everyone looks intent, lost in their own worlds, as the baby's heart pumps and whooshes its presence into the room. Sarah removes the Doppler, and the baby disappears back into its cocooned silence.

Sarah moves on with the exam, asking Sheila if she's going to do the AFP test. "What is that?" Sheila asks. Sarah explains that it is a diagnostic blood test. Abnormally high levels of alpha-fetoprotein (AFP) can indicate possible neural tube defects, multiple fetuses, low birth weight, or, sometimes, fetal death. On the other hand, abnormally *low* AFP levels can mean chromosomal abnormalities, such as Down's syndrome. Sarah goes on to explain that the test has what they call a "high false positive rate," meaning it is often wrong. This results in unnecessary anxiety and additional testing for the mother. Sarah explains that if Sheila gets a poor result on the AFP, they'll recommend a more detailed test, like amniocentesis. Sheila looks nervous but nods her assent to the test.

As Sarah measures Sheila's small bump of a belly, Sheila asks about ultrasounds. Sarah tells her that they only do them if they are medically needed, but it is a rare woman who gets through the system without one—not because so many women need them, but because they want them and the midwives try to oblige. "Most clients ask about ultrasound," Sarah comments. "A decade ago we did them routinely. But the cost to the system is high, and routine use has not been shown to improve birth outcomes," she explains. In situations where the doctor bills for every service and the patient's insurance pays for these kinds of tests, some doctors still order them automatically. In fact, I have one friend whose doctor ordered an ultrasound for every visit. When she asked why this was necessary, he brushed her off, saying, "Oh, it gives us important information," without explaining what that information might be or what they might be expected to do with it. In fact, the American College of Radiology recommends that ultrasound screening be done only when there is a "valid medical reason," and the World Health Organization finds that "routine ultrasound assessment has not been shown to decrease morbidity and mortality."[1]

One of the other Skyline midwives, Liz Donahue, put it this way: "In the fee for service model, where the provider, primarily the doctors, could charge for anything that they did, they did ultrasounds on a regular basis. They'd charge for them and make money on them. Now, we have to get pre-approval for any and all ultrasounds and they come out of our overhead. Women don't always understand that. So I get women in my office who say, 'When I saw doctor so-and-so on the other side of town five years ago for my other baby, I got six ultrasounds.' Of course, they were completely unnecessary. But he made a lot of money doing them. Unnecessary from a medical standpoint. From an emotional standpoint, a lot of people derive a lot of comfort from getting an ultrasound. It's not well founded, but it's very frustrating to try to explain that to people."

Sarah tells me, "When we did them routinely, we actually had some who refused out of concern for the fetus. I used to have patients who didn't even want the Doppler because they didn't want *any* ultrasound exposure. I haven't had that request for two or three years." Such concerns largely derived from the fact that there were no long-term studies on the effects of ultrasound on babies. "Now it's sort of an entitlement to see the baby," says Sarah. After discussing Sheila's diet and general state of health, Sarah says good-bye and we head to the small office she shares with another midwife.

Two large cardboard cutouts showing cross-sections of pregnant bodies lean against a wall in Sarah's office. Books and videotapes on childbirth, midwifery, and medicine overflow from her bookshelf. A bumper sticker that reads "Celebrate Life: Call a Midwife" is pinned to the bulletin board. Two prints of early Native American birth scenes hang on the walls. One has the caption: "The mother holds poles for support during labor in this Kiowa birth in a teepee." The other depicts "A goddess figure giving birth in a squatting position."

Also on the walls are three beautiful black-and-white photos of Sarah. In the first, she is standing in front of a window with the light shining through a thin nightgown, revealing her very pregnant body. The second shows her silhouetted, naked, holding her pregnant belly. The third is a close-up of her nursing an infant. I comment on how much I like the photos. She smiles, sighs, and says, "Every year, the hospital administrators ask us to take down those pictures, even though they are not even in the examining rooms, but in our private office where clients rarely go." It turns out that management objects to the images on two grounds: first, offensive nudity, and second, that breast-feeding pictures offend those who have not chosen to breast-feed, even though Skyline's position is that breast-feeding is preferable. While midwives have long held that breast-feeding is best for mother and infant, even the American Academy of Pediatrics (AAP) now recommends that women begin breast-feeding within an hour after birth, that the newborn should stay with the mother throughout the recovery period, and that the mother breast-feed for at least a full year, with other foods and fluids unnecessary in the first six months. The World Health Organization and UNICEF recommend that women breast-feed for at least *two* years.[2]

As justification for their position, the AAP cites research showing that when compared to formula-fed infants, breast-fed babies have generally improved health; a boosted immune system; less diarrhea; and fewer infections of the respiratory system, the gastrointestinal tract, the urinary tract, and the middle ear. A number of studies also show a possible protective effect of human milk feeding (it doesn't have to come straight from the breast, but can be pumped and fed if necessary) against sudden infant death syndrome, insulin-dependent diabetes mellitus, Crohn's disease, ulcerative colitis, lymphoma, and allergic diseases. Breast-feeding benefits to the mother include less postpartum bleeding, more rapid return of the uterus to normal, speedier loss of weight gained during pregnancy, and a reduced risk of ovarian and pre-menopausal breast cancer.[3]

Of course, not all mothers are able or choose to breast-feed. Some have medical complications that prevent them, some have babies who have persistent difficulty latching, and some suffer terribly from damaged nipples, or mastitis, or other problems. Unfortunately, as author Natalie Angier points out in her witty and informative book, *Woman: An Intimate Geography*, women who aren't able to breast-feed, or who choose not to, are all too often made to feel guilty. Angier writes, "It may be natural for a woman to nurse her baby, but it is not guaranteed," and points out that "the more we look at breast milk and the more we find within it, the more we are driven to marvel that anybody can survive, much less thrive, on its wretched artificial substitute. Yet many have. The majority of baby boomers were reared exclusively on infant formula." And yet, even she concludes that "any interval of breast-feeding is better than none at all."[4]

Sitting under the taboo picture of herself breast-feeding, Sarah shakes her head, raises her eyebrows, and points out, "We manage to keep these pictures up here in the private office, but in the examining rooms we have innocuous watercolor landscapes."

Clearly, a culture clash is occurring at this HMO, despite the administration's decision to have midwives, rather than obstetricians, care for patients during most prenatal exams, labors, and deliveries. Just because the administration has made the switch doesn't mean they are fully comfortable with the traditions and practices of midwifery, even though those very practices have proven to be advantageous to patients and administration alike. Many of the attributes of midwifery care that result in their excellent birth outcomes are often antithetical to the contemporary medical establishment. The increased time midwives spend with clients (the average prenatal exam with an obstetrician lasts six minutes, while the average prenatal exam with a midwife is fifteen to twenty minutes at a hospital-based practice and close to a full hour for home-birth midwives),[5] their personalized care, focus on women's social and emotional health in addition to their physical state, and faith in the ability of healthy women to birth without technological intervention can make midwives a hard pill for medical administrations to swallow.

Most midwives insist that a significant factor in their low caesarean rates and high rates of maternal and infant health is that they know their patients well, both emotionally and physically, and, thus, are more able to accurately assess the health of their pregnancies and the state of their labors. Clinic visits with a midwife tend to be friendly and informative, with lots of time to talk. Certainly, their in-depth prenatal exams are a major factor in patient satisfaction. My own prenatal exams were high points in my pregnancy. They were a time when I could air all of my fears in the company of someone who was both congenial and knowledgeable. They were also a time when I could focus wholly on the changes happening in my body, in my marriage, in so many aspects of my life, and I loved having the attention my midwives lavished on me during our time together.

⌒

It is time for Sarah's next patient, or client, as midwives often prefer to say as a way to avoid both the hierarchy of traditional doctor-patient terminology and the implication that a pregnant woman is in some way sick. As we walk down the hall, I ask Sarah if the administration's failure to understand some of midwifery's culture and traditions is galling. She shrugs and points out that the midwives themselves find ways to support each other, outside of work when necessary. She tells me that they make each other quilts with birth themes as well as other personalized gifts, and they hold a women's circle called a healing mandala when one of them has a difficult birth experience or an issue that the group can address.

We reach the examining room and meet Sarah's client Gail. She is a teenager. Sarah asks her how childbirth classes are going. Gail says that she felt pretty uncomfortable in the regular class that consisted primarily of adult couples happy to be starting a family, so she switched to the hospital's special class for teens and is doing much better there.

Sarah asks if she has any questions. Gail lifts her shirt to reveal a belly embraced at the edges by tentacles of dark red stretch marks. She asks what she can do, since they're not fading. Sarah smiles sympathetically and says, "No, they won't while you're pregnant. What we know about stretch marks is that we can't prevent them. You can use aloe vera to stop the itching. But the stretch marks won't fade until well after the baby's born." Gail looks decidedly disappointed. Sarah measures Gail's belly, feels for the baby, and listens to its heartbeat. Then, she asks Gail if she wants natural childbirth or anesthetics. "Natural," Gail says, "unless the pain is too bad. The epidural has side effects, right?"

"Yes," Sarah responds. "Headaches and backaches. Certainly if you are thinking about natural, you have chosen a good hospital. We have lots of alternative pain-reducing options: the bathtub, the big rubber balls to lean on or sit on, and the walking track. We can talk a little more next time about natural childbirth and epidurals after you've covered that in class."

The nurse comes in and says, "You've got three at once now." Sarah acknowledges her but remains unruffled, and I don't see any sign of her rushing through her subsequent exams.

Her next client is Angela, a teacher at a middle school, who is having her first baby. She has spiky, short hair, and wears a plaid top with a blue skirt. Sarah asks how she is.

"Okay, I guess, but a little problem," Angela says. "Last week I started bleeding. It felt like my period coming down and I had some cramping."

"Tell me what it looked like," Sarah asks. "What color?"

"It was red with some clots and then the next day it was pale pink and then a little brown."

"I'd like to look at you and do an ultrasound to look at the placenta. What you've described doesn't overly worry me. But I want to be careful. Is the baby moving okay?"

"Yes, it moves a lot."

Sarah does a vaginal exam and explains that the jelly is sort of cold. "You'll feel me touching here. Take a deep breath in and out. Keep breathing deeply while I do the exam. You'll feel my fingers going in."

"Ah!" Angela gasps.

"That's your cervix I'm touching. You're not dilating. The bleeding is not from dilating," Sarah reassures her. Sarah then checks her belly, saying, "Let's see how this baby is growing. Mmm. You've had a nice growth spurt since last time. You've really blossomed." She listens with the Doppler and says, "Its back is right there. Well, Angela, I don't think the bleeding is from pre-term labor. You can continue to work. It may just be part of your normal third trimester. I would like to do that ultrasound, and you need to call if you start bleeding heavily, like you're having your period. Then you need to call right away." The exam is over, but Sarah lingers a moment waiting to see if Angela has anything more to say. She does.

"Sometimes I feel like I'm doing too much. At school there's some stress."

Sarah nods, asks if she could cut back a little, and gently suggests she talk to her principal about this, reminding her, "You can continue to remain productive, but it is also important to listen to your body and to slow down a little." She asks Angela if she's planning to take childbirth classes. She's not. Sarah comments later that fewer and fewer of the moms she sees take classes. Some don't have money; many don't have the time. Now, she makes sure Angela has some books about labor and birth and urges her to start reading them and to check out a video about birth, too.

The next patient has a history of sexual abuse and requests privacy, so I don't go in. After her, a woman named Bonnie arrives for her annual exam. Her hair, slightly kinked and tinted a dark red, reaches halfway down her back. Her bangs are funky and short, and a row of earrings outlines her left ear. She has two children and has had a tubal ligation.

Sarah asks her if she works outside the home, careful to be clear that being at home is work, too. Bonnie works full-time as a veterinarian's assistant. Sarah asks if she's in a relationship, and Bonnie tells her she's been married for nine years.

"And that is monogamous as far as you know?" Sarah asks. At first, this seems like prying to me, but Sarah says it in a decidedly nonjudgmental way, and it opens up the possibility of discussing the touchy subject of her client's sexual history and exposure to STDs. Bonnie says yes, her relationship is monogamous and no, she has no history of herpes. Breast cancer? No. Sarah continues, "Any history of sexual abuse?" Again, Bonnie says, no. Sarah pauses, then offers, "And you don't have anything you want to chat about?"

Bonnie says no, but Sarah tells me later that many women use this opportunity to seek all kinds of advice from their midwives.

"Just want that pap smear, huh?" laughs Sarah.

"Yeah." Bonnie grins.

"Okay!" Sarah says, laughing. She washes her hands and begins the exam, checking Bonnie's breasts for lumps, telling her that the best time to do breast exams is right at the end of her period. She listens to her heart and comments on the snake Bonnie has tattooed on her belly. Bonnie smiles and says that she waited to get the tattoo until after her pregnancies, "Otherwise it would be a python by now, all stretched out." Sarah has her scootch down and does a vaginal exam, telling her, "You're doing a really nice job relaxing." She takes the pap smear, discusses the possibility of Bonnie using some extra lubrication, and gives her a sample tube. "It's possible you have a slight hormonal imbalance, nothing major. That's all. You just need to come back in a year."

Next, Sarah sees a woman who is using Deproprovera, a form of birth control administered by injection, and is experiencing some blurred vision. Her name is Nicole, and she, like Bonnie before her, is seeing the midwives not because she's pregnant, but for her well-woman annual check-ups and to get her birth control updated. She has a spiral perm in her long black hair and wears an oversized Nike T-shirt. Sarah asks if she's been on the Deproprovera for a while. Nicole says yes, for five years. Sarah asks her about the blurred vision, and Nicole says it doesn't happen all the time. Then she adds, "Though sometimes it's every time I'm going to come in for a shot, every three months." Sarah notes, "Sometimes we worry about headaches and Deproprovera. Do you want to think about getting some other form of birth control?"

"I want to," says Nicole. "But I don't know. I'm used to this."

Sarah tells her she can get her shot today, but that the headaches might be a side effect. "They're not dangerous, but . . . with the blurred vision, I'm a little concerned. I'll give you some information on other forms of birth control." Sarah tells her about birth control pills, Norplant, IUDs, the diaphragm, and condoms. "I always like to review that Depro is good at preventing pregnancy, but it does not prevent against sexually transmitted diseases," Sarah adds. "If you have a new partner you should use condoms, male or female. Do you have any questions for me?"

"Does the Depro make you tired?"

"It can do that."

"And I get so grouchy—is that from not having a regular period?"

"It can also be lifestyle things. Like stress."

"Yeah, I'm a single mom."

Sarah nods in sympathy and chats with Nicole for a few more minutes before wrapping up her appointment and moving on to her next client.

She'll see close to twenty women today. Sarah tells me that the midwives in this practice see most of the pregnant women who come through the door, but some women do "risk out" of their care and are sent to an obstetrician. Risk factors include anyone with a history of cardiac problems, those who are HIV positive or have cancer, or women who have diabetes and are on insulin (although women with pregnancy-induced diabetes can have a midwife delivery after seeing a doctor for their clinic visits). A woman carrying twins can be "co-managed" by a doctor and midwife. Breeches (babies whose heads are not down at the end of the pregnancy) are referred to an obstetrician who will try to turn them. If the baby doesn't turn, the doctor will either do a C-section or, occasionally, refer them to the doctors at a local teaching hospital, where they will deliver certain babies who are in a favorable breech position. The midwives do almost all of the vaginal births after caesarean, also known as VBACs.

While lacking the drama of birth, the prenatals, postpartums, and well-woman check-ups Sarah does are as central to her work as catching babies. Most, if not all, of what she deals with in the clinic will be routine. Her days here have a certain sameness. And yet she tries to make a personal connection with each woman as an individual and says that although she sometimes yearns for the closeness that can develop between home-birth midwives and their clients, who don't face the time pressures she does, even her relatively curtailed and mundane clinic work can be deeply satisfying.

Over the next few weeks, I visit a number of different Skyline midwives at their clinics, where I see firsthand how their different personalities affect their practices. Some urge their patients to do prenatal testing to look for fetal anomalies; some lean away from it. Some give a lot of information; others are better listeners. The procedures they do are, for the most part, all the same, but the experience of being their client varies. I had thought of writing about a single, representative midwife, but I realize that there is no one "typical" midwife.

Among the midwives I observe, one of the more openly holistic in her approach—a woman who recommends herbs as well as epidurals and who prescribes journal writing as a therapeutic practice—is Nancy Elder. Nancy has an open face and an easygoing, relaxed manner. As I enter the office she shares with several other midwives and nurse practitioners, I am immediately struck by how incredibly messy it is. Stacks of paper are everywhere. Two tall piles of file folders rise from the floor and are about to topple over. Both the desk calendar and wall calendar are graffitied with appointments. Dozens of baby pictures protrude from the edges of a framed photo of a beach at sunset, a white lab coat is tossed over the back of a chair, stacks of video-tapes tower in the corner, and shelves brimming full of medical reference books are bookended by a box of whole-wheat Ak-Mak crackers and a Magic 8-Ball. A stainless-steel coffee mug, a desk-top computer, and more papers fill Nancy's desk.

Clearing a spot for me to sit, Nancy says, "As you can see, we're a little busy here." When I arrived today, a nurse told me that they are overbooked to 145 percent of their capacity, adding, "That's pretty light for the midwives."

Nancy, who is a white woman from the midwest, tells me about the cultural diversity of their practice. With many Hispanic and Native American clients, she says she has learned to look be-yond some cultural assumptions she held when she began her profession. "I've learned a lot as a nurse and a midwife," she says, "for instance, the value of being quiet and just listening, and watching, and feeling. A lot of Native Americans are quieter than a lot of Anglos. I come from a very verbal background, and I've learned that talking is not always the best thing to be doing." Nancy flips through a file and checks her calendar. "On the other hand," she continues, "a lot of people make stereotypes about Native American people, that they're quiet and so on. Well, they're quiet when they want to be and," she laughs, "they can have a good time and talk a lot when they want to, too. And you know, a lot of people say that Native American women in birthing tend to bleed a lot, and quite frankly, I don't think that is neces-sarily so. Some of them do, and some of them don't. I was told, 'You always need to start an IV for a Native American who's going to have a baby.' And its like, 'No you don't.' It just depends on the situation."

Nancy stands up, "Well, enough talk. Let's go." She's halfway down the hall by the time I've gathered up my tape recorder and bag.

Nancy's first client today is Carla, who had a baby girl five weeks ago. Nancy asks how her other child, a three-year-old girl, is adjusting. Carla says her older daughter is doing okay but has had some potty training regression, or accidents, and also cries a lot more now that the baby is at home. Nancy asks how Carla deals with it. Carla shrugs and says, "When I get mad, I count to ten or leave the room."

Nancy nods in sympathy and approval, then asks, "Do you have friends with children?"

"No. We're pretty isolated. My sister lives close by but has no kids."

Nancy shakes her head and says she doesn't think it is natural to be all alone with kids, and suggests Carla try to network with other women. She tells her about a local nursing-supply store that has a mothering support group. Nancy also suggests that Carla try writing in a journal, encouraging her, "Sometimes that helps to process things, because what you're doing is not easy." Carla nods and smiles at the recognition.

Nancy asks how the nursing is going, to which Carla responds with a sigh, admitting that she has some problems and that she finds it difficult that her baby wants to eat every hour. She asks if it is possible the baby isn't getting enough milk at each feeding.

"Well, it's possible, but not likely if she's growing fine," Nancy replies. She tells Carla she can get some fennel and make tea or buy a commercially prepared "mother's milk" tea at a local grocery store. "But also," she says, "you can just try drinking more water. That can help."

While Nancy writes in Carla's chart, Carla chats with me, saying that a midwife delivered this new baby, but that her first was delivered by a doctor who had her on her back with her feet up. "I tore badly." Of course, this position might not be the reason she tore, but it isn't a great one for keeping an intact perineum, and doctors are less likely than midwives to be versed in the art of preventing tears. "This time," says Carla, "I pushed in a similar position, but when it came time, the midwife said when to push and guided me through it. She would say, 'Real hard this time.' Or, 'Not so hard.' And this time, I had no tearing. Also, this time I had the freedom to try more things because the midwives suggested more things—like I walked around more, and soaking in the bath helped."

Looking up briefly from her chart, Nancy responds to Carla, "That's great." Then she turns to me and adds, "But, you know, I don't see doctors as our enemies. I see the system that divides us as a problem. I've worked with private physicians and with public health physicians, and basically I see people trying to help other people across the board."

Later, when I ask Nancy to compare midwives to obstetricians, she is similarly diplomatic, saying, "What I like about midwifery is that I am able to promote what's okay, to look at what's right about the woman in terms of her ability to have a baby. Women are, for the most part, built to have babies. We're designed to give life. So how can we facilitate that process? And, I have to say, doctors don't get trained that way as much, and it affects how they deliver care. However, for any doctor who's been in practice long enough, I think his or her success still depends on being able to assess what's going well for a particular family and to ask, 'What can I do to help them recognize what's good and to recognize where they need help?' So I think both of our trainings have merits. When we do have a problem, and it doesn't happen often, but if you have a patient with, say, a uterus that simply isn't functioning normally and she's going to need a C-section, well, midwives don't know how to deal with C-sections. So it's good the doctors are there. There are also a few people with medical illnesses that affect their birthing. Most of our training has been not as in-depth as the doctor's has been in actual illnesses. Don't get me wrong, midwives have to look for problems, and we do. We're able to see malpresentations or dysfunctions in labor; we're able to recognize when something like preeclampsia is occurring. So we do have to be able to diagnose and consult, but our main focus is on health promotion. And with childbearing women, that's where our focus needs to be, because most of them are healthy. For the ones who aren't, I'm glad I can refer them to a doctor who has studied these problems."

As Nancy and I walk to the nurses' desk to pick up another chart, I ask her if suggesting fennel seed tea or mother's milk tea to help with Carla's breast-milk production is the kind of thing she does with most of her clients. Nancy grins and says, "Well, that is another thing that I like about midwifery—that we really try to individualize care. I might have a woman from a fundamentalist background who I might not suggest herbs to, because you have to be able to reach that woman in a way that is respectful of her, no matter what. And you know," she chuckles, "in terms of when to bring up alternative stuff and when not to, you have to be really careful. I am very sensitive to it. There are a lot of women who want to use herbs and other forms of complementary medicine, and then there are a lot who think that's Satan's work. So you gotta be real careful."

Nancy takes a look at her next client's chart, then continues, "Some things, though, are becoming more mainstream. It's pretty common for our patients to be taking red raspberry leaf tea during pregnancy. It's actually very common for people to be using mother's milk teas for breast-feeding. But I've recently had some patients complain about my pushing alternative medicines, and so I'm more reticent about bringing it up. I try to feel them out. I've used aromatherapy during labor, and still do at times, and, um," she hesitates and purses her lips, "I guess some other midwives got some complaints, like 'What's up with these people at Skyline? All they want to do is use aromatherapy, and they don't want to use epidurals.' I've even had a complaint letter put in my file about it. And that is *not* something you want getting around in a competitive hospital environment, you know!" Nancy raises her eyebrows, laughs, and shakes her head as she walks in to her next appointment.

This client is a teenager who asks that I not observe her. When Nancy is finished, I ask if she sees many teen moms. "Yeah. We see a fair amount. I think there's a lot of disdain for teen mothers right now, and I think it's unfortunate. I think it hurts them. I think, as midwives, we—and I'm not saying doctors wouldn't do this—but I think in general, midwives would approach this woman with, 'Okay, so what's right about having a baby when you're a teenager?' Well one thing is that your uterus usually works a lot better than when you're older. And you have a lot more energy," she says, rolling her hips in a mock-teenage dance.

"It's also important," she adds, "to empathize with the family of a teen, who may have some disappointment about how this is going to change the young woman's life and cut her childhood short. Sometimes we get pregnant at a time that's not ideal." Nancy shrugs. "I feel very strongly that, depending on the situation, it can turn out just fine or it can turn out to be abysmal. But you know, you can say that for any adult who walks in the door. Maybe the teenager's not married, but maybe she's got a mother who's 100 percent behind her. Then you can help engage the young woman's valuing of her mother and support the client's mother in her role. Meanwhile, you might see a pregnant adult who has money in her pocket and a little bit more confidence, and you might not notice any challenges, but she may have tremendous problems raising that kid down the road. You just can't assume anything."

After three-and-a-half hours of seeing patients, Nancy says she has another one waiting but that she needs to take a five-minute break. In fact, she takes about three minutes. We go into a conference room that doubles as a lunch room where she wolfs down a bowl of pinto beans and yellow rice. While I am still finding a place to sit and put hot sauce on my beans, Nancy dashes off to see her client, saying, "Catch up with me on the next one." Her long hair streams behind her as she jogs down the hall.

I meet Nancy fifteen minutes later, as she begins a prenatal exam with a woman named Dominique. Dominique is from France, and she has a one-and-a-half-year-old daughter, Elise, at home. Dominique is thirty-three weeks and five days pregnant. She is fair-haired and sun-tanned and wears a chartreuse T-shirt and black bicycle shorts. Nancy checks her chart and asks, "Baby moving okay?"

"Mmm-hmm." Dominique nods, stroking her belly, sitting perched on the end of the exam table.

"Did you start fetal kick monitoring? Are you getting four to six movements within an hour, twice a day?"

"Yes." Dominique answers, as Nancy has her lie down and measures her belly to see if she is growing close to the one-centimeter-per-month rate that most practitioners in the United States look for. "Oh, you know," Dominique reports in her thick French accent, "my daughter loves to put her finger in the nostril. She thinks she is having a baby, too."

There is a long pause.

"The nostril?" asks Nancy, clearly puzzled. "Hmm. Do you mean the belly button?"

"Oh, oops! Yes." Dominique says.

We all laugh.

Nancy asks if she has thought about pain control during labor. Dominique says she doesn't plan on having an epidural but that she is concerned about fatigue.

"Well, do you think you want to do it differently from last time or the same?"

"Let's see how it goes," says Dominique. "If it is easier, I don't want drugs. If harder, then maybe an epidural."

"Okay," says Nancy, "You know there are some risks associated with the epidural, right?" She goes on to explain that the risks include spinal headaches, respiratory arrest, temporary loss of movement, sometimes permanent losses, some delayed bladder function, some loss of ability to push, and a higher risk of a vacuum- or forceps-assisted birth. Also, it can lower the baby's heart rate, which can, in turn, lead to more interventions, such as a caesarean section. Finally, epidurals can give the mother a fever, which—since the staff can't be sure whether it is a harmless "epidural fever" or one caused by a potentially serious infection—can lead to a complete septic workup for her baby, which can mean placement in the newborn intensive care unit, intravenous antibiotic treatment (carrying its own risks), and a spinal tap.

On this final item, Nancy's statements are backed up by research done by Dr. Ellice Lieberman of Harvard University and published in the journal *Pediatrics* that shows epidurals are indeed associated with a hugely increased frequency (fourteen-fold) of fevers in birthing mothers and finds that the resulting "neonatal sepsis workups and administration of antibiotics are not necessarily benign." Lieberman points to complications that can arise from the antibiotics and psychological disturbance for the family when a mother is separated from her newborn. She concludes, "Given the cost, risk, and pain to the newborn, the higher proportion of sepsis workups that may be attributable to epidural use is cause for concern."[6]

When Nancy finishes going over the risks, Dominique wrinkles her nose and grimaces. Nancy nods and adds, "But, as a drug, the epidural is safer for your baby than other drugs we use. If you give a mother Demerol, you give her baby Demerol. So an epidural is usually safer for the baby, but not for the mother. As nurse midwives, we get kind of blasé about it—drug use that is—but there are risks." Dominique nods and says, "I understand." Nancy goes on to tell her that there are other things they can try first. She suggests walking around, aromatherapy, a warm bath, massage, and using different positions such as getting on hands and knees. Dominique listens and nods, then asks whether Nancy has any children.

"Just one. I stopped after him. He's grown up now. I had him at home with a family practice doctor. In retrospect, now that I know so much, I think that I was not managed very well and a midwife would have been better. But," she shrugs and smiles, "I had my home birth and no medication, which was what I wanted."

Later, Nancy comments more on epidurals, saying, "Epidurals are a great form of anesthesia for a woman who cannot tolerate pain. And there are quite a number of them. Maybe more and more, and I'm not sure why. It may be partly the media, you know, if someone on TV says 'Get yourself an epidural'. . . ." Nancy also cites the hospital's promotion of epidurals as part of their own "economic drive—the competition for patients."

She thinks for a minute, then says, "I think increased epidural use might have something to do with the fact that we don't think that we should have pain in this modern world. Most of the women we see don't generally challenge themselves physically. They are sedentary, and they aren't familiar with physical pain. But I think a lot of it is that we're all so stressed out that we just can't handle any more pain. It's funny, at a time when there are so many conveniences, why are we all so stressed out? Women are so stressed that even the thought of having intense physical pain is so scary that they would prefer—if its basically a safe procedure—not to experience the pain of childbirth. And you know, that sounds fairly reasonable. The only problem is that every form of intervention carries some risks. She may suffer back pain, have problems with her ability to urinate, or have problems with mobility. Yes, it is rare, but are you willing to take that risk? Usually, with normal labor, you have ten to twelve hours of extreme pain. And then it's over."

It's not just the birthing mother's stress that is a factor, Nancy adds. Sometimes the caregiver's stress levels play a role, too. "The increase in analgesia and anesthesia use may be related to our own pain as midwives and caregivers. It would be interesting to do a study that tried to see if epidural use was in part because we, and the nurses, too, don't want to deal with mothers' pain. I'm not proud of this," she says, "but it is true. When you're with a laboring woman, sometimes it is hard to bear her pain. And we see so much, volume-wise. It gets to you. So now, with epidurals, we don't have to bear their pain." She pauses, then continues, "There is an endless human need for comfort. The care provider herself needs some balance in order to help her clients with their pain and to promote women's health." Nancy shakes her head, "And managed care does *not* promote that balance for the health-care provider."

The issue of managed care's impact on midwifery is pretty much the same issue as managed care's impact on health care in general. Midwifery is just one site in the ongoing conflict between for-profit medicine and the healing arts. For midwives, this conflict tends to focus on the time available to spend with clients, both during labor and delivery and at the clinic. The higher-ups in the hospital administration mandate the number of patients the midwives should see each day and, thus, the number of minutes per patient. In fact, in the next few weeks, word will come down that the Skyline midwives need to change their scheduling templates in order to squeeze in several more patients each day, around twenty total, reducing the time of each prenatal or postpartum visit by a number of minutes. A nurse-midwife in another practice in town told me, "I'll see between fifteen and twenty-five people a day. I used to think, 'those people are not midwives,' but now I regularly jam four people into an hour. It's not optimal."

It is the start of another day at one of the Skyline clinics, and midwife Liz Donahue is getting ready for work. Liz wears a lab coat over a long purple and blue print dress that accentuates her tall, slim frame. She gathers up a pile of manila folders and checks in with the nurse, Michelle Owens. Michelle taps at the computer keyboard and reports that the clinic is 170 percent overbooked today. "Pretty typical," she says to me.

Liz nods in agreement and says, "We are getting pushed to be more and more productive. It's anathema to midwives." She shakes her head. "Well, off we go. Who's first?"

First is Maria Lucero. She looks very young, so I am surprised to find out that this will be her fifth baby. Liz listens to her heart, knocks on her kidneys, taps her knees, and checks her breasts. Then she teaches her how to do a monthly breast exam, showing her what to look for in the mirror and what to feel for, explaining, "cancer can feel like a little piece of rock, gravel, something hard." Maria nods. Liz feels her belly and asks if she has any problems. She doesn't. Liz oozes clear gel onto the head of the Doppler and says, "It will be a little cool. Sorry." She finds the baby's heartbeat and its sound fills the room. As we watch and listen, the baby kicks, interrupting the sound and making the Doppler shift. We all smile, and, once again, I find myself moved by such distinct evidence of the baby's presence, the sudden appearance of its sound in the face of its usual silence.

Liz says the heartbeat is normal, then does a pelvic exam and a pap smear. She checks Maria's chart and notes that Maria had some preterm labor with her last baby and is showing signs of doing the same this time. Because of this, Liz explains, she will have to come in more often than usual. Liz then refers her to a premature prevention program where a nurse calls every week to check in with her.

After checking her chart again, Liz pulls a chair up next to the examining table and says, "You probably remember that you had a positive antibody screen." During one of Maria's pregnancies, she formed antibodies against the fetal blood. It is possible that her blood cells could now attack this new fetus's blood cells. This can lead to a very serious illness for the baby and can even be fatal. It is rare, but if it shows up, Liz explains, sometimes they need to do blood transfusions in utero. "So," Liz continues, "we wanted to test your husband to find out his blood type and rh. Has he done that?"

"No," says Maria quietly, looking down. "He's in jail."

Liz doesn't miss a beat. She simply says, "That must be hard on you."

"Yes."

"Do you have help?" Liz asks. "Does your family help? Or his?"

"Yes. His family has my three oldest kids in Mexico now. They come back next week."

"So you just have Manuel Jr. with you? And he's two? Who is helping you here?"

"My mother."

"Okay. I'll check with the jail for the test. Now your other tests—spina bifida and Down's—those all look okay." Liz reads her the actual risk rates and tells her that they are low. Then she says, "Last time we gave you the booklet on tubal ligation. Did you read about it?"

"Yes," says Maria, looking straight at Liz. "I still want to do that."

"Okay. Are you doing okay? Are you working?"

"Yes, at home, piece work."

"No lifting?"

Maria shakes her head no.

"Good, 'cause you did have some problems before with preterm labor, so no lifting." Liz gives her two business cards with the midwives' telephone numbers and the hospital's emergency numbers, and tells her they are there twenty-four hours a day and that the signs of premature labor are on one of the cards. If she has any of those symptoms, she should call.

Before Maria leaves, Liz asks if she has a social worker and whether the social worker has enrolled her in the social service program for women with infants and children (WIC). Maria says no, she didn't. "Well, if you want to, I'll get my social worker to call you to help you get set up. She speaks Spanish. Also, we'll get you an appointment with one of the doctors for a tubal ligation consult." Maria thanks Liz with a warm smile and we leave the room.

I'm impressed with Liz's ability to seamlessly move from dealing with specific medical issues to checking on this mother's social and emotional situation. I'm impressed by her fluid response to the information that this woman's husband is in jail, and I'm impressed a little later when she takes thirty minutes to make the first of what will clearly be many phone calls to the jail to arrange for the blood test, then to a social worker on Maria's behalf, and, finally, to double-check that the tubal ligation appointment is properly set up.

The next client is Francesca. She is wearing a perfectly pressed white linen blouse. When she smiles, clear plastic braces glint on her teeth. Francesca is thirty-three years old, and this is her first baby. She is fourteen weeks pregnant.

Liz asks her how she's doing, and Francesca says being pregnant is both exciting and scary. She tells Liz that at her previous visit, another midwife told her about genetic counseling, which she's decided to decline. "I don't want the counseling, or an amniocentesis, or the blood test, because I wouldn't abort, no mat-

ter what." Liz nods, but then urges her to do the blood test because it can provide useful information on heart problems. If
something like that showed up, they could deliver at the local
teaching hospital with a pediatric surgeon standing by. Francesca
looks a little confused. Liz adds that such a problem is only a remote possibility. Francesca hesitates, then says, "Well, um, okay,
I guess, but just the blood test then." She pauses. "Well, if it is
positive, then maybe I'll do an ultrasound. Actually, I would like
an ultrasound." Liz gives her standard explanation that there
must be a medical indication, but she'll look for a reason to do one.

Liz asks if she has any questions or concerns, and Francesca
lets out a flood of worries. She tells Liz that she had been taking
an antidepressant, but she got terrible panic attacks, so she
stopped taking it. Now, she is worried that she might have been
pregnant at the time, and that the drug might have hurt her baby.
She adds that she often got bad premenstrual syndrome before
becoming pregnant and is often anxious. In fact, she cried last
night, she was so worried about the pregnancy. And she's starting
a new job as an assistant professor at the local university in just a
few months. Plus, she's writing a book that has a deadline coming up in just a few months. And she's still working forty hours a
week at the library. So she has a lot on her mind. I get exhausted
just listening to her, and I remember that in my own first
trimester, I was so tired I could barely do a fraction of the work
Francesca describes. Since I, too, was a budding academic at the
time, I feel a creeping sense of inadequacy. I remember sleeping
soundly in my study carrel instead of writing my dissertation.

Still, what she is trying to do seems like too much. She
shouldn't have to do all that while her body is going through the
exhausting first weeks of pregnancy.

Liz listens quietly to Francesca's mounting list of obligations
and pressures. Then she tells her that the midwives have had
other patients who were on antidepressants and didn't realize
they were pregnant, and they had no problems. She recommends
a counseling service that is familiar with women's issues such as
juggling career and children, and says that moodiness, depres-

sion, and ambivalence in early pregnancy are very common, especially for sufferers of premenstrual syndrome. Liz tells her that she is working too hard for somebody who is pregnant and that she should cut back at least for the next month. In her second trimester, she should get some energy back. Francesca nods at this good advice, but I wonder if she'll really work less.

Liz listens to the baby's heartbeat, measures Francesca's belly, and says, "Baby's doing great." She has already spent the eighteen minutes allotted for this visit, but Francesca has more questions, which Liz answers patiently. First, Francesca reports that she had some brownish spotting. She called the triage nurse, who asked if she had intercourse, which she had. There's been no bleeding since then and she has had sex again. Liz says that her cervix may just be bleeding a bit. "It's normal. We only worry about a lot of blood, or repeated episodes." Then Francesca says that she gets severe headaches. "Yes, that is a common problem," Liz says. "We think they're related to hormonal changes. Being dehydrated or not eating enough can make it worse. Have a snack and a glass of water and take a Tylenol. It's safe."

Francesca asks about anesthesia, saying, "I'm very worried that I will be hyperventilating and having a panic attack, and I think I might need an epidural." Liz says, "That is not a problem."

"Do you shave and do prep?" Francesca asks.

Liz smiles, shakes her head and says, "No, not since the 1950s!"

"Well, that's reassuring. There's so much to think about," she says and fiddles with her necklace. "Like, how do you tell colleagues that you are pregnant without looking like you are asking for a pregnancy leave? I've told almost everybody now, and my department was pretty supportive. I actually felt more support from the old boys than from the women, especially the ones who call themselves feminists, maybe because they had it so hard to get where they are. They think you're not going to be taken seriously. You know, it is very different in Europe. There, the mother gets three months paid leave, and the husband gets one month off. I think institutions here need to be more family-friendly." She shakes her head. It is pretty clear that isn't going to change during her pregnancy.

Liz and I leave. Liz is now getting behind schedule. Patients are starting to stack up. As we pass the nurses station, Michelle, the nurse, pulls me aside and says, "You should interview me about working with the midwives." She rolls her eyes and grimaces. The nurses often struggle with the midwives' tendency to spend more than the allotted time with each patient.

Liz's next patient is Pamela, who is thirty-two weeks pregnant. Liz asks how she is feeling. Pamela has been having contractions, but they go away when she lies down. Liz urges her to spend more time off her feet and teaches her how to count fetal movements. "Try twice a day when the baby usually likes to move. Drink something sweet. If there's no movement after another hour or so, you can call the hospital." Liz hurries through this exam; we're done in ten minutes.

For the next few hours, Liz sees clients back-to-back, keeping all of the exams close to fifteen minutes long. She does a postpartum visit for Roxanne, who had a C-section because of an infection in her uterus—after thirty-six hours of labor. Roxanne describes her birth, telling how she had an IV with Demerol for part of her labor and later had morphine and Percoset. "I've been on all kinds of drugs. I was totally out of it for days after the baby came."

Liz responds, "With the next baby, if the baby starts to look big, my preference is to induce a week early. You're so tiny you might have to have a C-section for all your babies. And the next time maybe we'll go straight to an epidural since you had such a bad reaction to the drugs." Liz's comment surprises me, since midwives rarely believe that "once a C-section, always a C-section," and they frequently take particular care not to label women as "too small" to give birth, because it is the relative size of the baby to the pelvis that matters. Roxanne nods but doesn't smile, she is clearly angry about her experience and is going to let Liz know. "They gave me pills 'in case you get an infection,' but it turns out they already knew I had an infection. I don't get it. It really sucked. I *do* know that I want a prescription for some birth control pills."

Liz says okay, does her pelvic exam, listens to her heart, and asks about her bladder and bowels. She tells her how to do breast exams, checks her caesarean scar, and gives her a flyer on parenting classes and on the pill.

Next up is Jamila; she and her husband are Muslim. I was in the hospital during her labor and delivery, but they did not allow me to observe. In fact, her husband was very upset every time the nurses or midwives wanted to touch or check his wife. There was some discussion at the nurses' station about whether or not Jamila had undergone female circumcision, but ultimately they thought not. The baby was face up, so her labor was longer and more painful than normal. Jamila got a very profound epidural, and Liz tells me that since her husband "freaked out when she felt pain, we kept the epidural strong right through to the end, instead of backing it off so she could push. Plus, Jamila was very afraid to push." So she ended up with a very difficult delivery. Liz cut a surgical incision, or episiotomy, and then enlarged it twice. Before we go in to see her today, Liz shakes her head and tells me that Jamila's bottom (a common euphemism here at the hospital for the vaginal and perineal area) was a mess from the high vacuum they ended up using on her and her baby got a bad hematoma, or blood-filled swelling, from the vacuum suction.

Liz greets Jamila, who is wearing loose black pants, a pearl-gray gauze tunic with black buttons, and a matching scarf. She has her long black hair in a single braid and wears dark wine-colored lipstick on her full lips. She is strikingly attractive, as is her tiny baby.

Liz coos over her baby, then asks, "How are you? Sore?"

"Yes." Jamila nods.

Liz asks if she is breast-feeding or using a bottle.

"Breast-feeding." Jamila replies.

"How's it going?"

"Good."

"How are your nipples?"

Jamila pulls a face.

"Use the lanolin cream. That will help them from getting too cracked."

Then Liz asks, "What does Hanif think about having the baby?"

"He's excited."

"Is he helping?"

"Yes, but um . . ." Jamila hesitates, then asks a seemingly unrelated question, "Will the baby get everything through the breast? It affects them, right?"

Liz says yes, what you eat or what medicines you take can affect the baby, "But the breasts are better filters than the placenta."

Jamila asks, "What about spices? Hanif says I should eat everything, that the baby needs to learn to like spices, but my mother disagrees."

Liz smiles and says, "Listen to your mom."

Jamila flashes a brief smile, sighs, and says, "He's driving me crazy."

Liz arches her eyebrows and says, "I can understand. He's a handful."

Jamila visibly relaxes and says, "Thank goodness he's at work eight hours a day."

Liz nods and asks about sleeping and feeding, then she comments that she's happy to see Jamila smiling again. Jamila nods. Then Liz explains to her that it is possible to get pregnant again now, and that they recommend waiting for two years to have another baby. She offers Jamila a handout on contraception, which Jamila accepts. As Jamila leaves, Liz gives her a hug, and Jamila says, "I couldn't have done it without you."

"Oh yes, you could," Liz reassures her. "Yes, you could."

⌒

Liz lucks out when two clients don't show up for their appointments and she is able to duck into the midwives' office to make the calls for Maria Lucero. The office has two old wooden desks and a futon with a wildly printed purple, blue, and black cover.

On the walls are two calendars, a framed picture of a woman cradling a baby, and a cross-stitch piece that says "The most rewarding job in the world is being a MOTHER—the second most rewarding is being a MIDWIFE." A tall bookshelf is packed with a range of books, from *The Physician's Desk Reference* and *The Textbook of Medical Physiology* to *The Womanly Art of Breastfeeding* and even *The New Age Herbalist* and *Hygeia: A Woman's Herbal.* Another shelf is heaped with videotapes on everything from choosing birth control methods to getting a hysterectomy.

One of the other midwives comes in to check her mail and to get the lowdown on the rumor that the hospital administration is planning to cut back the midwifery staff. She and Liz whisper about who they think are the most likely ones to be let go and express their disbelief that this can be happening to a department that is already so overworked and provides such savings over the obstetrical model. These are the first murmurings I hear of what will grow to a near roar of anxiety, frustration, and disbelief as the administration's plans become more definite over the next few weeks.

In fact, Liz is going now to meet with the chief medical officer about their financial problems and to offer ideas about how to resolve them. As she leaves, she checks in with the nurse, Michelle, who says, "Friday looks bad. You're 215 percent overbooked." Liz leaves looking tired and grim.

3

The Managed Midwife

I T is August. I am on vacation at my parents' house in the Finger Lakes region of New York State. They live on one of the lakes, a long, bent digit whose crook conceals its forty-mile length. The house is separated from the water by a set of railroad tracks on which a clanking old train carries coal in one direction and salt in the other, giving this otherwise bucolic scene a faintly industrial air.

It is early. I am the only one awake to see the dawn. I am watching the water, silent beyond the windows. The lake, always shifting hues, is now deep blue with just a hint of gold. As the sun crests the hill behind me, the windows of the houses on the far shore shine like gilded mirrors, a brief mosaic of iridescent, yellow tesserae. The surface of the lake is dimpled with tiny ripples, my view of it partly obscured by an incredible cottonwood tree— a tree so big it looks like an illustration from a children's book of fairy tales. It is impossibly massive, two or three times the size of the neighboring full-grown maple it towers over.

I am happy here in this scene, happy and excited because I think I might be pregnant. My period is only one day late, but already I am obsessed by the idea. I keep telling myself not to hope, but an instant later I find myself nearly giddy with the possibility it might be true. I am prone to flights of ecstasy. No doubt I am setting myself up for disappointment.

A Canadian goose flies by, its full bottom pulling its bottle-shaped body earthward. Its wings flap heavily. On the shore, a mother mallard and her five young peck among the pebbles. I hear only the refrigerator hum and feel cut off from the scene, the world. I rise to open the window and feel tired and nauseated. Nausea? Surely it is morning sickness! Or perhaps it's only too much coffee on an empty stomach. Still, I feel the edge of euphoria sneak up again, even though I have to admit to myself that this feels nothing like the nausea I had during my first pregnancy.

I go to the bathroom. No blood. I do an excited little dance, stop, and tell myself to get a grip. This is ridiculous. You are not pregnant. You have no other symptoms. You don't even feel particularly pregnant. Still, one thing is for sure, I do have a yeast infection. Yeast infection! The brochure with the yeast medicine says one common cause is pregnancy! I'm pregnant! Or maybe I've been hanging out too long in my wet bathing suit. Oh. This is also true.

I start to think I must be seriously unbalanced, but after breakfast I call my friend Elena, who is also trying to get pregnant, and she reassures me that such mania is normal. She tells me that last month she had a "hysterical pregnancy," a nineteenth-century medical term denoting a neurosis in which the symptoms are hallucinatory but the patient remains mentally calm. "Oh come on," I say. No, she swears, she had sore breasts and nausea and was completely convinced it was true until the day her period was due, and there it was. Okay, I confess, it sounds familiar.

All day, I dream up baby names.

In the afternoon, my husband, Richard, and I go downtown,

and I insist on stopping at the pharmacy where, as a teenager, I used to buy sickly sweet lip gloss and jumbo packs of purple flair pens. Today, I buy an instant pregnancy test. I stuff the kit in my bag, and we head off to a bookstore. The bookstore is housed in an old red-brick schoolhouse which also has a natural foods grocery, a guitar shop, a café, and a vegetarian restaurant. It has hardly changed since I hung out here as a child in the seventies. I used to take modern dance classes in the old gym. I loved those classes and the time I spent with friends here, so I am pretty sentimental about this place.

I duck into the public bathroom, which has not been renovated in the past twenty years and maybe not even cleaned either. It is filthy but familiar. And there in the dim light, surrounded by graffiti, I pee on a plastic stick. Immediately, two dark pink lines emerge—rosy signals of a tiny life in my womb. I can't believe it. I wait the requisite few minutes, but the lines only deepen with certitude. I am dumbfounded. Joy and wonder.

Dazed and grinning, I find Richard in the bookstore and tell him. He smiles and we kiss. He is pleased, but less ecstatic than I; his ambivalence about having another child to care for lingers. I am only momentarily deflated. I feel content and happy with the world. I am pregnant! I am pregnant.

Two weeks later, I call Addie, one of my best and oldest friends, to tell her my news. I'm a little nervous, because I know she's been trying to get pregnant for several years, and I think she might be jealous. I tell her and there is a long pause, followed by what sounds like a giggle. I'm confused for a minute and then I realize . . ."Oh my God, you're pregnant, too, aren't you?!" I can hear her smile a mile wide as she says, "Yes! I wasn't going to tell anybody right away. It just happened, but, yes! I'm pregnant, too!" We shriek with delight like school girls. I am so happy, for her and for us. We will be pregnant together, we will have children born within a month of each other, and we can compare notes now and for the rest of our lives. I imagine a long string of conversations reaching out from the tiny lives we carry today to the time when they will leave us behind. I feel like the luckiest person on earth.

Back home, I continue my observations of midwives in the hospital with renewed interest and a newfound purpose. On some level, from now on, I have to admit to myself that I am in search of the perfect birth, despite my understanding that there's no such thing, and that looking for it might mean asking for trouble.

Shortly after my return, I attend a midwives' staff meeting at the hospital. The meeting's agenda reveals that the administration is renewing their pressure on the midwives to be more profitable. In attendance are about half the midwives, including Liz Donahue, and their obstetrical ally on staff, Dr. Jeremy Kaplan. Dr. Kaplan is young and attractive with dark hair, glasses, and a short beard. He begins by saying, "The administration is looking for ways to optimize efficiency. And maybe they really should have only one midwife on at night, as they claim. At any rate, they don't seem interested in my opinion or Liz's."

One of the midwives, Elaine Romero, a heavy-set, middle-aged woman with a quiet demeanor, says forcefully, "There's a reason why the statistics here are good with the midwives. If they're going to change the situation by having fewer midwives, our time will be used differently and our statistics will be worse."

"The fifth floor [home of the administrative offices] doesn't seem interested in our dropping C-section rates and in our good outcomes," Dr. Kaplan responds.

"We went from a 22 percent to a 13 percent C-section rate when they switched from one midwife on labor and delivery to two," says Liz. "Basically, it was just a change in labor management. We were able to spend more time. Now they want to go backward?"

I recall how Sarah Walker-Adams had recounted the time in the early 1990s when the chief medical officer noticed that, despite their switch to midwives, the hospital's caesarean section rate was still close to 20 percent, lower than the rest of the country at the time, but still high when one considers that, as Suzanne

Arms reports, "The World Health Organization states that there are no known benefits to women or babies when a nation's caesarean rate rises to higher than 7 percent."[1] Or, as birth historian Robbie Davis-Floyd writes, caesarean sections are "supposed to be a life-saving procedure, resorted to only when it becomes clear that vaginal birth is not an option. By this criterion, the caesarean rate nationwide should be no more than 5 percent, as indeed it was before 1970." Davis-Floyd also points out that the National Center for Health Statistics has concluded that about half of the caesareans performed in the United States are unnecessary, "costing the public an extra $1 billion and uncalculated increases in maternal morbidity, with no discernible benefit to neonatal outcome."[2] So, Sarah, who was the head of midwifery at Skyline at the time, responded to the inquiries of the CMO by suggesting that their C-section rate was high because they weren't truly being allowed to practice midwifery.

"We were extending the physicians' practices and practicing more in a medical model," she says, "and I told him if he wanted to see the C-section rate go down, we needed to have more midwives to better attend women at the bedside. So we doubled our on-call staff at that time. And," as Liz Donahue reminds the meeting now, "we brought our C-section rate down the first year to 13 percent."

Of course, the drop in C-sections pleased birthing mothers and hospital administrators alike. However, it isn't just the reduction of costly caesareans that saves the hospital money; the midwives are less expensive all around. As Liz once told me, "We are cheaper on two counts. One is that, clearly, we earn less money than a physician, but the other is that we consume fewer health-care resources, therefore, health-care dollars." She explained, "If you have a midwife manage the same population as a physician, the midwife is going to order fewer tests, she's going to have fewer expensive interventions and procedures, and she's going to have better outcomes, despite the fact that she didn't throw all this technology at the patients."

Liz continues to address the staff meeting, saying, "Interesting that the administration wants to go to one midwife at night and two in the day, when we have more deliveries at night, and during the day at least there are often other people around." In fact, a recent study confirms Liz's concerns about staffing for nighttime deliveries. In August 2000 the *New York Times* described a study published in the *British Medical Journal* which reported that in four hundred thousand normal, low-risk deliveries, the death rate *doubled* for babies born at night. Even worse, the death rate quadrupled for night babies when the cause of death was asphyxia. The probable cause? Improper staffing. According to the researchers, "This may be the result of staff's increased physical and mental fatigue during the night," as well as nighttime "over-reliance on less-experienced staff."

Elaine Romero nods when Liz comments that cutting back at night is illogical and reiterates, "Whenever they cut us, it's not going to be true midwifery care."

"Yeah," midwife Joanne White says. "But I don't know how to make our case. You could probably make the best case in the world, but they say they're losing money like crazy."

"That doesn't make any sense," says Elaine.

"Some of the other proposals on the table to stop what the bean counters upstairs say is 'a hemorrhage of money' from this department include closing the White Hills clinic," Liz says, referring to a new clinic in a part of town that is one of fastest-growing communities in the nation.

Everybody sighs and laughs, but just barely. They shake their heads.

"And," continues Liz, "another proposal is to see more people. They want to go from eighteen to twenty-two people a day."

"Again, that's not midwifery care," Elaine interrupts. This time, she sounds angry.

"They don't care," Liz says, throwing up her hands.

Elaine continues, "And its not going to save money, because they're going to have more problems in delivery and with babies."

The tension in the room is mounting. There is a long silence, which Dr. Kaplan eventually breaks by raising the issue of how much money the midwives are actually bringing in. They currently bring in fifteen hundred dollars for a global package, meaning all midwifery services including prenatal exams and delivery. Five years ago the midwives' reimbursement was approximately $2,700 per birth. Sarah Walker-Adams commented later to me that this huge reduction was "pretty disrespectful," adding, "It's just another example of how women's health care is not taken very seriously." Some places haven't been as hard hit. For example, Dr. Kaplan points out now, "in New York State, midwifery reimbursement is $3,100." He adds, "No one will tell me what we get paid on the ob-gyn side. We need to go back and say, 'You guys have gone too far.'"

"Yeah," says Liz, "I feel like it's reached a point where we need to go to the wire. But it is not clear to me that we generate our salaries based on the number of deliveries we do. The managed care health plan clients are getting us really, really cheap, and there's too much competition in this area with the other hospitals. These people are looking at the bottom line—not how much work you do, just how many deliveries. We've got to do things like minimize how much we consult with specialists like the perinatologist. You know, people like us who practice preventative medicine are at the bottom of the pay scale. We've got to master whatever information and data we have and defend this department because we may be going down."

Everyone seems confused by the economic questions at hand. But even if they had a better handle on the numbers, the midwives in this practice are in a particularly disadvantaged position from which to negotiate, because Skyline is owned by a major insurance company. This means that the hospital administrators are not able to adequately back them against the demands of the insurers. An independent midwife in town once commented on the fact that the hospital is owned by an insurer by saying, "Talk about having the fox in the hen house!"

One of the midwives at the staff meeting, Connie, asks, "Are we just going to live with this over our heads?"

Again, there is a long silence. Finally Dr. Kaplan says, "The only thing you can know is they're talking changes." The meeting ends on this gloomy note.

Liz and I walk back to her office, where she reveals to me that she's actually been told to lay off four midwives. "They say we have a hemorrhage of money from this department. But I don't know how that can be true," Liz says, shaking her head. "The number of births we're doing keeps going up," she sighs. "But it's also true that we're getting paid less per birth now than we were five years ago." Her face is drawn, and she's very serious. She looks right at me and says, "I'm not going to do anything until they put a gun to my head."

A *few* days later the hospital is a changed place. Nobody is smiling. The usual relaxed, joking atmosphere at the nurses' station has disappeared. When people do stop to chat, it is in secretive little clusters in the hallway. Midwives and nurses stop talking abruptly when I walk up. It is clear that the word is out about the upcoming firings.

I am following Joanne White today. When I join her at the nurses' station around noon, the dark mood of the staff is further dimmed as Dr. Kaplan, who is in the hospital today, tells Joanne and the nurses about a couple who are thirty-five weeks pregnant and came in this morning with no heartbeat from their baby. Joanne winces. Dr. Kaplan also looks pained and says, "They're hurting." He confides that he's sad, and that this is one of the worst things about this work. He's clearly looking for some comfort from his co-workers, but no one is able to say anything that helps. A nurse attempts to make a joke but stops herself midsentence. Dr. Kaplan wanders off.

Joanne turns to me and says, "You'll hear a lot of gallows humor. We're all upset. Four of us are going. The administration is very shortsighted. And, of course, everyone assumes it is them. It might be based on seniority, it might not. There are lots of quiet phone calls going on, checking out job possibilities." The nurses at the station join our conversation, gossiping about who they think will be fired and who they wouldn't want to lose. Everyone seems edgy, nervous, and angry. Joanne frowns, rubs her forehead, and says, "It's hard, waiting for the other shoe to drop."

With the situation at the hospital simmering, I decide to take a Sunday off, a day I would normally use to observe the midwives because my husband is available to take care of our four-year-old son, Max. But it is August, and the heat in the city is brutal. The car's steering wheel is searing, and standing in the direct sun for more than a few minutes feels downright dangerous. On top of this, my morning sickness is really kicking in, and I am nauseated on and off every day. Plus, I have that first trimester exhaustion. You can't stand up in the face of it. Naps are no longer a luxury; they are unavoidable, involuntary lapses of consciousness. No doubt this situation is aggravated by the fact that when you're pregnant you're not supposed to drink much caffeine. I find myself napping with my head on the kitchen table, my single, daily cup of coffee still steaming in my hand.

So on Sunday we head off to the nearby mountains. Even at an elevation of seven thousand feet, it is blisteringly hot. But a stream in a small canyon is cold, so we wade for hours and finally feel refreshed. I chat with Max about what we should name the new baby. If it is a boy, he thinks we should call him Emrys. Max is fascinated by Arthurian legends, and Emrys was Merlin's name before he became a magician, when he was just a boy in Wales. He was named after a Welsh mountain. Max says that it would be a good name because Emrys was a boy with big dreams. I'm pretty taken with this. For a girl, he thinks for a minute, then says, "How about Ruby Red Lipstick Flower?"

Here, with my feet playing in the icy water and the distractions of daily life far away, it is easy to dwell on how amazing it is to be pregnant. With my first pregnancy, I was aware of it constantly. The second time around, I forget about it for long stretches. My life is busier now that I have a child, but also, there is something so endlessly fascinating and magical about a first pregnancy. Still, the second pregnancy can feel that way, too. I am struck by the way making a baby is at once such complex and yet effortless work. Beyond taking good care of myself, there is nothing I will actually *do* to help build the billions of cells that will make up my child—the heart with its flapping auricles and ventricles, the tiny, ballooned air sacs, or alveoli, of the lungs, the sculpted folds and lobes of the brain, plus any dimples, bowed-legs, double cowlicks, or other quirks of inheritance—all of which are growing in me even now. The end result will be at once mundane and mysterious. A baby. A new human being. A new soul.

I find that pregnancy reconnects me to my own, admittedly vague, sense of spirituality. In dwelling on how miraculous it all is, I can't help think that perhaps it couldn't happen if the larger miracle of some divine spirit wasn't also true. Certainly, pregnancy engages us in an act of faith. All I can do is take care of myself, arrange for as safe a passage to the outside world as I can find for my baby, and await his or her arrival. Oh, and I can remember to have a sense of humor about the fact that even while wading in a cool, mountain brook, a pregnant woman might have to ruin the pastoral scene with her persistent urge to vomit.

The next day, after a breakfast of Saltines and disgusting ginger tea (which is supposed to be good for nausea, but tastes so repulsive I can barely choke it down), I arrive at the clinic to observe midwife Nancy Elder. She sees her French client, Dominique, again today. Dominique looks more fit at nine months pregnant than I do in my first trimester. Still, she is getting close to her due date and as she gets bigger, suffers more and more from lower-back pain. Nancy is showing her a few tricks.

"Try this," she says, flinging her long hair back over one shoulder and unceremoniously hoisting one leg up on the back of a chair. She stretches forward gently. "This can relieve both back and pelvic pain." Nancy switches sides, saying, "Whoa, now I have to do the other side or I'll be unbalanced." She laughs, then adds, "Another good one is to lean on something and then push in on the hip. It realigns the sacrum. These are good during labor, too. And have your husband massage the area that's being torqued." Finishing her demonstration, Nancy pulls out Dominique's chart and settles onto a small stool. "So what else is going on?"

Dominique says that she's worrying a little bit, but doesn't give any details.

"Hmm." Nancy nods, and asks, "Do you do any art work? Or do you write at all? Do you have a journal? Sometimes those creative outlets can really help."

Dominique says she doesn't write in a journal, but that she has always wanted to record the changes she sees in her daughter, now a toddler. "I just haven't done it."

"You might want to pick up a nice journal and just start writing," Nancy says, "because as you get closer to labor so much comes up, and as you write, you'll unravel it and bring the unconscious to the conscious. You might even be able to work better in the labor having done that."

"Hmm." Dominique nods. "I think I will start."

"So," Nancy moves on, "the question last time was epidural or not. I think you should just go with what feels right."

"Yeah," Dominique responds. "But can I eat if I'm going to get it?"

"Well, it used to be that you had to have had nothing in your stomach for six hours. That has changed. As long as you haven't eaten much very recently, they'll usually still give you an epidural," Nancy says. "But there are certain protocols that the hospital does stick to. For instance, they'll put you on antibiotics eighteen hours after your water breaks, and you'll have to be in labor twenty-four hours after you water breaks, which means we'll give you Pitocin if you haven't started on your own."

Dominique nods and pulls a face. She's heard Pitocin hurts.

Pitocin is a synthetic form of oxytocin, the hormone your body releases that triggers contractions during labor, and is also responsible for letting down your milk flow and generally giving you feelings of calm and cuddliness. Naturally produced oxytocin gives you both the affection effect and the squeeze to your uterus, while intravenous oxytocin, or Pitocin, which can't cross the blood-brain barrier, doesn't offer you any chemically induced serenity.[3] Admittedly, oxytocin's mellowing properties don't hold up much in the face of a contraction that feels like a ten on the bodily Richter scale, but it's better than nothing at all.

Nancy finishes the day's physical exam, then tells Dominique that they should be able to talk more at the next appointment, as long as she doesn't go into labor early.

When Dominique leaves after a twelve-minute appointment, I joke that it was a "quickie." Nancy says, "Yeah. I think she's okay. Sometimes you do think a client might have more they want to discuss, but we just don't have the time." Nancy shakes her head and says, "I'm so distressed by the effects of managed care, the emphasis on volume. You have to see so many. There is not enough time to see most people, especially if they need to talk or break down and cry. And yet, midwifery care, by its very nature, involves assessing the psycho-social as well as the physical or medical."

Nancy estimates that at least 50 percent of any visit needs to be spent on some form of counseling in order to truly promote the mother's health, and she believes she can just about accomplish this in a twenty-minute appointment. "But if you start trying to do that in less time, or if a client is actually having a problem in those areas, you *cannot* get it done in less than twenty minutes," she says. As we walk down the hall to her next client, Nancy adds, "Asking us to see more and more patients per day is a big issue, and I think its affecting *all* health-care providers. I don't think we're a factory. I think we just haven't come up with a business model that somehow addresses both the financial and the human need." She points out that while some physicians might be able to provide appropriate care in a short amount of time, even they will suffer some duress by hurrying their practices. When it comes to hurrying prenatal visits with midwives, she is adamant. "That is not midwifery care. We midwives have strong opinions about what is the best of all possible worlds for child-bearing women."

In a break after her next appointment, a pap smear visit, I ask Nancy to talk a little about how she deals with the hospital's rigid time protocols regarding antibiotics and Pitocin, which she had mentioned in her appointment with Dominique. I ask if she feels these time restraints conflict with midwifery's traditional focus on honoring each woman's individual labor.

Nancy considers this for a minute, then tells me, "I think as a midwife you get a sense of women's ability to birth being innately within them. What might present as an inability or problem is often really just a different way and speed of birthing." She adds that there are some women the hospital is probably right not to wait on, women who really do need to be induced. But a healthy woman who is willing to wait a few days to go into labor on her own, or whose labor is just moving a bit slowly, who is told, without true medical cause, that she can't wait for labor to begin naturally is being overcontrolled. "We are taking over her way of birthing," Nancy says, "and I find that somewhat aggressive and insensitive to women's ways. And that gets to me. I would say that our hospital probably has more liberal policies than most places, and I will also say that we can be remarkable. When a woman puts her foot down and says, 'No, I don't want to get induced,' then we'll say okay. We'll do daily ultrasounds to check the fluid volume and daily nonstress tests, and we won't induce. And you know, then I'm proud of our hospital." Nancy points out that a number of women still don't go into labor even after waiting as long as possible and end up needing induction. "But they did it when they were ready to do it," she says. "I think that's respectful, and I think it helps the woman feel that she is an active participant rather than just a receiver of our management."

"You know," Nancy continues, "as an expert in normal birthing, the midwife is able to connect the woman's needs with the interventions. And usually that works pretty well. But over the years—and I've been here eleven years now—I'd say everything's been speeded up. We used to wait longer on people who hadn't gone into labor. We weren't in as much of a hurry to get them delivered. And I think a lot of it is the push for standardizing care, cookbook medicine, setting a standard of care that's based on both good intentions and intentions that are fear-based. I don't exactly know what the answer is, but I know it's bothering me."

Nancy's schedule for the rest of the day is too packed to allow for much chit-chat, so we agree to get together at her house on her next day off to continue our conversation.

A week later, we sit on a futon couch in her small, sunny living room. South American weavings decorate the walls, and there are shelves upon shelves of books. I begin by pointing out the irony that while managed care may be making it difficult for her to practice good midwifery, it is also managed care that is allowing her to practice midwifery at all. In other words, the cost savings midwives offer managed care have made them desirable enough to hire but has also plunged them into an environment that challenges their way of practicing.

"Yeah," Nancy agrees, shaking her head. "Let's face it, health care's in trouble, and we are cost-effective. We provide safe care at a lower rate than a doctor could. I don't know if you've heard about this, but Medicaid sets the rate for midwives at 65 percent of the rate that doctors get for deliveries. We'll probably spend more time sitting at the side of the patient, and we get paid less. I suspect that a lot of the reason why midwifery has flown so well is because of the cost. But that's okay. In the process, people get to experience support for their wellness."

Nancy pauses to stroke a big, gray cat that has wandered in, then adds, "But if we are bringing in 65 percent of what a doctor could for that birth, is that a good thing for the institution we're working for? And how does that affect the security of midwifery in hospitals? How does it affect their salaries?" She trails off, thinks for a minute, then says, "It seems that because cost has become such an issue in health care, all caregivers, but especially practitioners at a place like Skyline, which is part of a major insurance company, are being organized in a way that is determined

by management people who have only been trained in business."
Nancy acknowledges that this can mean significant savings for
the consumer. Birthing parents often pay a very reasonable
amount for their care. But, she adds, this might result in a compromise in quality and almost certainly proves more demanding
for practitioners. "It's a very difficult time, full of a lot of conflict
for everybody," Nancy says. "It affects the morale for both midwives and doctors, and this is where I see the hospital model of
birthing being somewhat compromised."

I ask Nancy if the situation might push her out of working for
managed care. She replies, "Well, I basically feel that midwifery
is a wonderful job, but within the managed care system it's becoming more and more difficult to practice. And Skyline is probably one of the best places in the country. So I will stay with it
part-time, but I'm looking to develop something else for myself,
because it is frustrating."

Nancy's sentiments about how the pressure to see more patients in less time detracts from midwifery care is echoed by almost everyone on the staff with whom I speak. The one exception
is a midwife who has been on staff longer than most, Alison
Davies. She tells me, "I don't agree with that. Because it's saying
that back when we started the practice and there were only a few
midwives here, back when we were really understaffed and saw a
lot of people and gave a *lot* of care, it's saying that those ninety-
six-hour weeks and seeing all those people wasn't midwifery care.
Well that isn't true," she insists.

Alison's short gray hair and grandmotherly appearance belie
the fact that she is a powerhouse of a worker. She works full-time
as a nurse-midwife, teaches at the university, runs a home-birth
practice on the side, and is raising two children. Her feeling is
that midwives bring a unique form of attention to birthing
women, even when their services are stretched too thin. "Before
we started the midwifery service here," she recalls, "there were *no*
midwives in hospitals. And there are some women who don't feel
safe at home, so having midwives at the hospital is important. My
philosophy is that every family should be able to birth wherever

they want, however they want. I don't care if I am in the hospital, or a birth center, or a home-birth setting. That doesn't matter. What matters is to work with families to get what they want. Options are incredibly important to me; and that's pretty much what drives what I do. So when I actually can work with a family and they get the end results that they want, that's the greatest pleasure, however and wherever that happens."

I find myself agreeing that the midwives, even with all the restraints they face and all the cutbacks they might experience, do still practice in a way that is significantly different from the obstetrical model. And yet, making the best of a situation is a far cry from making it the best situation. I am surprised to find myself so focused on questions concerning managed care, but they are central to the way women in this setting will birth.

When I began observing midwives in the hospital just a few months ago, I expected to be reporting only on the loving care of midwives, on the way that they reduce unnecessary interventions like episiotomies, and on the way they empower women. And while much of this is true, I can't help but feel that many of the hospital-based, certified nurse-midwives I have been observing often work with their hands tied, and that they are only beginning to approach the kind of care they are truly capable of and that women truly deserve.

Finally, the ax falls. Four midwives lose their jobs as part of the administration's effort to cut costs. Morale at Skyline Hospital is abysmally low. The midwives feel betrayed and overworked. Instead of having two midwives on each shift, their new schedule has three midwives on every twenty-four hours. Each midwife does a twelve-hour shift. For their first four hours, they overlap with another midwife, then the middle four hours they are on alone, and during the last four hours they overlap with the next midwife coming on. While quiet days are manageable like this, it can be stressful on a busy shift. A busy shift, at its worst, can mean as many as eight to ten births in a row.

I arrive at the hospital in the middle of the day shortly after the new schedule has gone into effect. The midwife on call, Liz Donahue, is on the solo part of her shift. She's with a client, so I wait for her at the nurses' station. There is a staff meeting today, so a number of midwives drift past the nurses' station on their way in. I chat briefly with Joanne White, who says people are "freaking out" about their new twelve-hour shift schedules. Alison, the senior midwife on staff, stops by the nurses' station during our conversation and comments that the ones who are freaking out are "the same whiners who never want to work Saturdays."

I ask Alison about the stresses the midwives feel and why she doesn't seem to feel them, too. She says, "I go home energized. I may be physically tired, but most of the time I'm energized. I see myself as part of a huge picture, and so I don't resent what needs to happen as part of that. Some of the others are very individualized. There's a section that's for work, there's the section for play, there's the section for . . ." she trails off. "I'm really concerned that people are not seeing their lives as a whole. They don't get the free flow of everything, and it's discouraging. See, I'm not segmented. I see it as a whole way of life. I play at work." We are interrupted by a nurse and Alison bounces up, smiling, as if to prove her point.

A few minutes later, Anne Eliason-Ward, a bubbly, younger midwife, comes by, and while she waits for the staff meeting to begin says, "I've got a story for your book," gesturing at my note pad. She proceeds to tell me a story about catching a baby that shot out of the mom and became airborne. "She was barely pushing, she just rolled over, and . . ." Anne demonstrates the position she was in by holding her hands up in front of her like a quarterback awaiting the hike. "I yelled, 'Whoa!' and caught the baby in mid-air," Anne laughs and heads off to the meeting, smiling.

While I wait for Liz, I check the patient information board and comment to the nurses that it looks pretty full. All three nurses agree and say they're glad they're not midwives and they have no intention of going that route. One says, "If I'm going to go back to school and I still have to work nights, and take on that much work, and with that liability . . . No way!" Liz sits at the nurses' station and catches up on some charts. Although nobody is in labor right now, it is too busy, once again, for me to pursue any of my questions. Liz and I agree to get together later.

⌒

As *soon* as Liz and I begin our interview, she blurts out, "I think women's health care in the United States is criminal." She looks and sounds angry as she says, "It has been relegated to male O.B.s for one hundred years. Our morbidity and mortality rates are awful. I'm very resentful that medicine has made obstetrical care or prenatal care and birthing a moneymaking process. If you look at the statistics in Western European countries where they've maintained midwifery over the last hundred years, their outcomes are so much better, and the women there believe that pregnancy is a normal process. Women in the United States believe that pregnancy is a diseased state and that only the almighty physician can save them from that. You know, every physician who's got any intelligence whatsoever will admit that they've dug themselves a big hole because of that. That's why we have the kind of malpractice that we do, because if you promise somebody that everything's going to be okay and it's not, well. . . ." Liz pauses in her impassioned outburst to drink some water, and I check to make sure my tape recorder is working, since I'm stunned to hear Liz being so forthright. The last time we spoke at length she had said that, for all its faults, the hospital system is a reasonably good one and had emphasized how much improvement she thought Skyline was bringing to birthing women.

I assume the recent downsize is triggering some of Liz's response, so I ask her about the layoff. She sighs and says, "They downsized the physician group as well. It's not just us. Unfortunately, you're kind of seeing us at our worst right now. It's not been easy, because our births are actually going up. And now that it's done, they're finding out that maybe they weren't allocating some of our billings correctly and things like that. This year we're going to surpass last year's births by several hundred."

I ask if there's any concern that people won't be properly attended for their births, with the number of births going up and the numbers on staff going down, and if that isn't a potential liability for them. "It's the way they've done it in private medicine for many, many years," Liz says. "Having somebody actually with you through second stage is considered a luxury. Because in private practice, an obstetrician will manage labor over the phone. They'll have the nurse manage the labor, and then the nurses call when the top of the baby's head is crowning."

"But if you do that, then you step away from the midwifery model and all the outcome benefits that the model was providing in the first place, don't you?" I ask.

"Right. Right," she nods.

"So will it take them a year of bad statistics for them to realize this?"

"I'm not sure they'll care. What they're going to care about is billings vs. overhead."

Liz sounds bitter and a little defeated. She tells me that the administration's short-sighted cuts are nothing new. When they remodeled their department, the midwives were very vocal about wanting deep bathtubs in every room. They were told it was too expensive. "But then they put in a lot of crappy stuff like the fancy wall paper, the paintings, and the artwork, and they could have spent it on a decent tub," Liz groans. "It didn't even have to have jets—most people don't even use the jets. Just to be able to immerse yourself in the warm water. The deepness is really what gives you the pain relief. It gives you some relief from gravity, and then you get relief from the hot water." Liz shakes her head and tells me about a client who has decided that she wants a water birth and is going to rent a tub and have the baby at home. "I can't imagine not being in a tub if I was having a baby. I mean just for relief from the cramping."

I ask Liz what changes she would like to see on a national level, and she replies, "Well, on a social level, I'd like to see the United States recognize the cost-effectiveness and the good outcomes that midwives have and move to having midwives manage

80 percent of the pregnancies and births in the United States. Because you don't need to pay a physician three hundred thousand dollars a year to do that. If you take the same patient population, the physician will use more technology, consume more resources managing that same pregnant population, and have worse outcomes. So if you just look at it purely from a cost-effectiveness standpoint—and it doesn't even have to do with salary, just with consumption of medical resources—increased use of midwives makes sense."

When I ask her about the specific impact of managed care—as opposed to for-profit or corporate health care in general—on women's health care, Liz explains that with managed care the practitioners get a fixed amount of money for the people who are in their group. "You get away from the fee for service, as in, 'I just did a coronary bypass and I'm billing you for it.' If one member of my group gets a coronary bypass, the cost of that comes out of the money I've collected on the per-member, per-month amount I get. So in theory, people who do preventative medicine and minimize unnecessary surgeries and unnecessary interventions should come out ahead. Curiously enough, in the cardiology department, their reimbursement has gone up. At the risk of sounding like a flaming feminist, cardiology is primarily a rich-white-man's disease—you know, quadruple bypasses and that kind of thing. I recognize that that's a gross generalization," Liz shrugs. "But at the same time, the reimbursement for a global package for prenatal care and delivery of an uncomplicated pregnancy and vaginal delivery has gone down by two-thirds over the last ten years."

Two-thirds is a shockingly large reduction. When I ask how this can be, Liz says, "Because insurance companies don't give a shit about women." She pauses, looks up from her lunch, and adds, "That's my jaded conclusion. It's very frustrating."

As it turns out, one of the midwives who was let go is Nancy Elder. I don't get a chance to speak with Nancy until many months after the layoffs. We finally meet at her house, where we sit in her kitchen and drink a cup of cinnamon tea. Since she was laid off, she's finished massage therapy school and has opened a private practice. She talks at length about how much her identity was tied up in being a midwife. After the layoffs, she says she found herself asking, "If I'm not a midwife, who am I?"

Nancy misses the actual practice of midwifery as well and wishes she could attend a few births a month by working part-time. However, "That's not really available," she tells me. She sighs, then says, "I still have dreams about delivering babies."

When I ask Nancy how she felt about the layoffs, she begins by saying fiercely, "We're just employees of a big corporate world," but then backs off a bit, grinning and admitting that this might sound like sour grapes from a disgruntled former employee. "My ego got bruised," she says. "I'm still bitter. I've had to experience what it is like to lose face, but I try not to internalize the layoff as rejection. I think I have good clinical skills, and I didn't want there to be any insinuation about my skills. They did acknowledge that." A few of the other Skyline midwives I spoke with at the time of the layoffs felt that Nancy's frequent focus on natural or holistic treatments might have put her at a disadvantage when it came time to decide who would be let go. I wasn't privy to any of the layoff decisions, so I'll never know for sure why Nancy was one of the four selected.

When I ask her to talk about being laid off, she says, "I was having a hard time fitting into the increasingly autocratic hospital management. I was having a hard time with the decreased time spent with patients, and with patients being allowed less time to labor. Even if they were making small progress, the midwife was told to start Pitocin. But the more you push a woman's labor, the more you create problems. It's not going to keep the cost down. Also, there was less time in clinic. I like the teaching part of midwifery and listening to the women's take on things. You can't do that in fifteen minutes. I always wanted some time to educate, and if I only have fifteen minutes, I can't tell all of them all the risks of an epidural, or what an AFP really shows, fetal movement kick-count wasn't always explained, and women were not getting all the information about risks." Nancy shakes her head at this litany of shortcomings.

Nancy's comment about not being able to give women all the information they need reminds me of a conversation I had with Professor Leah Albers, a certified nurse-midwife who also has a doctorate in public health. We were discussing "informed consent," and Albers said, bluntly, "Informed consent for epidurals is a big fat joke." While Professor Albers was quick to make it clear that she does not oppose epidurals per se, saying, "there is no question that epidural analgesia has a place in modern obstetrics," she agrees with those who feel we are in the middle of what is often called "the epidural epidemic" and was adamant that women rarely get the full picture about the risks of epidural use.

Albers asserts that although most hospitals attribute the rise in epidural use rates to "maternal demand," most women lack sufficient information to make a knowledgeable decision. Often, women will have received little information about the procedure's risks during their prenatal exams. Then, when they are in labor, in pain, and not in any position to weigh evidence and opinions, says Albers, "a practitioner will come and say, 'Are you ready for your epidural now?' Well, where is the informed consent in that?" Albers describes big labor units where she's seen women who are having their second or third baby, are eight centimeters dilated (nearly complete), and are having an epidural inserted. "That is the biggest abdication of professional responsibility," she says.

No doubt this is true for a number of reasons, some having to do with a long-standing tradition of medical practitioners being the keepers of information and the authority to whom the patient defers (a situation that may, in some cases, be justified by the practitioner's education), some perhaps having to do with sexist and classist attitudes about women's abilities to make important decisions, and some having to do with the kinds of time pressures practitioners face that Nancy Elder has been discussing with me.

Nancy's opinion is that the "sheer number of people" practitioners have to see when they work for large institutions prevents them from truly "connecting with individuals." She elaborates, saying, "A majority of patients take care of themselves, but for the ones who need it—the institutions cannot rise to their needs. Then they just go along with the system; as in when a patient says 'Whatever you think is best.' There is an abdicating of responsibility to the institution; patients have good faith that the institution will do right by them. But because of the sheer pressure of the numbers, the institution and providers *can't* do that. They also abdicate, saying, 'Well, I can't do that because I have to see the next patient.'"

Nancy pauses, then adds, "The role of managed care has been to manage midwives and clients instead of promoting their health. I think that, depending on how many clients you had, you could or couldn't practice true midwifery care. True midwifery care is limited by managed care but can still exist if time is provided. But the less there is, the less you, the midwife, are attached to it. I remember sitting with a woman and breathing with her—spending hours—and then she could tolerate her pain. Some women don't want that attention. But for the ones who do, if you have other patients in labor and you are frustrated, you can't provide that kind of care."

This is precisely my worry for myself as a pregnant woman. What if someone else needs my midwife at the same time I do? If I were only expecting her to show up at the end and catch the baby, this wouldn't be much of an issue. But if I am expecting her to help me through my labor—and let's face it, I am—I may end up disappointed, just as I was with the birth of my first child. Those stretches when I labored with only the support of my well-intentioned but overwhelmed husband were nothing less than torturous for me. They may have been only for a half-hour or at most an hour, but they felt eternal. Should I just lower my labor support expectations and go with a doctor?

I ask Nancy this and she looks startled. No, she shakes her head. Despite the problems the profession is facing, she says, midwifery is vital. "The midwife is there at the birth to protect the woman from unnecessary interventions like episiotomies, and she is there to make sure the woman is not treated roughly, physically or emotionally," she reaffirms. "When people say what we do at the hospital is not midwifery care, I say it's not ideal, but it's better than if there was no midwife there. We want to protect and promote the natural ability of the woman to birth. I still think Skyline is a good place to have a baby. The labor-delivery-recovery rooms are good. The midwives are good," Nancy insists. She gives me a tight, sad smile and says, "Midwives will muddle through."

PART TWO

First Trimester

4

Medical Midwives

IT is one o'clock on a late August afternoon at Skyline Hospital, and Vicky Martinez is having her fourth baby. She is lying in bed on her back, moaning, holding her husband's hand. "Oooh, Steven," she groans to her husband, "Ohh. My back is killing me." Vicky's midwife, Robin Hern, a young, athletic-looking woman with a medium build and short light brown hair, asks if she wants to push because she feels the urge. Vicky says yes, she feels the baby. Yes, she wants the baby out. Robin tells her that her position, on her back, is one of the worst she could be in and and asks her to roll over, but just then a contraction hits her and she can't move. Robin gently traces her fingers over Vicky's pregnant belly and holds her hand until the pain subsides.

"Okay, you want me on my side?" Vicky asks.

"If you can," says Robin, helping her over. Vicky is a large woman, and turning is an effort, even between contractions. Thirty seconds later, another contraction bears down on her and she yells, "Ow, ow, ow, shit. Oh my God, my back, oh Steven."

Robin pushes on Vicky's back, massages her sacrum with her fingertips, and gently rubs her thigh. The contraction passes, and Vicky says, "No more babies after this one."

Robin smiles, pats Vicky's thigh, and tells her she has to see another patient and she'll be back later. I follow her out into the hall. Given that Vicky has just said that she wants to push, I find our departure surprising. This is the second time I've seen a nurse-midwife leave her client at this stage. When I ask her about this issue later, Robin says, "It's difficult. Nobody enjoys leaving an active patient unattended. Yet there are other things that have to be done and attended to. We try to compensate by having a nurse attend them."

While the American College of Nurse Midwives, the main professional organization of certified nurse-midwives, states in its list of "Core Competencies" that one of the "Hallmarks of Midwifery" is the "therapeutic value of human presence" in the hospital, the very real pressures of attending several laboring mothers at once can undermine a midwife's ability to provide this kind of care.[1] I recall another nurse-midwife at a different hospital telling me, "Sometimes we're so busy that we don't get to do midwifery care. I can't labor-sit. I hardly know what labor-sitting is anymore!" The frequent, maybe even chronic, interruption to the midwives' labor-sitting might also erode their determination to do so even when it is possible.

We walk down the dark, green hallway, past a series of tastefully framed artworks, to Mandy Herrera's closed door. Robin tells me that Mandy is in labor, but the pain medication the previous midwife on call gave her has apparently slowed down her contractions and stopped the progress of her dilating cervix. Outside Mandy's room, Robin stops to check her chart and talk to the nurse. "I already broke her water earlier," Robin says, "I should probably offer Pit," meaning Pitocin. At which the nurse chimes in, "and an epidural." Robin nods, but sighs and says, "If we give her more meds it might knock out her labor."

We step into the room to talk to Mandy, who, like Vicky Martinez, is also lying on her back with her head only slightly raised. Robin checks her cervix, while Mandy cries, "Aiiii! Oooh!" Robin pulls out her hand, shakes her head, strips off her rubber glove, and says, "Well, you haven't changed in three hours." Mandy groans, "Ohh, baby."

"If I just give you pain medicine you will probably still be pregnant because the pain medicine does diminish the contractions," Robin explains. "We can offer you Pitocin to stimulate contractions. You can have medicine with that, and we can do an epidural. Our next step should probably be the Pitocin, with no pain meds, or with them, or with an epidural."

While Mandy considers her options, Robin tells her that she's in the worst position possible and asks her to move, saying, "Lying on your side can hurt more, but that's because the contractions are doing more work." Mandy nods but does not change her position. She agrees to do Pitocin and more pain medication. We go out, leaving her on her back.

In the hall, Robin checks her chart again and says, "Wow. That is a huge meds dose. No wonder her contractions died down." The mind-altering effect of the narcotics may also account for Mandy's inability to rouse herself and change her position. She needs someone to insist she change her position or simply roll her over. And because she is drugged, Mandy's ability to decide about Pitocin and further medication is inevitably impaired. This is a dilemma many hospital patients face—having to make decisions about their care while under the influence of drugs. It is a tricky situation. Even if Mandy had outlined a birth plan prior to accepting the narcotics, and even if she had a support person there to remind her of it, her midwife would still need to respect her wishes in the moment, impaired or not.

Robin goes back to the nurses' station and confers with a doctor about another patient, Emmanuela Sidoli. This is her first baby and she's in labor, but her contractions are low. Robin asks the doctor to recommend Pitocin to her "since right now, one of the nurses is suggesting nipple stimulation." Nipple stimulation is a fairly common natural method that has been shown to effectively increase contractions,[2] without raising the incidence of instrument-assisted deliveries in the way that intravenous oxytocin does. But Robin and the doctor both roll their eyes, and Robin says, "Do you want to pinch your nipples or have a baby?"

The doctor moves off, and Robin sits down to do paperwork while Vicky in Room 121 screams. Robin doesn't move. Vicky's screams are piercing and insistent. It is 1:25 P.M. Twenty-five minutes have passed since we checked on her. Three minutes later, Vicky and Steven ring the emergency bell. Robin, the nurse, and I all run to their room.

Vicky is in the bathtub. She is crying. "I need to get out," she moans. As the nurse helps her out, Robin says, "We thought you were going to have a baby in the tub!"

"I'm sorry," Vicky apologizes, through her tears. The midwives here say they'll deliver you in the tub if you're stuck there, and Vicky certainly seemed stuck. But before I can dwell on this, the nurse says to Vicky, briskly, "Dry yourself off *now*, before you have another pain." Robin says jokingly to the nurse, "You should have been in the military. You cut right through!"

Meanwhile, Vicky is moaning, "Oh, my back! Oh, it feels like I have to go shit." The nurse maneuvers her close to the bed, where she ends up standing, holding on to her husband. Robin is saying, "You're doing a really good job. This is hard work," when Vicky suddenly yells, "Oh my God, something's coming out!"

"Sit. *Sit* on the bed," the nurse commands.

"I can't," protests Vicky. It looks like she will give birth where she is, standing and holding on to her husband. But after a brief pause, the nurse and Robin urge her over to the bed and pull her up onto it, where she lies down.

While many of the midwives at Skyline Hospital encourage all sorts of positions during labor (on all fours, standing, walking, kneeling, leaning against the bed, etc.), when it comes time for the actual birth, every birth I will eventually see will be in a sitting or semi-reclining position where the woman has her knees bent and held back either by her own hands or the hands of others simulating stirrups. Some sources call this a sitting squat and praise the way having the legs flexed thus increases the diameter of the pelvic outlet, but others are concerned that perineal tearing may be more common in this position.[3] Skyline Hospital doesn't have a firm policy that women must birth this way, but some hospitals do restrict the way midwives work with their clients' positions. For example, a nurse-midwife told me that at one large American hospital, the midwives are not allowed to have women walk around during labor and are not allowed to deliver in any position but in stirrups. The director of the department apparently said any midwife who squats a woman to deliver would be fired. This nurse-midwife said to me, "Then you're not really a midwife, you'd just be a technician."

As Vicky lies down with difficulty, Robin reaches over and puts her hand on the baby's already-emerging head. "It's right here," she says, then turns to me and asks me to call for a baby nurse and open a sterile package of instruments. I rip open the package, run to the door, and yell "Baby nurse!" as I've heard nurses do before. Immediately, another nurse down the hall takes up the cry, yelling loudly, "Baby nurse! Room 121!"

I duck back in the room and see that the baby's head is all the way out: a black-haired ball resting between its mother's thighs. Vicky turns to Steven and says, "I love you," and then, a single beat later, "I want a Coke *so* bad!" We all laugh, as the baby still isn't all the way out, just its head! "Big shoulders," comments Robin as the body begins to emerge, and Vicky asks urgently, "What is it? Is it a girl?" Vicky and Steven have three boys at home, ages seven, five, and three, and they are hoping for a girl. But the baby still isn't all the way out. A few seconds later, at 1:34 P.M., the baby is born, and Robin says to Steven, "You look."

He barely glances at the baby before saying, "It's a boy." Right away two nurses and Robin all correct him, saying loudly, "NO! It's a girl!"

Silence.

Then Vicky exults, "Oh! It's a girl! A girl!! Oh, I have daughter! I'm so happy!" She is beaming, she is so pleased. We all smile at her joy and excitement.

In another minute or two, Vicky delivers her placenta and Robin briefly massages her belly to get the uterus to contract. Without a word to Vicky, the nurse jabs her in the thigh with a shot of Pitocin, routinely given to speed contraction of the uterus and, thus, prevent excessive bleeding. Vicky whips her head over to see what's happening and says, "Ow! You wanna give me a heads-up on that needle?!"

As Robin cleans up, she asks if Vicky is bottle- or breast-feeding. Vicky says bottle, and Robin tells her she can breast-feed if she wants to now and it doesn't commit her to that. She's careful to encourage breast-feeding without overtly criticizing Vicky's first choice. Vicky nods, stroking her baby's head, but she doesn't move the baby to her breast.

It is 1:50 P.M. Less than an hour has elapsed since we first checked on Vicky and so much has happened. But Robin still has six other laboring women she's in charge of. She turns to me and says, "I've got to get one thing done; I've got to do this chart." We stop by the lounge to grab a piece of someone's birthday cake and then head back to the nurses' station.

⌢

Back at the nurses' station, Robin tells me, "Vicky was so much fun! I love this job!" The "baby nurse," Renata, a big-boned, beautiful woman with flowing black hair, olive skin, and a no-nonsense demeanor adds, "I'm glad she had a girl. I was really touched, and I don't get touched. I'm so jaded." Robin nods in agreement and tells me that she had ordered the shot of Pitocin Vicky got right after the birth because there is a higher risk of hemorrhage with a precipitous, or rapid, delivery, which this was—the nurse says that Vicky was only four to five centimeters thirty minutes prior to the birth—and with a fourth baby. Robin says, "I think fundal massage" (where the fundus, or top of the uterus, is massaged through the belly) "is ten times worse than Pitocin. It hurts."

As Robin continues to fill out Vicky's chart, she works in silence and I look back on what I've seen so far today. I recall that only an hour or so earlier, when Robin was going over the patient status board with me, she told me that Vicky Martinez's water had been broken at 11:40 A.M., adding, "This was the most bogus breaking of water. With third and fourth pregnancies you have so much false labor from thirty-five weeks on, and the moms worry.

She *is* contracting, and her cervix has changed, but she's not in active labor. By breaking her water she might have the baby sooner, since it usually results in the baby's head pushing more forcefully on the cervix. It probably reduces her from twelve to three hours. But now she risks infection and a prolapsed cord, plus she is committed, she's on the clock." And yet, when we checked on Mandy Herrera, Robin said she herself had broken her water, or ruptured her membranes, thus committing her in the same way as Vicky.

"On the clock" is a phrase I hear a lot in midwifery circles. It means that the mother's labor and birth will be affected by hospital protocols. The management of her labor will be based not just on her specific condition, but also in accordance with a strict set of rules based on mathematical averages determining how long she can go without antibiotics after her water has broken, how long she can labor, how long she can push, etc.

Ideally, these rules exist to serve the best interests of the mother and child, but in practice, they often serve to protect the legal needs of the hospital. Again, ideally, each birthing mother would have her case treated individually, with "the clock" serving only as a guideline—one that would have some flexibility. For instance, if a woman's water has broken but no internal exams have been done (thus keeping the risk of infection low), and her labor is progressing well, most practitioners suggest that antibiotics might not necessarily need to be administered at precisely eighteen hours. But the hospital does not allow for such individualized care, because of the chance that should a problem arise (and an infection in a newborn can be serious), a patient (and their lawyers) could then say that the hospital wasn't following the recommended labor management practices.

The administration of antibiotics is actually one of the lesser interventions brought about by the set of time-based protocols that put patients on "the clock." And yet it is not entirely benign. One midwife told me that when mothers have been on antibiotics, she sees a higher incidence of yeast infections,[4] an often agonizing condition that can hang on for weeks. This same midwife told me that a yeast infection she herself shared with her own newborn after being on antibiotics got so bad that one day when she was breast-feeding at a staff meeting the other midwives were horrified to see that blood was rolling down her infant's cheek. The blood had come from her cracked and bleeding nipple, a condition any nursing mother with sensitive skin or a baby who isn't latching on properly can face, but which was greatly aggravated by her yeast infection. Additionally, hospitals' routine use of antibiotics contributes to our society-wide problem of growing antibiotic resistance. Plus, giving a woman IV antibiotics has the simple but powerfully adverse effects of tying her to an IV pole that can limit her mobility and sending the message that she is a sick patient. Still, from the hospital's point of view, it needs to be evident that they have done all that they could to prevent more immediate, and potentially (even if remotely so) more serious problems.

"The clock" can also bring more significant interventions, from the administration of Pitocin, to induce or augment contractions, to vacuum suction- or forceps-assisted delivery, to a caesarean section. Pitocin is often used to induce labor, a practice that has risen dramatically recently, doubling from 9 percent in 1989 to 18 percent in 1997.[5] Pitocin is most frequently given when the hospital feels the woman is not making adequate progress according to a set of standards based on what Dr. Emmanuel Friedman found to be the average rate of cervical dilation in the 1950s.[6] Hospitals generally interpret this data to mean that a woman *should* dilate one centimeter per hour, despite the fact that studies show the Friedman standard fits less than half of all laboring women, and despite the fact that Dr. Friedman himself has expressed dismay over this use of his research.[7] Just because a woman's labor deviates from the *average,* doesn't mean it is no longer *normal.*

Two recent studies, published in *Obstetrics & Gynecology* and the *Journal of Perinatology* (and picked up by *Glamour, Redbook,* and *The Today Show*) looked first at 1,500 women, then at 2,500 women, and found that the normal course of labor, without any interventions, is nearly *twice* as long as the Friedman norms still used by most hospitals. The studies also found that, contrary to what some textbooks state and many obstetricians have long believed, extended labors are *not* associated with worse outcomes such as hemorrhage, infection, or complications with the baby, and that "active management" of labors with Pitocin, often recommended as a way to prevent such complications or prevent a caesarean, does neither. Confirming the *Guide to Effective Care in Pregnancy and Childbirth's* statement that use of Pitocin to augment labor, and in fact all steps that constitute "active management" are actually "forms of care for which the effectiveness is unknown,"[8] these two studies found that the only thing active management does is speed up labors.

Professor Leah Albers, one of the study's authors, notes, "When women's labors slow down, it often begins a cycle of overtreatment. We start an IV and give them drugs to speed the labor, then they're hurting more and are more likely to get an epidural, and then they're confined to bed. A leads to B leads to C leads to D. So the question of how long is a normal labor speaks directly to the beginning of the 'cascade of intervention.' Now we know we don't need to be so focused on time. We need to focus instead on how the mother and baby are doing."

Nonetheless, most hospitals persist in using the convention that women should dilate one centimeter per hour, and if a laboring mother deviates by much, "Pit," as it's known, is the next step. Some research shows that if too much is administered, Pitocin can endanger the baby by causing excessive pressure on the blood vessels that supply the placenta, thus decreasing the blood supply to the fetus.[9] And, in a cruel irony, some research shows that "most cases of 'prolonged' or 'arrested' labor do not result in fetal distress except as an effect of the use of Pitocin."[10] As Professor Albers notes, most women who have Pitocin report that labor is made more stressful and more painful, so the administration of Pitocin usually leads to the need for pain medication, either analgesia or anesthesia, both of which can then slow labor down again, as in Mandy Herrera's case, making it more likely that the woman will reach the end of the window of time allowed for labor and delivery.

To what degree epidurals raise the risk of caesarean section is still being debated, but a number of sources find a correlation.[11] One study found that the earlier in labor a woman was given an epidural, the more likely she was to have a caesarean. One randomized trial was actually halted because the correlation between epidurals and caesareans was so high that it was found to be unethical to continue the randomization. And a meta-analysis of six randomized studies found that the caesarean rate was 14 percent higher for women with epidurals.[12] Frequently, women with epidurals can't feel enough to push effectively, thus necessitating either a vacuum- or forceps-assisted delivery often accompanied by an episiotomy. Genital trauma from tearing is also increased with an epidural, because the anesthesia relaxes the pelvic muscle floor, allowing the baby's head to become untucked, so the smallest diameter of the head is no longer coming through first at birth.[13]

During my observations, I met one woman, Doreen Brown, who told me that she felt her need for a caesarean birth was caused by the cascade of interventions that resulted from the care she received. Doreen was attended by a certified nurse-midwife at another local hospital. After reaching eight centimeters in seven hours—rapid progress for a first birth—she was exhausted, in pain, and asking for help. Doreen didn't want to tell me her story at first, saying it was too upsetting to go over it all again. I encouraged her, and she recalled, "Well, the midwife said, 'You're tired, you're hurting, you can have an epidural.' I thought, okay. I had been told in my childbirth class not to let the hospital deny me my epidural if that was what I wanted. Nobody ever told me that the epidural could slow my contractions down or even stop them. And that's what happened. I got pain relief, but my contractions died down to nothing. I got Pitocin, but my contractions never got strong enough again to bring out the baby. This went on and on and finally I got a C-section for failure to progress." She pursed her lips, shook her head, looked right at me, and said bluntly, "I'm still mad."

Given that even the American College of Nurse Midwives defines one of the first characteristics of midwifery as an "advocacy of nonintervention in the absence of complications,"[14] the clock and its symbiotic partner, "the cascade of interventions," are two of the most powerful ways in which midwives' cultural traditions and professional objectives are challenged, eroded, or compromised by those of the hospital.

⌒

Robin puts away her charts, and I ask her whether she thinks Mandy Herrera's Pitocin dose will increase her pain. "Probably, though I'm not sure," she says. "But your body does lose some control of when and how it is contracting. It does take your control away."

"And is that a problem for you as a midwife, as someone who is theoretically less interventionist than a doctor?" I ask, a little afraid I'm going to offend her. But Robin takes no offense and says bluntly, "I'm not the most interventionist, but I'm not the most granola. I don't think there are any silver medals for going natural. I don't care if they get Pitocin, epidural, episiotomy, forceps. Some midwives want their patients to have *their* ideal births. I don't feel that. Some midwives like to use their bias and either push Pitocin or not. I try to let the patient decide." She pauses, "Me personally, I'd like to have a home birth."

Robin's decision to allow her patients to choose the care that most suits them makes a certain sense. For instance, nobody in pain wants to be denied a pain-killer based on their caregiver's vision of the ideal birth, unless, of course, that vision is based on an opinion about what is healthiest for mother and child. Mothers may beg for drugs when they're at nine centimeters, but if it is withheld, it is generally understood that it was a decision made in the best interests of mother and infant. On the other hand, is urging Pitocin or not the result of a "bias," as Robin says, or is it the result of a clinical opinion? Is it a prejudice or a position? In letting the patient in labor decide, is the caregiver allowing the mother to retain control, or is the midwife abdicating her responsibility? How well-informed about birth technologies must parents be in order to make the right decision? Can parents in the middle of the unfamiliar and often disorienting experience of labor make good decisions? I can't help but recall that this is the same midwife who earlier today asked a doctor to urge Pitocin for a patient who had opted for a natural form of labor stimulation.

I'm also reminded of the time another nurse-midwife said to me, "Women with epidurals are just lying there like stuffed whales from four centimeters on, and then you get the baby not coming down, or not turning face down because they've been in the same freaking position for twelve hours. So I tell them the risks of epidural, but I also tell people, it's your birth, and there's no wrong way to have a baby. And if your way is an epidural with your legs up in stirrups and somebody vacuuming your baby out, well hallelujah, everybody's happy." This midwife, like most of the half-dozen midwives in her private practice, had her babies at home.

Epidurals and the so-called "epidural epidemic," are touchy subjects for midwives who are torn between an ethic of care that tries to avoid unnecessary interventions, including anesthesia, and a belief that each client has a right to choose the kind of birth she is most comfortable with. It is an uncomfortable contradiction that comes up repeatedly in my interviews and observations. Most midwives feel that epidural rates are higher than they should be, and that low-intervention births are best for the baby and the mother, but they don't want to tell any individual woman how she should birth. Hearing Robin assert that she wants a home birth leads me to wonder. If low-tech is better for her, she must have some pretty good reasons. It is her business after all. I haven't followed Robin at her clinic visits, but I have followed four other Skyline midwives, and not one of them has ever mentioned this option to their clients. And yet, all of the midwives I spoke with, even those with the most medicalized practices, said that they would choose natural childbirth for themselves, and almost all of the midwives I followed who had children, had them at home.

"So you feel home birth is safe?" I ask, trying not to sound too astounded.

"Absolutely," Robin replies. "For a self-selected population, yes."

Up until now, I had thought of home birth as a romantic, vaguely appealing, but potentially dangerous and definitely fringe idea. But here is someone in a lab coat, someone who has attended medically managed births every week for years and years, telling me she thinks it is safe. I can't decide if I'm more interested in pulling apart the apparent internal conflict of her position or grilling her more about home birth. I opt for the latter, and Robin tells me, "I think loss of identity and loss of control in the hospital increases the pain. At home, mothers perceive less pain. When I worked in Texas at a birth center, I often did underwater birth and the mothers got naked and had a higher comfort level. When you're in the hospital it is harder to reach that comfort level."

As Robin and I sit talking, the next midwife on call, Anne Eliason-Ward, arrives. Anne is tall with short-cropped, reddish-blond hair and wears small gold-rimmed glasses. She is easygoing and friendly. She, Robin, and the doctor review the patient status board. Robin says Anne should take care of Isabella Canova, the woman who is in early labor with her first child and doing nipple stimulation, and that Anne should tell her she's got to have some Pitocin. The doctor says, "Examine her. And when you do, give her Pit. Let's get things rolling, 'cause I don't want to do a C-section at three o'clock this morning."

The next patient on the board, Maureen Riley, was just induced with a drug called misoprostol and is contracting regularly. (Misoprostol, also known by its trade name, Cytotec, is not approved by the FDA for use in induction of labor. It was approved as a treatment for stomach ulcers, but obstetricians found it effective at producing cervical contractions and began experimenting with its use in labor. Since the time of this reporting, Cytotec has been linked with numerous cases of horrific uterine rupture, a number of which resulted in the death of the baby. Its manufacturer issued a warning that it should not be used with pregnant women, and yet a large number of obstetricians continued to use it because it is extremely cheap and very effective at producing shortened labors. Eventually, the manufacturer revised its labeling in order to accommodate the views of these obstetricians. Yet many women who receive misoprostol are not made aware that it isn't FDA approved for use in labor and that it carries certain risks for uterine rupture. Thus these women cannot give informed consent to their becoming guinea pigs for this potentially dangerous drug.[15] Referring to Maureen, the doctor says, "I would rupture her," meaning he would break her water. "Let's commit her," he adds abruptly, and walks off.

Both of the women the doctor made recommendations for are midwife patients who have probably never seen this doctor and probably never will. Nevertheless, he made important decisions affecting the course of their labor, decisions that the midwives could theoretically oppose, but are unlikely to, given the power structure at the hospital. I wonder if they'll even tell these clients that it is the doctor who is now making their labor management decisions, so I leave Robin and follow Anne to Isabella Canova's room.

Anne puts her hands on Isabella's belly and says, "When the contractions come I can feel them quite well, but . . . what are your feelings about starting Pit?"

"I'm not looking forward to it since I know what's going to come with it," says Isabella, looking nervous.

"Think of it as getting labor off the ground," says Anne.

"I was hoping it would start itself, but I guess it's not . . ." Isabella trails off.

Anne smiles and nods, saying, "Well, you are in labor, but . . . I think you're here and we should just do it." Anne does not mention the doctor's opinion or his desire to avoid a late-night caesarean.

In the next room, Anne meets with Maureen Riley, who is being induced, and goes over her options, telling her it will probably be best to break her water now. Again, she makes no mention that it was the doctor on call who has recommended they rupture her and, thus, "commit her" to labor according to the hospital's schedule and not her body's. Both Isabella and Maureen are clients of the midwives, and yet, unbeknownst to them, their cases are now being co-managed by a doctor.

⌒

The next time I see Robin Hern, Labor and Delivery at Skyline Hospital is hopping again. The board is full of red ink, indicating patients in labor. I follow Robin to Gloria Edmonds's room. She is eight to nine centimeters dilated and has had Pitocin and an epidural. When we walk in, Gloria is already pushing. She looks like she's in her early forties, has light brown skin, and has a mass of dark hair. Her mother and two sisters are with her. She's on her back, her head slightly raised, her feet up on the squat bar. A nurse is sitting on the end of the bed between Gloria's legs, her gloved hands at the ready.

"How long has she been complete?" Robin asks the nurse.

"Forty minutes."

"Oh. I wasn't that busy, I was just out there drinking coffee," Robin says, sounding a little embarrassed and defensive. She turns to Gloria and says, "You go girl! Great job. Are you comfortable with that epidural?"

"Yes. A lot better," Gloria replies. She is fairly chatty and coherent. She has had an epidural, and doesn't have the distant Laborland daze of someone coping with intense pain. She has little to no pain with her contractions but clearly feels enough to push. "I'm ready," she says, and then groans with the effort of a big push.

"The baby has meconium, which means he pooped inside," Robin explains. "So when the head comes out we'll ask you to stop pushing and we'll suction him so he doesn't breathe it in on his first cry, because that can cause problems with his lungs and can be dangerous."

Two more pushes and the baby's head starts to emerge. Gloria's two sisters and her mother are all taking pictures or videotaping. "You okay, sis?" asks one.

"Yeah," Gloria grunts.

"Here he comes! Oh my goodness," says her sister, lowering her camera momentarily, "We as women are amazing. I'm serious."

Gloria grimaces and cries out, "Oh my God!" The head emerges and Robin yells, "Don't push!" She suctions his nose and mouth and then says, "Okay. Whenever you're ready."

"Ow, ow!" cries Gloria as she births a very large baby who is immediately passed up to her. She holds him and cries. "His name is Hakim," she tells us, smiling.

Within a few minutes, Robin asks, "Who wants to cut the cord?"

Grandma says, "Let me in there," and snips vigorously through the umbilicus, which is twisted in curly loops like a telephone cord.

Robin puts what is known as "traction" on the cord, pulling it down toward the bed, keeping tension on it. Two minutes later, Robin says, "Okay. Here comes the placenta. Scary for a minute 'cause it feels like you're having another baby, but there are no bones." The placenta emerges and Robin says, "Its a big, beefy one." She shows it to Gloria, telling her, "Its the only disposable organ our body makes. Do you want to keep it?" It is not uncommon for mothers, especially mothers attended by midwives, to keep their placenta and plant it with a special tree or flower for their child. For years, one of the Skyline midwives tells me later, a local midwife kept a thriving rose garden fed by her patients' placentas.

"Keep it?!" shrieks Gloria's sister, "No! No."

Robin cleans up, puts on her lab coat, and leaves.

At the nurses station, I ask if Robin was surprised to find Gloria pushing when we went in. "Yeah, but you know, if they have an epidural, I don't feel compelled to labor-sit. If they're in active labor with no epidural, I'll sit next to them. I tailor it a lot to their needs. Some women never need me."

Then she tells me that because Gloria already had an IV in she called for Pitocin to be administered through the drip following delivery of the placenta. "If they have an IV already in, I do it. It does decrease the bleeding, and hemorrhage can interrupt their bonding. I don't find any harm in giving it. I routinely give it. I know it's not going to happen very often, but I'll do anything to prevent hemorrhage and having to hurt women either with fundal massage or having to go in with my hands, either bimanual compression or massage. It is so painful. If you put that in your book, other midwives will think I'm a quack. I can hear them now," she says, then mimics a high-pitched, smarmy tone, "Just put the baby to the breast—that will stop the bleeding." She chuckles and pulls a face.

Robin practices what is known as "active management" of the third stage, which includes giving Pitocin when the baby is being born, early clamping and early cutting of the cord, and putting controlled traction on the umbilical cord when delivering the placenta. Several midwifery-led studies have shown that such active management does help prevent hemorrhage and is thought to be appropriate when the mother has had previous postpartum hemorrhage or a very long labor.[16] But many midwives do not like to practice such active management and have anecdotal evidence supporting their position. Robin tells me, "after midwifery school, I practiced passive management of the third stage and now I do active. I had more hemorrhaging with passive management. My blood loss is way down since I started doing active management of the third stage. At the birth center it was a mess and awkward; it looked like a massacre in there with all that blood. I don't think passive management necessarily causes the bleeding, but it doesn't prevent it either." Robin's relatively aggressive management of placental delivery is common but also somewhat controversial, even within the hospital. Later, another midwife tells me she had to reprimand a student of Robin's for causing a massive hemorrhage by overactive third-stage management.

Sarah Walker-Adams, the other midwife on call, arrives at the nurses' station and Robin asks her, "Sarah, do you do active or passive management of the third stage? Do you do any traction?"

"Only after signs of separation," says Sarah, pulling her long dark brown hair back into a loose ponytail while she talks.

"How long until the placenta?" Robin asks. "I'm usually five to eight minutes."

"I'm usually under ten, sometimes longer. I do very gentle management." This doesn't surprise me because Sarah has a reputation for being noninterventionist and laid back in a way that is in accord with her generally spiritual demeanor.

"I put the weight of my arm on the cord," Robin states. "My time to delivery of the placenta is less than it was, and my bleeding is less than when I just waited. I feel like I'm a medical management midwife now, but I hate fundal massage."

Sarah turns to me and says, "Something very real about working in a hospital is what the nursing situation is. My care can depend on who the nurse is, whether I have someone who is very attentive in the recovery phase or someone more concerned with charting. If I have an attentive nurse, I won't give Pit. Having had after-pains myself, I feel if you're not bleeding, you don't really need anything." She turns back to Robin, who says, "Sarah is the birth goddess; she doesn't get postpartum hemorrhage."

Sarah shrugs and smiles but doesn't deny it. I find myself curious about what makes her "the birth goddess" and why her clients don't get postpartum hemorrhage. Surely it has to do with her practice and not something more mystical, although perhaps one could argue that there is an element of the mystical in any truly attentive practice.

Robin starts talking about possible baby names for the child she is trying to conceive when a nurse interrupts with the news that Sarah's patient, Wendy, is pushing.

"She's pushing? Wow. Okay," says Sarah, clearly caught off guard that Wendy has progressed so far while she, like Robin earlier, was chatting at the nurses' station.

Wendy, like every other woman I've observed at Skyline, is giving birth on her back with the back of the bed raised and her knees bent. She is young, maybe in her mid-twenties, slim despite her pregnant belly, with long golden brown hair and gold earrings. Sarah puts on a sterile paper gown and asks the nurse when Wendy started pushing. It turns out she was getting the test dose of an epidural twenty minutes ago when they checked her and found she was complete. Now she's moaning. She closes her eyes, pushes, and lets out a high-pitched squeal.

Sarah says, "That was great. I could see the top of your baby's head," and puts a warm cloth on Wendy's perineum.

Wendy opens her eyes and says, "I'm not feeling anything anymore."

"It's okay, it's just a little break," Sarah reassures her.

Wendy pushes again and right away a head peeps out. Wendy squeals and bursts air out between her lips.

"Beautiful. You're doing very well. Maybe a few more contractions," Sarah says, cupping both the emerging head and Wendy's bulging perineum with her hands.

Wendy suddenly screams and turns red. Then, just as abruptly, she stops and rests, even though the head is on the perineum. It seems like a long pause, although it is probably less than a minute. Wendy's entire body tenses up, she breathes heavily, then pushes.

"Okay. Slow. Take a breath," Sarah instructs her.

"It hurts!" Wendy cries. "Oh my gosh it's hurting!" and at the same time the baby whooshes out, covered in blood. Before passing it up to her, the nurse covers it with a blanket, saying, "She's really wet," and tries to wipe some of the blood away.

Wendy rubs the baby dry as it lies on her chest, while the father, who has been quiet the whole time, looks on, his brow furrowed as if he wants to cry. Sarah does a brief suction on the baby and asks, "Does she have a name?" "Eliza," Wendy replies.

"Welcome to our world, Eliza," Sarah says gently to the baby and then to Wendy, "You did such a beautiful job."

The father is stroking Wendy's bare shoulder. Sarah asks if he wants to cut the cord, but he declines. Wendy says, "Do it." He shakes his head.

Sarah tells him, "It's not hard, you can do it," at which he relents and cuts the cord. He has to use quite a bit of force to get the scissors to sever the thick bluish-white twist of umbilicus, but he manages. "You did it!" Sarah laughs and Wendy smiles broadly. Sarah explains that the cord stump will fall off and that the way he cut it doesn't affect the belly button. He looks relieved and gives back the scissors. Slowly a smile spreads across his face and he wipes a tear from his cheek.

Sarah clamps the cord and puts some traction on it. She uses her hands to keep it taut, just as Robin did with Gloria, although not quite so soon. Then she asks for a push. One push and the placenta slides out. "I'm going to cut some trailing membranes," Sarah reports, snipping several long, pulpy, red tentacles that make the placenta look vaguely jelly-fish-like. Her comment triggers a sudden memory of lines from a poem by Wordsworth, "Our birth is but a sleep and a forgetting: / The Soul that rises with us, our life's Star, / Hath had elsewhere its setting, / And cometh from afar: / Not in entire forgetfulness, / And not in utter nakedness, / But trailing clouds of glory do we come." I like the idea that we come into this world with some wisp of another clinging to us; trailing clouds of glory and trailing membranes, too.

The television has been on the whole time, and now a woman on a soap opera is screaming bloody murder, but Wendy doesn't seem to notice. Her body is shaking violently, which Sarah explains is normal. Wendy contentedly strokes her baby. Sarah writes in her chart, while the nurse puts Pitocin into Wendy's drip bag. Afterward, I ask Sarah about this since she had just said she doesn't usually use it. Sarah explains, "Oh, she had Pitocin from the induction," and when I shrug as if to say, "So?" she adds, "And when I mentioned cutting the trailing membranes, the nurse knew to give her some Pit because sometimes a little gets left and it can bleed."

Back at the nurses station, I ask Sarah why none of the midwives at the hospital seem to wait for the umbilical cord to stop pulsing before cutting it. I had read that midwives like to do this both because it can ease the baby's transition to breathing (since the pulsing cord is still providing oxygenated blood) and because the final pulsing can help shrink the placenta, thus allowing it to more easily separate from the uterus.[17] Many doctors, on the other hand, are trained to cut the cord earlier, as a way to speed up the process.[18] Sarah tells me that, "The cord usually stops pulsing around the time of placental separation, but our pediatricians like us to do it sooner rather than later. Some think that at this high altitude they're already at risk for polysythemia, a high number of red blood cells, and clamping cuts the number, which has indications for jaundice." When I ask if she agrees with the doctors she says, "I wouldn't have a problem waiting."

Sarah has attended more than one thousand births, she was trained in midwifery at Yale University, and she's been practicing for more than ten years. But when she's in the hospital, her practice and that of the other midwives often has to conform to the doctors' approach. And as I saw today, sometimes the doctors are calling the shots, while the patients are left to think that their care is being managed by a midwife who is supposedly going to treat their labor as a normal, nonmedical event that only needs intervention when there are complications.

Several weeks later, I will see this happen with another patient of Sarah's. It proves a harsh reminder of the limitations on midwifery in the hospital.

⌒

It is the middle of the afternoon. Sarah arrives for her shift wearing her small wire-rim glasses, loose black pants that look vaguely Asian, and a white lab coat. Her hair is pulled up in a silver barrette with a Celtic design on it, and she seems tired. As she goes over some charts, a nurse arrives, looks at the board, and says, "Oh my God!" It is busy again.

The midwife who is just going off call comes to fill Sarah in, and tells her about laboring mother Tracy Hoffman. Tracy is a cross-country track coach who predicted that she wouldn't go into labor until after her team's last meet was over. Minutes after their final race, her water ruptured spontaneously. Her latest ultrasound showed that her baby may be quite large, but Tracy is a very large woman, tall and big-boned. She's contracting every five minutes, she's had an epidural, and her blood pressure is slightly elevated. Janelle Kolesky, the midwife going off shift, passes all this information on to Sarah and says, "I'm not sure what that high blood pressure is all about. It might just be positional. She's on her back. She's 90 percent effaced, at five centimeters, with an anterior cervix." She adds, "She was a prenatal client of mine. I think you'll have a really nice baby in there." Janelle looks around the nurses' station, then beckons Sarah to follow her down the hall to a more private room, where she confides that she had several clashes with the doctor on call tonight and warns her that he is being incredibly rude. This is pretty unusual, since the midwives have good relationships with most of the doctors, but it isn't unheard of. A few minutes later, one of the nurses pulls me aside to tell me that the doctor was so domineering that he actually made Janelle cry. The nurse shakes her head and says, "What an asshole."

Sarah gathers her charts and goes to Tracy's room. She introduces herself, checks Tracy's blood pressure, and asks how she's doing. Tracy says she's okay—better now that she's received the epidural. Tracy is very athletic-looking; she has muscular arms, and she's deeply tanned. Sarah asks her to roll onto her side to see if it brings her blood pressure down and urges her to get some rest in order to save some energy for pushing. Tracy agrees. Then her husband asks if there is a bucket around since Tracy is feeling nauseated. Sarah brings her a basin and Tracy immediately throws up into it. Sarah gently wipes her face with a washcloth and asks if the nausea is passing. Tracy nods, says, "Yes, I'm feeling sleepy. I think I'll sleep now," and closes her eyes.

"Well, you get some rest and then wake up and have a baby," Sarah tells her. "Sounds good," says Tracy and drifts off.

Sarah heads back to the nurses' station. In a little while, she checks Tracy's blood pressure again. It has dropped since she rolled onto her side, and Sarah seems relieved. She goes to take care of a number of other patients, and the afternoon begins to pass. Tracy sleeps on and off for the next few hours. Just after dinner, her husband walks by the nurses' station and Sarah asks him if Tracy's awake. "Yes, she just threw up again," he says.

"I think I'll check her then," Sarah says.

There are now two nurses and one set of soon-to-be-grandparents crowded into the darkened room. Sarah checks Tracy's cervix, closing her eyes as she reaches far in, feeling for change. "Your cervix is still about five or six centimeters," she reports. Apparently, the epidural has allowed her to sleep but may have diminished the strength of the contractions. But Sarah says there is also the possibility that this baby is too big to fit, a condition known as cephalopelvic disproportion or CPD. Although CPD is known to occur, its actual incidence is probably far lower than the incidence of its diagnosis, which, according to Henci Goer's *Obstetric Myths Versus Research Realities: A Guide to the Medical Literature,* is often inaccurate.[19] Goer cites a number of studies, including one that found women in the United States were six times more likely than women in Ireland to be diagnosed with CPD, prompting the authors of the study to comment on the "strong subjective element" in these diagnoses.[20] According to leading midwifery authority Judith Pence Rooks, Goer's research shows that "most women are capable of delivering even very large babies vaginally, if they are given time and adequate support."[21]

Sarah tells Tracy that she and Janelle, the previous midwife, had agreed that if Tracy didn't dilate more, they would like to put in an internal monitor to see how strong the contractions really are since the external monitor she's on only measures frequency and duration.

Tracy has been hooked up to the electronic fetal monitor since she got her epidural, a standard procedure due to the increased risk of fetal distress with an epidural.[22] Without the epidural, she would have been more likely to have had monitoring done only intermittently for twenty-minute intervals, although most hospitals routinely use continuous electronic fetal monitoring (EFM) on all laboring mothers. Continuous monitoring, where the woman is strapped to a machine from start to finish (keeping her immobilized), is now used at the vast majority of births, despite the fact that study after study has found that in low-risk cases it is no more effective than intermittent monitoring, providing *no* medical advantages to mother or baby, while increasing the risk of forceps and vacuum delivery by 20 percent and caesarean delivery by 40 percent.[23]

In her meticulously researched book, *Midwifery and Childbirth in America,* Judith Pence Rooks reports that "twelve prospective, randomized controlled trials involving more than 55,000 births in many countries have found higher rates of caesarean sections and forceps deliveries but no fewer fetal or neonatal deaths associated with electronic monitoring." Rooks further asserts that one 1993 study found that "increased use of EFM has not been associated with reduction in the overall national incidence of cerebral palsy in infants born at term, and explained that most cases of infant brain damage are not related to events during labor."[24] One study in the *New England Journal of Medicine,* which looked at continuous electronic fetal monitoring's ability to predict or prevent cerebral palsy, found that it had no benefit over intermittently listening to heart tones, that it increased the caesarean rate, and lead to no decrease in the incidence of cerebral palsy. In addition, EFM had a false positive rate of 99.6 to 99.8 percent, meaning "the proportion of pregnancies erroneously identified as at-risk because of these monitoring abnormalities (the false positive rate) was extremely high."[25]

Dr. Fredric Frigoletto, chief of obstetrics at Massachusetts General Hospital in Boston, agees that although the monitors are meant to screen for perinatal hypoxia or asphyxia, or damage from low oxygen levels and build-up of acid byproducts, they often wrongly suggest distress when it is not there, leading to unnecessary caesarean sections.[26]

Phyllis Rattey, CNM, of Special Beginnings Birth and Women's Center in Arnold, Maryland, explains that increased interventions associated with EFM come from "inaccuracies in interpreting the monitor strip, or simply seeing a bad strip and not looking for ways to help the baby do better, but instead jumping to an intervention to deliver the baby right away." She adds that by relying on the machine, instead of personal observation and attentive care, decisions to use interventive technology might be made too quickly, "instead of looking for simple ways, such as changing the mother's position, to provide improved oxygenation for the baby."[27]

As far back as 1988, the chairman of the Department of Obstetrics, Gynecology, and Reproductive Biology at Harvard Medical School called EFM a "failed technology," but foretold that it would be "difficult for obstetricians to stop using it in the absence of a substitute, in part because of the fear of being sued."[28] He was right. In fact, the use of EFM on laboring mothers went from 62 percent in 1988 to 84 percent in 1998.[29]

Tracy is now going to be switched to an internal monitor, which will measure more accurately the strength of her contractions. Sarah explains that if the internal monitor shows that her contractions look strong enough to bring forth the baby and she still doesn't progress, it could be a sign that the baby is too big to fit. On the other hand, if the contractions look weak, the baby's size might not be the issue at all. Sarah puts in the monitor and a nurse straps its trailing cord to Tracy's leg. Tracy is lying in a forest of tubes, wires, blinking monitors, and running IVs. I am reminded of something Seattle midwife Heike Doyle, who works in a birth center and attends home births, once said to me about labor and delivery suites like this one, decorated to look like nice bedrooms. "I have some choice words for those rooms," she said. "I call them the 'fooled-you rooms.' The pictures turn around and there is all the medical equipment. Just because you put pretty wallpaper on the wall doesn't mean you've changed the protocols."

Later I'll ask Sarah how she feels about being a midwife in a highly technologized scene like this one and she says, "I think you have to be wise about technology and certainly have an understanding of it in order to know when it would truly be helpful. But you also have to balance that with a trust that women's bodies have been birthing babies for all of human time, and it's generally something that doesn't need to be altered. But when it does need to be altered, I think the midwife has powerful responsibility to do that wisely." She tells Tracy that it takes thirty minutes to be able to get a good reading off the internal monitor and heads off to check on her other patients.

⌢

Tracy's blood pressure continues to creep up whenever she lies on her back but comes down each time the staff roll her onto her side, suggesting it isn't a sign of something serious like preeclampsia. Sarah asks the nurse to see if Tracy has any protein in her urine. A few minutes later, the nurse reports that there is no protein in the urine. Sarah admits to being a bit anxious about Tracy's baby being too big and her blood pressure being high, but when, after fifteen minutes, she checks the reading on Tracy's contractions, and finds that they don't look very strong, she tells me that it is possible that the baby is not too big, just that her contractions haven't been strong enough. So Sarah has the nurse bump up Tracy's Pitocin. "Still," says Sarah, "I'm going to have to order a panel of tests to check for preeclampsia, and I'm going to have to consult the doctor."

Unfortunately, the doctor who made the previous midwife cry is still on call, so Sarah is treading carefully around him. She doesn't want to rock the boat by not consulting and then have him say she should have done so. She groans and says, "Get ready to run mag," meaning magnesium sulfate, which is sometimes administered for toxemia or preeclampsia and which Sarah feels sure the doctor will recommend. I ask how this will make Tracy feel. "She'll feel flush, and hot, and yucky, and then I'll have a doctor breathing down my neck," Sarah responds, clearly reluctant to hand over control of Tracy's case. As it turns out, Tracy's bloodwork comes back normal, thus she avoids the nasty side effects magnesium sulfate would have brought, and is able stay under the care of a midwife—for now.

"This is when it is hard sometimes," Sarah says with a sigh. "On top of everything, I can tell when Tracy looks at me that she's disappointed I'm not Janelle, who was also her midwife for her prenatal clinic visits." At Skyline, with seventeen midwives on staff, the chances of having your birth attended by the same woman who did your prenatal care is fairly slim. For some women this is an issue, but many don't question it, and the midwives themselves express mixed feelings about the trade-offs of this system. While most of the Skyline midwives have told me that they don't think it is important that their clinic patients get the same caregiver for their delivery, and recent studies show beneficial effects from continuity of care, including outcomes for both infants and mothers.[30] Many of these same midwives have also told me of patients who seem to stall their labors until "their" midwife comes on call. And when I asked them directly if it would be *ideal* for women to have continuity of care between their prenatal visits and the delivery, most of the midwives say "yes," citing the wealth of subtle, yet important, information they acquire about their patients over the course of seven or eight months, and something they refer to as a "therapeutic relationship" that grows out of trust.

I ask Sarah if her inability to provide that kind of continuity to her clients is troubling for her. "It was a huge problem for me early in my career," she says. "And I would come in a lot when I wasn't on call to attend my clients' births, but my life now, with children of my own, doesn't allow for me to do that as much. Also, having birthed my children now, those prenatal visits were far more important to me than who was there to catch my baby. I'm pretty oblivious to that. So there's been a little shift inside of me about how important that really is." I can see how, for some women, it might not matter whether they have their midwife of choice at the birth, because they may be so deeply into their own world during labor. But I can't imagine that for myself, and Sarah's answer doesn't truly address the importance of continuity of care for her clients.

Later, another certified nurse-midwife working with a large hospital-based practice tells me, "I remember, in school, people were just like 'oh, the shift midwives,'" she shudders. "'How horrible. Could you imagine leaving somebody when they're pushing?' and I thought that, yeah, that would be horrible. But even though it sounds terrible, I need to compartmentalize my job and my family. The way that I keep my own health and harmony is to have that separation. So one of the reasons I chose to work in the hospital was because of working in shifts. I need to find a way to do this for a long time so that I'm not going to get burnt out; I want to be sixty years old and still be catching babies. I think that that would be phenomenal—to have that history and that expertise. And so, I feel like, yes, the mother is short-changed, but if you need more, you should find it, and you won't necessarily find it in this kind of practice. I have people who, when you talk to them after their birth about the care they received, say, 'Gosh I really thought that I was going to be midwifed more.' And I think that's a legitimate complaint." She adds that she often recommends that her clients hire a doula, or private birth assistant, since so many of them have a lot of anxiety about not knowing which midwife will help them with their birth. "And you know," she says, "that would never have been acceptable to me, for my own births. So I chose differently. I knew from the get-go that I was going to have a home birth."

I tell Sarah what this midwife said. She nods in agreement, having had both of her children at home. Now I ask her if Tracy's disappointment at having her own midwife go off shift could affect her progress? Sarah nods, "It could. The mind is powerful, but also her epidural is probably slowing down her contractions."

Just then a nurse reports that Tracy's blood pressure is way down, plenty low, and everybody sighs happily. Things are a little less busy now, and when a passing father-to-be relates how he was nauseated the first four months of his wife's pregnancy and is now feeling sympathy pains (a documented psychosomatic condition known as couvade), this prompts one of the nurses to tell a related birthing joke. It goes like this: A doctor invented a machine that transfers labor pains to the father. The mom goes into labor and the doctor puts it on low because he thinks the dad won't be able to handle it. But the dad says, "No problem." So he cranks it up. The wife's pain goes down even more, but still the dad says, "No problem." So the doctor sets the machine on full power. Still no problem. The mom gives birth, they go home, and find the mailman dead on the porch.

We all laugh.

It is a brief moment of ease. Shortly after this, at 9:15 P.M, the doctor walks up to Sarah, points to Tracy Hoffman's name on the patient status board and says gruffly, "If she's not at seven [meaning seven centimeters dilated] by 10:30, then she's going to be post-op by 11:45." It takes me a minute to realize he's threatening a caesarean section. Sarah looks at him with raised eyebrows.

"That was a statement," he says snidely. "We need to be more aggressive with the Pitocin."

Sarah retorts, a little edgily, "What do you want us to do differently?"

"Well, I just want us to be more aggressive," he practically barks. "You can take the Pit up every fifteen minutes." His tone and his demeanor are decidedly bullying and nasty. Sarah agrees tersely and leaves. The nurse bumps up Tracy's Pitocin again, but nobody mentions to her that a doctor down the hall is threatening to section her.

I find myself thinking of the several studies I've read that show how the chance of having a caesarean section can be reduced by up to 50 percent simply by being continually attended by a support person with relevant knowledge and skills, usually a woman who provides soothing encouragement.[31] Tracy does not have such a person. Labor and delivery nurses have not been shown to have a similar effect; studies show that, on average, they spend only between 6 percent and 10 percent of their time providing actual support to women in labor.[32] Tracy's midwife is too busy to stay with her, and she hasn't hired a doula whose services, unfortunately, are almost never covered by insurance companies.

A half-hour later, at 10 P.M., another midwife shows up and takes over some of Sarah's patients, but Sarah says she'll stay with the two mothers the doctor is hovering over. She and the arriving midwife roll their eyes while discussing his behavior, and Sarah says, "He has these tantrums, and they bother some people more than they do me. But you know, its sort of like being the mother of a three-year-old," (which she is) and then adds, grinning slyly and speaking sotto vocce, "It's also like, 'I have a penis! I have a penis!'"

She gestures with her hands in front of her, swinging her hips and an imaginary penis from side to side. Everybody at the nurses' station cracks up and some of the tension of the moment dissipates.

But at 10:25 P.M. the doctor returns and silently watches Tracy's contraction pattern on the computer monitor at the nurses' station. He comments that Tracy's pattern is not looking great. "Do you want to go in and check her?" Sarah asks. He doesn't respond, simply grunts, "Hmm," shrugs his shoulders, and continues to watch the computer screen.

Sarah waits for a few minutes and then goes to check on Tracy herself. She says Tracy has a little bloody show, and that's a nice sign. Her cervix is at six centimeters. Sarah and the doctor consult in the hallway.

"I have some concern," Sarah says, to which the doctor retorts in a nasty tone, "We've had some concern for some time. How long since she hasn't progressed?"

"Three hours by my count, more by Janelle's."

"Enough!" he snaps. "Let's call it a day and go to Plan B."

Back in the room, the doctor introduces himself to Tracy and says, "You certainly get high marks for effort, but so far it hasn't been for much. In days of old they would just let you labor and labor, and eventually you would deliver. In some places in the world they still do that, and some of those women's uteruses rupture. Here we don't let that happen because we go to Plan B, which would be delivery by caesarean section." He goes over the risks, including the risk of bleeding, infection, and the risk of injury to the ovaries and bladder. He informs Tracy and her husband that the expected recovery time is about six weeks, to which her husband says, "Okay. Let's do it. The sooner the better." At 11 P.M. Tracy Hoffman gets a C-section for failure to progress, and at 11:45 she is post-op, just as the doctor said she would be.

⌒

Skyline Hospital has a reputation for being the least-interventive care center in town, and I don't doubt it. Their epidural rate is much lower than their competitors', as is their caesarean rate. (I want to make it clear that while overly high caesarean rates are of great concern—rates in the United States reached 22.9 percent in 2000, an 11 percent increase over the previous four years with nearly 50 percent of those thought to be unnecessary—midwives as well as doctors recognize that there are times when caesareans are life-savers for mothers and babies. No one wants to eliminate caesarean birth.)[33] Yet, while I have seen many respectful, supportive births at Skyline Hospital, many of these births have been attended by far more technology than I would want for myself. As my mounting fatigue and morning sickness keep my own pregnancy front and center in my consciousness, I find myself increasingly concerned with hospital protocols and the way they shape not only a woman's experience of her birth, but the birth itself.

I ask Liz Donahue if she thinks the conventions and practices of the hospital undermine the midwives' ability to consistently focus on birth as normal. She says, "I think that the midwives who practice in a setting like this are very aware that it requires changes in some behaviors and perhaps some clinical practice changes. But I think that, for the most part, we're capable of changing hats. I can be very medical and I can direct a very medically managed labor, and I can also stand back and not do pelvic exams, and put a woman in a bathtub, and tell the doctor why she needs to push for longer than two hours. It's true that it can be hard on us sometimes; we kind of forget which it is we're supposed to be doing. And we walk a fine line in terms of meeting the demands of the system. This is a medical system, and it's medically driven, but we see ourselves as go-betweens; we soften the medicalness of the system a little bit for people."

When I ask one of the senior midwives on staff, Alison Davies, why she thinks there are so many interventions, even at this self-avowedly low-tech hospital, she says, immediately and as if it were obvious, "Oh, because we have all young doctors who have been trained with technology. It's scientific, you know," she says with mock seriousness. "Few of the new doctors have been trained that this is a natural process. Also, they have not been trained to recognize when the process may be getting off course and how to get it back to normal. Fifteen years ago, the doctors who worked with us were, well, old." Alison chuckles. "They were old, so they hadn't had the technology." She pauses, then adds, "And then, the medical-legal atmosphere has made a huge difference, too. We are all more likely to use technologies that we think might protect us from law suits."

Of course, there are times when it is medically advisable to use technological interventions—to speed labor along, to hasten a delivery, to do caesarean sections, and sometimes even for failure to progress. I do not mean to suggest that women's lives should be put at risk. But I wonder about the ways hospitals might actually work to exaggerate the risks of childbirth and certainly to reduce one's experience of childbirth as a normal process which usually goes right, particularly when the "cascade of intervention" gets rolling, as it does with some frequency. The interventions begin benignly, but soon they are piling up like wrecked cars on a foggy highway until the idea of normal childbirth is gone, gone, gone.

I say "normal" childbirth and not "natural" childbirth for several reasons. The first is that even a birth that is not completely natural can still be normal. I am not categorically opposed to any interventions or assistance per se. A sense of normalcy can be maintained even when interventions are necessary, it just takes more effort. Second, the word "natural" is a slippery little adjective. For example, both herbs and pharmaceutical drugs are substances foreign to the body, so what do we mean when we say one is more natural than the other? Third, and most important, the phrase "natural childbirth" has become so loaded, and sadly, even divisive among women. A recent article in the *New York Times Magazine* attacks the "persistent tut-tutting of the natural childbirth community" for making a "fetish of the perfectly orchestrated birth experience" and for fostering "the illusion that women themselves can exert complete control over what is, in fact, a notoriously unpredictable event, and that those who ask for pain relief have failed a test of character."[34]

Although I agree with the *Times* article that childbirth is unpredictable, as unpredictable, in fact, as the ways of love that get us there, it is not my impression that perfect orchestration and complete control over birth are truly the main tenets of natural childbirth. And yet, many women believe this is so, and, unfortunately, there is often some sort of insidious moral judgment associated with women's decisions regarding pain relief. How unnecessary and infuriating. As if we didn't already have our hands full making difficult decisions without adequate information and while suffering incredible pain.

When the same article goes on to attack the natural childbirth movement's claims that unmedicated birth can be "hugely empowering," that "with anesthesia, a woman misses out on the peak experience of her life," and that birth can be "an opportunity to define the self," I find I cannot join in scoffing at these claims. Instead, I am curious and sad about what I may have missed with my first birth, and sadder still to find that I live in a culture that finds such concerns laughable, or aligned with the forces of moralizing oppression, or worst yet, placed in opposition to having a healthy baby. The article ends with a position I have heard many times; "What matters, surely," it concludes, "is not how you get through labor but what you get through it. What matters is a healthy baby." Well, of course, a healthy baby is paramount, but can't one have a transformative experience, too? And, in fact, according to statistical evidence, natural childbirth is actually more likely to produce a healthy baby, free of the side effects of analgesia and the risks associated with anesthesia. True, my own baby didn't seem to suffer any negative consequences from the drugs I took, but I would rather not have taken the chance, and my own drug-hazed birth experience was far more depressing than elevating or empowering.

I am left wondering why the physical and the spiritual aspects of childbirth must be pitted against each other. Haven't we finally come far enough with the treatment of women to provide opportunities for childbirth that are at once safe, humane, and at least potentially empowering? I know in my gut (my extremely nauseated and quickly expanding gut) that this is possible, and I am determined to find access to it.

I remember meeting, not long ago, a young woman who was

living a back-to-the-land lifestyle in a remote mountain community in rural New Mexico who had given birth on a wooden platform under a dizzying ocean of stars. At the time, I was shocked as well as intrigued. I know I am not ready to birth so far outside of my own cultural expectations, and yet I am envious of the splendor of her birth setting, so far from the conventions of the hospital. I yearn to have even a trace of her experience.

I had thought that having a midwife was the way to ensure this, but now I am not so sure. Although midwives are likely to care about the spiritual aspects of pregnancy and childbirth, or at least be willing to talk about them with their patients, this is not universally so. There is an incredible range of personalities and practices among the certified nurse-midwives I have met. At Skyline, there is no one midwife who typifies the group. Some are more attentive than others, just as, I am sure, is the case with obstetricians.

While I am considering all this, I get a call from a friend in New York who used a midwife with her first birth. She is pregnant again and tells me that at her first prenatal exam with the midwife who attended her the first time, the midwife had said brusquely, "Well, I don't remember you or your birth." Then, during her exam, she suddenly called out to her assistant, "Hey, come look at this cervix. You won't see another like this one." My friend felt violated. Since there weren't any other midwives to choose from at her practice, she is having her baby with a more sensitive obstetrician. Midwifery's goals are humane, but the profession itself is no guarantee of the individuals who practice it. Even the certified nurse-midwives who try hardest to protect a sense of normalcy during birth often find themselves tilting against the constraints of the hospital itself.

And yet the mere existence of midwifery's professional goals has been critical to the improvement of birthing women's health care. Midwives have made great strides in bringing respect to birthing women and lowering the incidence of unnecessary medical interventions. If my pregnancy stays low-risk, I will still choose a midwife over a doctor.

5

Balancing Acts

I WORKED in an extraordinary setting in New Zealand for several years. I was on a tiny island doing home births," certified nurse-midwife Joanne White tells me as she gets ready to begin her shift at the hospital. "And am I there now? No. Will I ever do it again? No."

I ask why.

"Oh my God, see this gray hair?" She holds out a hank of her salt and pepper hair. "It was brown when I went there."

Joanne is always very forthright with me, but she's also likely to make light of difficult situations, so I am a little taken aback by how unsmiling she is even as she makes the crack about her hair. "Being a home-birth midwife is exhausting and really hard on your family," she says. "There's lifestyle and there's making a living. The home-birth thing almost has to be like a hobby, because you sure as heck can't make this kind of money in a home-birth practice. Eventually home-birth midwives are divorced, or broke, or whatever." Joanne pauses to pull her hair back into a ponytail, momentarily silenced by the rubber band she holds between her teeth. "Although I should tell you that the two midwives who are there now love it."

I ask if they have children of their own. "No." Joanne laughs.

"Funny you should ask. No, they don't. Working there was tre-mendously hard on my family, mostly because of the meltdown that was happening to me. I have two children, and for me, fam-ily comes first. Period."

This is a common sentiment among midwives. It is perhaps unsurprising that women who become midwives are often women who are both "adrenaline freaks—people who like to live on the edge," as Joanne describes them, and women who want children and feel committed to family life. Being a midwife who has to drop everything when a client goes into labor and stay with her for as long as she needs is not easily compatible with parent-ing. This is where midwives have to make a personal trade-off. They can choose to work in a private home-birth practice with its freedom from the medical culture of the hospital, its intensely re-warding personal relationships, and its demanding schedule and uncertain financial viability. Or they can choose to work in a hospital with its predictable schedule, decent financial compen-sation, and often frustrating limitations on the way they can prac-tice midwifery. Either way, they are faced with a career, like many, that involves a delicate balancing act.

For Joanne, shift-work in a hospital looked pretty appealing.

"Hospital work is how you sustain what you do," says Joanne. When she first made the switch, she had a hard time leaving a birthing woman when her shift ended, but she soon realized that handing her client off to another midwife was, for her, preferable to staggering home in the wee hours of the morning. "At some point," she says, "it occurred to me that they wouldn't give up their families for me, so why was I giving up my family for them?" This argument seems a little specious to me. I mean, do firefight-ers say they won't risk their lives for people who aren't doing the same for them? If everyone only made sacrifices or went the ex-tra mile in their jobs when they knew the act would be recipro-cated, we'd be in a lot of trouble. Nevertheless, I understand what Joanne means when she says, "Boundaries are something midwives have to learn. And I truly feel the good midwives have learned boundaries. The new midwives haven't, you'll see that. You have to learn boundaries, because it's very seductive to become part of these women's lives."

From a professional standpoint, this makes a lot of sense, but I feel my perspective as a pregnant mom creeping in when I ask, "Don't women need you to be part of their lives, at least temporarily?" Joanne concedes that, yes, midwives do need to connect with their clients, but assures me that it is possible to do that and also trust that someone else in your practice can pick up where you left off. She adds that she feels lucky to work in a practice where she knows she can trust everyone else to do a great job, even though continuity of care is sacrificed.

Joanne believes that continuity isn't everything. "Your clients see you at the end of a twelve-hour shift, and you don't look so good," she says. "I tell my patients, 'You want the fresh horse. This horse is tired. You can see what happens here when the fresh horse comes in.' Maybe she'll adjust the lighting or fluff the pillows—whatever—but the energy changes. We all acknowledge that this is a good thing, and that other midwife just couldn't have done that anymore. She may be excellent, but she's gotta go home because she's tired. It's not because the last midwife was bad; she's just spent."

One of the downsides to a hospital practice is that sometimes, even at the beginning of her shift, the midwife can't attend a birthing woman properly if it is a really busy night. Then, Joanne says, the midwife needs to draw on all her interpersonal skills to make the woman feel as supported as is possible, and the birthing woman might need to rely on someone other than the midwife as well. "You walk the line in this setting because we're not generally able to be there," Joanne says. "You try to tell the patients early on 'Your family is going to be essential here; they're really important, so use them.' I tell patients 'I'm not going to be there breathing with every contraction. I *will* be with you when you're pushing.' I'll also tell a patient, 'I've got four people going, but when I'm with you I'm completely with you, okay?' And I don't necessarily have to be physically in the room to give whatever it is she needs. It's all coming from her. All we do is just tweak it a little. We give her a little confidence; we give her a little hint. We're out of there, we come back, we might be there for three minutes, but it doesn't mean you have to go into O.B. mode. You never have to do that. You always go into it from a midwifery perspective."

For Joanne, this means being able to offer some loving words of encouragement, or a foot rub, or whatever seems right for the woman and her family. "I can be as groovy as you want me to be," she says. But it also means teaching family members how to be supportive when the midwife can't be there. "It is my best resource to midwife a family," says Joanne. "I'll suggest, 'Why don't you rub her here?' If I do that all myself, if I am physically as well as mentally exhausted, how long can I do this job? Not very long. But if I can midwife the *family* through the birth, then that's a greater gift, because that gift is going to go on after labor as well. It's sort of that 'teach a man to fish' thing."

Sometimes, though, she admits that she misses the connection that comes from staying with a woman in labor from start to finish or from attending a woman who she's come to know well throughout the course of her prenatal exams. Every now and then, Joanne will come in for a certain mom or a certain couple, even if it isn't her shift. "Coming in special is the way we pay ourselves back," she says. "So occasionally, I'll put a yellow sticky-note on the chart saying they can call me at home for this patient. And everybody goes 'Whoaaa!' because that's so rare for me. I mean, for me to do that." She rolls her eyes, "Well, ask my colleagues how often that happens. Like never. Because that puts you back on call, and the reason I took this job was so I wouldn't have to be on call. Again, it's a question of boundaries."

Ultimately, Joanne suggests that while her presence as a midwife can be crucial to a woman's positive birth experience, her personality and a long-term relationship with the woman are not so important. I'm not convinced by this argument, but I understand that it may be true for some women, and that for midwives working in the hospital, it is a point of view that allows them to do the best they can, given their circumstances.

⌒

Joanne and I have been chatting at the nurses' station before her shift begins. Now she goes to check the big white patient-status board and, beckoning me to join her, says, "Let's check on Kim in room 129."

Kim is thirty years old, working on a degree in social work, and having her first child. When she was last checked, she had dilated to between five and six centimeters. As we walk down the hall, Joanne tells me, "Her baby's o.p.," meaning the baby is occiput posterior, or face up, which, because the baby's skull is putting pressure on the spine, often results in extremely painful back labor. "She seems to be moving along pretty quickly. She prefers to lie on her side, and she's had some pain meds, Fentanyl. It's in and out of the system quickly."

We enter the room and find Kim lying on her side, moaning. Her husband, Chris, is sitting next to the bed, talking on the phone. He is trying to get the right paperwork sent to their room so they can have some of the blood from their baby's umbilical cord saved. The procedure involves harvesting blood from the cord immediately after birth and freezing it, because it can be useful in treating certain future cancers. Chris and Kim heard about the procedure at a hospital orientation visit but have just decided to pursue it now, so Chris is busy setting it up, leaving Kim on her own to deal with what is clearly a good deal of pain.

"It's so bad," moans Kim, her loose hair covering her face. "I want more drugs."

Joanne has Kim change her position so she is up on her knees leaning into the raised bed. Joanne checks her and then gets up on the bed herself as she administers another dose of Fentanyl. Kim asks how much she has dilated. Joanne says, "Oh, it's stretching out. You're not quite seven centimeters."

Kim starts to moan again. She sounds close to tears. A contraction mounts, she cries out slightly, then it passes. A trickle of blood runs down her leg. Joanne gets off the bed and motions to Chris to take her place. He does and rubs Kim's back. "Harder," she groans. Joanne stands by her head and gently rubs her shoulder. Kim says, "Here comes one."

"Just ride it out," Joanne says.

Kim moans.

"That's right, keep it low," says Joanne, referring to the tone of her cries.

After the contraction passes, Chris and Joanne help Kim roll over. Joanne asks if Kim wants her to break her bag of water now and "see if we can get that baby to move along." Kim says, "Yes. Let's do it."

Unfortunately, after a woman's water breaks (whether it does so naturally or is broken manually), because the force of the baby's head is no longer dispersed over the cushioning sack of amniotic fluid, it can really add to the pain. Chris looks so anxious. Two nurses come in and check the monitors. One nurse hands Joanne a long, yellow plastic stick with a flexible hook at the top. "Like a crochet hook" Joanne says.

"You'll feel some pressure," Joanne tells Kim. "We're just going to get the membrane out of the way." She inserts the stick, moves her hand slightly, and says, "Beautiful!"

"I'm having a contraction!" Kim cries out. "Aaaaah!" she shrieks in a high pitched voice. If her contractions hurt before, it is clear that they've now ratcheted up a notch.

"Keep your throat open, nice and low," instructs Joanne, reminding her that a lower tone will help relax her throat and diaphragm thus reducing unnecessary tension.

Kim lowers the pitch of her moan. She rolls over, and there's a lot of blood between her legs.

At this point, Chris asks Joanne if she can help him get the cord blood procedure set up. She says she'll look into it, and we leave Chris and Kim on their own so Joanne can go to the nurses' station to make some calls. It takes several phone calls and around twenty minutes for Joanne to locate the right information.

While she works on this, she writes a letter to a friend and chats with some of the nurses. I can't help wondering how Kim and Chris are coping on their own. When we get back, Kim is still moaning. Chris is standing by her side, still looking anxious.

"Ooohhh. Push on my back. Rub there," she says, and then the contraction passes. With the next contraction, Joanne pushes hard on Kim's back, leaning her whole body into it. Kim breathes hard through her mouth and says she's cold. Joanne covers her with a blanket.

Another contraction. "Aiiiiii!" Kim screams.

"Breathe through it," Joanne says, stroking her arm.

"Uh," grunts Kim, "Here's the pushing feeling."

"Ride through. Ride it out."

The urge to step in and help is strong. I want to do something. But it is not my place, and I'm not sure what I would actually do, anyway. Then, as if she has just read my mind, Joanne says she has to step out to check on some other moms and would I stay here with Kim and Chris. Without waiting for an answer, she pops out the door. Chris has now practically disappeared; he is silent and slumped in a chair in the corner. I take over pushing on Kim's back. It feels like hours, but I actually spend only twenty minutes or so alone with Kim. During that time, I feel helpless and wonder whatever happened to my sitting in the corner, taking notes. And yet it also feels good to do something for Kim. Even if it is just to provide counterpressure on her sacrum. I find myself thinking that I better learn more about how to help laboring women if I'm going to keep hanging out with them for another six months or more. I also find myself thinking that a half-hour seems like a very long time when every third minute or so brings an intense bout of pain. Surely, the regular disappearance of the midwife to attend someone else affects the laboring mom's ability to cope.

Finally, Joanne comes back. As she arrives, Kim has a huge contraction and totally loses control. She's yelling like a little kid now. Wailing. Joanne gets in close to her face and whispers in her ear. After the contraction passes, Joanne puts on her gloves and slips her fingers in to check Kim's cervix. She's still only seven centimeters dilated, but the baby has moved down more. With the next contraction, Kim is shrieking again. Joanne says, "Catch your breath and relax. Yes, good." When this one passes, Kim asks if she can get an epidural. Joanne says yes, if she wants to, but does she want to try the bath first?

"Okay, but that's my last try," Kim says. Another contraction hits her and she changes her mind. "I want an epidural. Let's skip the bath," she says. Joanne nods her assent and goes to get the anesthesiologist. She has already offered a natural alternative, and she's not about to deny this woman more powerful pain relief if that's what she really wants. While one could argue that Kim might feel better if she were more adequately attended, it is also true that honoring a woman's choices is one of the hallmarks of contemporary midwifery.

I push on Kim's back through another contraction. A few minutes later, Joanne comes back and reports that the anesthesia guys are in a C-section, so it might be a while.

"Oh nooo. No. No!" Kim yells.

Joanne smiles weakly and says, "Want to try the bath while it's warm?"

"I don't think I can move," Kim replies.

"We'll help you," Joanne offers.

Joanne and I lift Kim up to a sitting position. As she gets up, she has another contraction at the edge of the bed. She's sobbing in a guttural, heavy, child-like way. The noise she makes sounds like it must hurt her throat. There is a brief pause, followed by another contraction.

"Pressure!" Kim calls out. "Put on the pressure!" she screams. In the next pause, Chris walks her slowly to the bathroom. Kim gets into the tub, going down onto her hands and knees, the warm water barely reaching her belly. While they are in the bathroom, a nurse asks them to fill out the paperwork for the epidural. The form gets soggy and tears; Chris curses under his breath. Joanne says quietly to me, "You're kind of like a flight attendant in the voyage of life—fluff 'em up and make 'em comfortable."

I sit on the floor by the door to the bathroom, watching as a nurse checks the baby's heartrate with a Doppler. I wonder why nobody is getting Kim more comfortably settled in the water and wonder if I should stop being a mere observer here. Kim asks again for the epidural. Joanne asks a nurse how long until they get out of the C-section. The nurse doesn't know and goes to check. Joanne takes a few minutes to write in Kim's chart, then leaves the room.

When Joanne leaves, I decide to give up my plan of being a "fly on the wall" journalist in favor of being what anthropologists call a "participant observer." I get Kim to sit down more comfortably in the tub. She turns and, from behind a veil of loose, dark hair, asks me, "Why does it hurt so much? What's happening?" Chris, too, anxiously asks me, "Is something wrong?" They seem to think that now that the hospital staff is gone, I will reveal some awful truth that is being concealed from them. They both seem terrified. I tell them that this is totally normal; that childbirth can be excruciating, but that it won't last forever. "Yes, it hurts," I say, "but your baby will be here soon." I smooth Kim's hair back into a ponytail. She lies back and relaxes a tiny bit. Even though I have found something good to say, I still find myself wishing this would just end for her and wishing that she and Chris hadn't had to come into this event so obviously unprepared. I wonder what, if anything, could have prepared them. I know my own childbirth classes still left me struggling though my first labor like a sailor going down at sea. Maybe simply seeing other births would help, but only good, normal, well-attended births. This is a tall order for the average new mother and father.

When Joanne returns, I go to the lounge to wolf down a burger, fries, some salad, and an apple. It is almost 3:00 p.m., and this is the first time I've eaten since a breakfast of crackers, nibbled during a wave of morning sickness. I know I must really be pregnant because my body is oscillating between hideous nausea and ravenous hunger. I take a few minutes to call my friend Addie, who is due just a few weeks after me. She's suffering from outrageous nausea but says, "I console myself by telling myself that it's a good sign. I hear morning sickness usually means the baby's doing okay. But . . . this stinks. When's it going to stop?" I tell her I've heard that by the fourteenth week it usually subsides, but my mom was sick her entire pregnancy. Addie groans. I tell her I just heard that my friend Elena is pregnant, too, and I'm so excited that we are all doing this at the same time. Then I've got to run, since I've got to call my family, finish eating, and get back to Kim before she gives birth. Right after I hang up, I hear a nurse say the C-section patient is bleeding and the doctors just went back in, so it will be a while before the anesthesiologist is free to give Kim an epidural. I feel sorry for her.

When I get back to her room, Kim is back in the bed, still with no epidural. It turns out she was nine centimeters dilated when the "epi guys" as Joanne calls them, finally got out of surgery. She was completely dilated just a few minutes later, and so she was too far along to get anesthesia. Joanne strokes her arms and says, "You have really done it all by yourself. Are you ready to do some pushing?"

"Yes," Kim says weakly, bears down, and groans.

"Great pushing! Good, good, good," Joanne says.

"Put your chin to your chest. There you go. Look at that. Excellent."

Kim pushes with each contraction, with Joanne urging her along, saying, "Come on little one." Joanne's voice gets very high pitched and excited, "Yes, yes, come on baby. Come around the corner. Good."

After half an hour or so, a little patch of black hair starts to show. It is a shock; I'd almost forgotten there was an actual baby in there. Kim's bladder is very full, so Joanne inserts a catheter and drains her bladder to give the baby more room. With the next contraction, one of the nurses joins the chorus of "Push! Push!" I can see how it is hard to resist the urge to be a vocal cheerleader for pushing as the baby hangs on the verge of birth. The room heats up and starts to smell a bit rank. Kim is now on all fours on the bed.

Joanne puts her hands just inside Kim's vagina and says, "Right there. Don't let it out through your mouth. Push there." As she pushes, we listen to the baby's heart on the monitor. It sounds like horses' hooves galloping through wet sand. On the next contraction Joanne says, "Okay, let's have a baby. Push into it." But Kim's not quite there yet. Joanne asks Kim to turn over onto her back with her legs up on the squat bar. There it is, *the* hospital birth position. Joanne is still offering encouragement, saying, "Oh Kim, good girl. Go, go, go, come on baby, come on little one." Joanne explains that the baby is facing off to the side, trying to turn, and that it probably will. Kim is grimacing and pushing, holding her breath. Joanne asks her to hold onto her thighs, but she doesn't.

Now we can really see the top of the head. It is 4:25 P.M. I find myself holding my breath with every push. Finally, with baby's head staying on the edge of the perineum, Joanne and a nurse put on sterile, blue paper gowns and wheel in a table lined with instruments. Intermittently, they put the flat monitor on Kim and check the baby's heartbeat. It is always fine. Joanne asks Kim to touch her baby's head, but she won't do it. Joanne says, "Wait . . ." puts a gauze pad on the baby, tells Kim she's put a hat on it, and Kim agrees to reach down. The baby starts to crown, and Kim yells, "It's burning!" The baby has turned facedown now. As it begins to emerge, fluid comes gushing out with it. Joanne suctions the baby as its face appears saying, "Your baby is here!"

"I don't care. I just want it out," Kim says.

Chris cries out, "The face is out." Then, suddenly, the baby is fully born. Joanne passes him up to Kim saying, "We don't have a name for you," meaning it is a boy, as they had only picked a girl's name, Leanna Grace.

Kim turns her head and says to Chris, "Take it. I don't want it now. Take it. I'll take it later." I'm a little taken aback to hear her refer to the baby as "it" and by her rejection of the infant. And yet, I'm not entirely surprised. If I'd gone through the pain I saw her go through, I might feel that way, too.

With just a hint of reproach, Joanne says, "It's a him, not an it."

Chris smiles tentatively as he cradles the baby.

Kim asks anxiously, "Did I rip?"

"I don't think so," says Joanne, "We'll see after the placenta is out."

Kim grimaces and pushes out the placenta. A nurse turns on the overhead light and Joanne looks for tears. "No tears on a first baby! Awesome." Kim is still bleeding, so Joanne pushes on her belly, saying, "I can't let you bleed too much. I need to find out what's bleeding. We're going to give you a shot of Pitocin."

"Will I contract?"

"Yes, you will."

"Ohhh no. Can I get some pain medicine?"

"Yes. Some Fentanyl," Joanne says, and the nurse gives her yet another dose along with the Pitocin.

Kim is bleeding quite a bit. "We've got to stop the bleeding," Joanne says, and presses on her again. Kim groans. "This is as bad as giving birth." After a few minutes, Joanne reports that the bleeding appears to have stopped, "but we'll watch you pretty closely."

Chris looks at the baby, who is now lying on the warming table. "He's so big," he says. "I was picturing a G.I. Joe doll, but he's so big!" I say good-bye and apologize if I intruded at all. Kim glances at me and says, "Oh, I didn't even notice you."

⌒

Kim's birth brings up a number of issues for me. First, I think about how Joanne's obligations meant she wasn't able to be with Kim as much as Kim seemed to need. Second, I found Kim's pain deeply disturbing. I wanted her to get some relief, whether it came from human support or drugs. Despite my belief that natural childbirth avoids unnecessary risks and is more likely to allow birth to be a spiritual experience, I can't help but think that, given her circumstances, Kim might have had a better experience with the assistance of drugs. If that's true for her, it can be true for anyone. Even me.

I find myself reliving my own labor with Max and remember how great a toll the pain took. How angry I was at the world and at him for weeks afterward. I knew it was unreasonable, but I couldn't shake the feeling. Given that I wasn't going to get any additional emotional support in that hospital at that time, an epidural might have been good for me. Though not my first choice, I would much rather have had someone's loving touch and constant support. But without that, I can see how an epidural might have helped. Seeing Kim helps me accept that although I may not have toughed it out with a natural labor with Max, I did what I could. Sure, it would have been better to have set up more support for myself. Kim, too, would no doubt have benefited from more loving care. But there's no going back. Neither she nor I can change those labors. For myself, all I can do is look to the future. I can accept that if I get medical pain relief at my next birth, it will be because I truly needed it, and I decide right now to look into having a doula there.

I had heard of doulas before my first birth, but thought it was an unnecessary expense. I also thought it would disrupt the bond between my husband and I. I had the crazy notion that birth would be romantic. It isn't. Or at least mine wasn't. And even if it was, a kind, well-informed advocate would have done nothing to lessen the bond between my husband and I. If anything, she might have helped strengthen it. She could have helped my husband so he could help me. Certainly, she could have helped me to relax and to understand what was happening both with my body and my care. A doula can help fill in the gaps that hospitals bring to midwifery care. As Joanne writes up Kim's chart, I ask her what she thinks about using an on-call doula, or suggesting a couple hire one, if the situation seems to warrant it.

"Oh, I think they're great," she replies. "We don't utilize them enough. Personally, I just got tired of dealing with them. And that's sad, because there are some really nice ones out there. So when we need them or when somebody requests them, great, but I tend not to do it. Our nurses are pretty good about checking in. The truth is, I just can't be bothered."

Thinking about doulas, it hits me that if I were to train to become a doula myself, I would gain some skills in being with laboring women, skills that would have come in handy with Kim, and no doubt will again during the course of my research. Also, I've been worrying about how to convince women who are planning home births that they should allow me, a writer, a stranger, into that intimate scene. Maybe if I'm a doula myself, that would help smooth the way. So as I drive away from the hospital that evening, I decide to become a doula.

Doula School:
How Birth Attendants Soften the Blow

Pam England rises to pour her assistant, Courtney, a cup of tea from the pot she has made for the first session of the doula class they are teaching. As Pam pours, Courtney raises her hand to indicate that she has enough. Oblivious, Pam continues to pour, even as the teacup overflows. Hot tea is suddenly streaming over the sides of the cup and down onto the floor. Courtney yells, "Whoa!" and pulls back. Pam says calmly, "Oh look, your cup was already full." Before any of the gathered students can jump in to help clean up the mess, Courtney breaks into a grin and Pam reveals that this was a well-rehearsed scene intended to teach us a lesson. She explains that it is a Zen master's teaching, a metaphor in motion, about the necessity of approaching new experiences with an empty cup, an empty mind.

Pam England is a thin, wiry, and energetic woman in her mid-forties with shoulder-length light-brown hair. She is a former midwife who now focuses on doula training and childbirth education. Her assistant, Courtney, is in her mid-twenties with short, spiky, brown hair, a delicate face, and funky, little oval glasses. As Courtney mops up the spilled tea, Pam tells the circle of seven women students, ranging in age from their early twenties to their late sixties, that it's essential to be open to a variety of ideas about how to best help birthing women. In her wonderful book on childbirth, *Birthing from Within,* Pam expands on this, saying, "In birth preparation, your first task is to empty your mind of expectations and judgments that narrow the possibilities for coping with pain, surprises, and the hard work of labor." Now, she turns to us and reiterates, "When you work with birthing parents, you must empty your cup first, so you can accept what they want and what they are offering. You'll need to keep emptying your cup, so you can really hear them."

The class is being held at Pam's Art of Birthing Center, which includes the offices of a two-person midwifery practice. The center is housed in a small and sunny stucco bungalow. In the entrance porch, a handwritten sign asks visitors to please take off their shoes. Underneath the sign, a row of gathered sandals stretches out along the wall; the imprint of their owners' feet a Rorschach-series of darkly rubbed toes and heels. Today, one pair sports a trendy, zebra print and platform sole, but most are Birkenstocks, sport sandals, or other "sensible" shoes. At the end of the porch a small fountain burbles.

The center's restful, cream-and-ocher-colored walls are decorated with art made by participants in the childbirth classes that are also taught here. A plaster cast of a pregnant belly painted in a yellow, orange, and red sunburst motif hangs in one corner. Pastel drawings of pregnant bodies or babies are accompanied by quotes from the parent-artists describing their experiences of pregnancy and birth. One photograph shows a baby being born in a pool of water, and another reveals a very pregnant woman belly dancing with veils and cymbals. The décor is deliberately quiet and peaceful, yet upbeat. Gentle music plays in the background, and a votive candle burns on the mantelpiece in the main room.

In the circle of women gathered here to become doulas sits a young mother of four who had her first baby when she was a teenager, an older woman minister, a childless college student majoring in women's studies, a grandmother who is the wife of a retired military obstetrician, a therapist and mother of two in her mid-thirties who lives on a Navajo reservation (where her husband is a doctor), a woman who teaches childbirth education classes, and myself. Pam asks us to take a few minutes to write about why we want to become doulas.

The word *doula* has come to refer to a woman with training and experience in childbirth who provides continuous emotional and physical support to a mother during labor and birth, advocates for her rights in the hospital if necessary, and assists postpartum as well.[1] According to most sources, the word *doula* comes from a Greek word meaning "female helper" or "caregiver" (my *Greek-English Lexicon,* however, just says "slave")[2] and was coined for labor assistants sometime in the 1970s by anthropologist Dana Raphael.[3] Becoming a doula seems like a pretty tall order to me, and as I watch the other women hunch over their journals writing their reasons for wanting to join this order of commendable servitude, I feel a bit like a mole, a spy.

After all, I'm a journalist. Maybe I'm just here to gain a cover, to better disguise myself as nurturing mama-type. Convincing birthing women to allow me to observe them in the hospital has been relatively easy, but I know that doing the same with women who have chosen to birth in the privacy of their own home will be more challenging. If I become a doula, I can more readily persuade them to let me tag along at this incredibly intimate event, because I'll be able to offer some help, some professional nurturing. But maybe becoming a doula isn't just a sneaky tactic for infiltrating the world of moms. On the more legitimate side, it is true that I'm here because I need some skills to put both myself and the birthing mothers I'm observing at ease. Being a doula really would help me help birthing women cope with pain. And I do want to be useful when I can; I owe the moms and midwives I'm writing about at least that much.

I notice that I'm feeling a little ambivalent about the whole doula business, probably because I have such ambivalence about women who devote themselves to the nurturing professions, raised as I was at the feminist teat. I was taught that women should liberate themselves from the underpaid and undervalued "caring professions." I tell myself that I'm just becoming a doula so I can keep writing my book. And yet, if I am honest with myself, I have to admit I am drawn to this doula class by more than just careerist utility. Doula work is good work.

When Pam asks us to share our thoughts with the group, I mumble something sanctimonious about wanting to make birth a better place. Then, I confess that I am writing a book that has exposed tremendous shortcomings in my ability to simply be with people in difficult circumstances. One excuse I offer is that my family is from England, so physically touching strangers is pretty alien; plus, I've spent most of the last decade doing library research, which doesn't require a lot of interpersonal skills. I blush and stammer as I say this, apparently eliciting the group's sympathy since nobody points out that journalism is a poor excuse to enter such an important sisterhood of sympathy. At the last minute, I realize I have an ace in the hole. I decide to play it. I tell them that I also want to feel more comfortable with labor because, well, I'm pregnant. That does it. I'm in. Everyone in the room lights up and smiles at me as Pam moves on around the circle.

The first thing we cover in class (this is the first of a three-day intensive portion, followed by six weekly classes) is a set of statistics on the effectiveness of doulas. They are fairly amazing. Women attended by doulas have been shown to have a 50 percent decrease in caesarean sections, need fewer pain-relieving drugs, have fewer instrumental deliveries, less augmentation of labor, babies in better condition at birth, shorter hospital stays, fewer perineal tears and episiotomies, major reductions in the length of labor, and report less pain during labor.[4]

Not only are the statistics impressive, but so are their sources. These aren't allegations made in a bunch of alternative mothering magazines (although I get a lot of great information and parenting support from those publications), but the conclusions of at least eleven randomized, controlled tests that have been published in places such as the *New England Journal of Medicine,* the *British Medical Journal,* the *British Journal of Obstetrics and Gynecology,* and the *Journal of the American Medical Association.*[5]

The most prominent researchers in the field are Marshall Klaus and John Kennell, whose book, with Phyllis Klaus, *Mothering the Mother: How a Doula Can Help You Have a Shorter, Easier, and Healthier Birth,* is a birth attendant's bible. In it, they publish the results of several of their studies comparing doula-attended and "no-doula" births. In one hospital in Guatemala, the average length of labor for the no-doula group was nineteen hours, while the doula group's was less than half that, at nine hours. When they repeated the study at a hospital in Texas, where the routine administration of oxytocin to augment labors lowered the average length of labor for the no-doula group to 9.4 hours, the doula group still came out ahead at 7.4 hours.[6] Even a two-hour reduction in labor is a godsend when every minute can feel like a season in hell.

Perception of the birth experience and postpartum issues are also helped by the presence of doulas. The doula group reported less pain twenty-four hours after the birth, fewer doula-supported mothers considered the labor and delivery to have been difficult, fewer thought it was much worse than they had imagined it would be, and more believed they had coped well during this experience. Additionally, at six weeks postpartum, 63 percent of the no-doula group reported feeding problems, compared with only 16 percent of the doula-attended mothers.[7] By the time we are done reviewing the studies, I'm convinced that no matter where or with whom I give birth—at the hospital or at home, with a midwife or a doctor—I am definitely saving my pennies to hire a doula.

The rest of this day's class is spent in a series of mini-lectures and role-playing sessions intended to introduce us to the art of listening to parents, providing soothing support, and negotiating with hospital staff. Our assignment for the night is to put together a doula bag, which will contain a set of items that include a change of clothes, tampons, breath mints, extra money, a snack, the mom's chart, back-up phone numbers, a children's book on birth to entertain siblings, a water bottle, a pen, a toothbrush, massage oil, cough drops, a pillowcase to cover annoying monitors, ponytail holders, lip balm (with Q-tips to keep it sanitary), a heating pad, drinking straws, a handheld fan, and a mini–Crock-Pot in which to place water and essential oils (lavender, citrus, or peppermint are recommended) for aromatherapy. I go home feeling a bit overwhelmed.

The next day of doula class is jam-packed. We cover some basic anatomy, go over the stages of labor, review a long list of assigned readings, discuss appropriate behavior for home visits, watch a video on doulas, then break for lunch. In the early afternoon, we learn a few relaxation and massage techniques. One is called called "touch breathing," in which you move your hands up the laboring woman's back as she breathes in and down her front as she breathes out. As you bring your hand down, you can tell her things like, "Let it all go," or "Shower it out," or "Let yourself release all the way down to your vagina." Courtney demonstrates this for us and says, "That's all you have to do."

The students pair up and practice on each other. It is harder than it looks. Sure, if the woman is breathing loudly you can follow her lead, but if not, it turns out to be a challenge to time your movements with her breath. There is some giggling and chattering as the class struggles to get it right, but after a few minutes the tension in the room dissipates and you can once again hear the fountain burbling in the background. Another technique we learn is simple breath awareness. Rather than the patterned breathing of Lamaze, many childbirth educators now advocate a more relaxed approach where the woman is simply reminded to "follow her breath." In doing so, she will often slow it down herself and find a measure of focus. As we practice, Courtney circulates through the room, reminding us not to command women to "Relax," but just to suggest that she become aware of her outward breath.

"Remind them that their bodies will often work better than their minds during labor," says Courtney, "and that they don't need to control their breath. Simply noticing it can give them a way to get centered. Tell her to bring her focus to her outward breath, since the inward one is often too quick. So watch your outward breath from beginning to end; put all of your mind and body into that. And doulas," Courtney exhorts with a smile, "Be enthusiastic. Jump right in and tell them to notice the space after the breath and before they inhale. And don't forget to urge your moms to work on this prenatally." Some of us are looking a little dizzy from all the heavy breathing. I'm surprised to find that something so basic is clearly going to take a little practice.

Next, we learn to give foot massages using scented oil and small basins of warm water. Again, it takes a while to get it right, but, in the meantime, we all get to experience just how great even an amateur foot rub feels. While we are doing this, Pam returns and tells us that another thing laboring moms often like is to have warm water poured over their bellies from a cup as they lie in a bathtub while the doula says something like, "Follow the water down." We don't practice this one.

After drying off our feet, we shift gears a bit, with Pam leading us though an imaginary interview and prenatal session with a set of clients. Throughout, she models certain types of behavior, then leads us through a role-playing session where we take turns being the doula or a parent. Pam says, "One place to start is by suggesting to the mom and dad, 'If you could predict that you'll have a four-hour labor with no hitches, then you might be able to count on your fantasy of a romantic birth. But you could get a twenty-four-hour labor, or it could start at midnight. Since you *can't* predict what you'll get, it's good to have someone who knows a lot about birth there, because you probably don't know birth that well.'" Pam pauses to get our attention, then continues, "Make sure that they hear from you, during your first meeting, that the doula is *not* there to take the place of the father, but to fill whatever gaps open and to help the father as well. You might tell them that a lot of men *thought* they wanted to do it solo, but when they found out about what doulas can offer, they changed their minds."

Pam coaches us on ways to get the couple to visualize how the doula will be helpful and how to add pictures to their image bank. Repeatedly, she reminds us never to be critical, only supportive. Parents, she tells us, are often worried that the doula will say "no drugs" when the mom really wants them. That is not the doula's role. Don't defend drug-free labor if they resist the idea. However, she points out, we should try to assess early on if the parents actually have different points of view about pain in labor. Then, we need to honor the mother without alienating the dad.

While Pam makes it clear that we shouldn't impose our ideal birth on parents, she doesn't hide her own desire to help parents and doulas understand the pathway to what she calls birthing in awareness. "I've just seen too many moms who had really medicalized births and then felt disappointed," she says. "People have grief about their bad experiences." So her position is that drug-free labor should be supported, rather than mercilessly pushed. "For example," she says, "If a client says, 'Shouldn't we avoid pain?' You can tell them, 'In general, yes, but in labor it is a little different. In a really long labor, yes, anesthesia is useful. But in a normal labor, pain can actually be useful, and the trade-offs you make with the anesthesia may not be worth it.' Here's a list you can turn to," Pam says, posting a piece of paper on the wall behind her. It reads:

1. Pain is natural to the process of labor and birth, and it can help you and your caregiver gauge how things are going.
2. Pain-relief medicines are often bad for the baby. They can result in decreases of early response, nursing ability, and early bonding.
3. Epidurals can have serious side effects for the mother.
4. Pain releases endorphins, which help labor and birth become a positive experience, and may help with the forgetting of the pain afterward.
5. Pain is part of a rite of passage.

I find myself raising an eyebrow at the idea that endorphins can help you forget the pain. Most women I know I have startlingly clear memories of their labor pain. But it is number five, pain as a rite of passage, that really surprises me. In a culture where epidurals are routine, I can just imagine the resistance with which this would be met. And yet, for me, it is also the most convincing item on the list. The other reasons for natural child-birth could be countered with arguments about how machines can gauge your progress as well as your sensations, how rare problems stemming from medication are, and how much more effective strong drugs are than weak endorphins. But it is a fact that pain has long been associated with rites of passage, and either you're into the idea or you're not. I'm intrigued for myself, but skeptical as a budding doula. I ask Pam to talk about this issue.

"Well, our idea *is* that if you miss the pain, you miss the rite of passage," she says. "But you're right, not all couples will be interested in that. I would never bring it up early. But on the other hand, if you never bring it up at all, who will? And aren't you denying them a chance to at least consider it?"

I nod. This seems fair.

Pam adds, "You want to motivate without using guilt. And never forget to really listen to what the mother has to say. Keep emptying your cup. After all, you are not there to rescue them. Even from themselves."

She moves on quickly—we've still got tons to cover. Next up are some prenatal visualizations for the mother concerning positions she might birth in. Pam encourages us to get mothers thinking about upright positions and squatting, since they'll have the force of gravity on their side and nice open hips. She says, "Sometimes you really have to work to help them see the possibilities. If they can only see doing it on their back, tell them 'Imagine you can't be on your back because you have a slipped disk. Good. Now visualize another position.' You might even have to demonstrate some." Pam jumps off her chair, squats down low to the ground, and grunts in mock labor. Then she's up, one leg hoisted onto the seat of her chair, her hands on its back. Now she's down on all fours, groaning. Finally, perched on the edge of her chair, legs spread wide, she says, "Always try sitting on the toilet. Oh, and tell your clients that they can ask their caregiver, 'How do most of your clients give birth? What is the most unusual position you've seen?' Their answers may be very telling."

Pam winds up the day by telling us that she wants us to spend some time thinking about the distinction between pain and suffering. "You can experience every sensation, even pain, and not suffer," she says. "Start trying to make that distinction for yourself, and then you can make it for others." I remember that another nurse-midwife once told me, "The whole concept of suffering is something that should not be in a birth vocabulary. Pain does not equal suffering. Suffering is when you have no hope, when there is no end in sight. That's torture, that's suffering. But the pain of childbirth has an end point, so there is hope and there is pain, but it doesn't have to equal suffering."

Adrienne Rich, in her book *Of Woman Born,* says that French writer Simone Weil made a similar distinction, although she said that suffering was "characterized by pain yet leading to growth and enlightenment," whereas "affliction [is] the condition of the oppressed, the slave, the concentration-camp victim forced to work endlessly and to no purpose." Weil stressed that affliction occurred where pain was associated with powerlessness and disconnectedness. When pain was inevitable, it could be "transformed into something usable, something which takes us beyond the limits of experience itself into a further grasp of the essentials of life and the possibilities within us."[8] I start to consider the distinctions among pain, suffering, and affliction and find my lingering dread about my own upcoming labor begins to shift.

The next day we begin by howling like coyotes. Then we grunt like gorillas, and finally, we make the short, loud barks of a powerlifter. Pam is cruising the room, getting in our faces and saying, "Louder! What are you, a baby chimp? I'm looking for a mama gorilla, and she's mad! Come on! Let's practice our noises!" She pulls a fierce grimace and lets loose an enormous roar.

We've reached the labor portion of the class, and we're learning how to encourage birthing moms to practice making noises *before* they go into labor, since some of them will never have done this before. I think of the tiny little whoops some aerobics instructors make, and, compared with the power-lifter shout, I think Pam's probably got a point.

Pam tells us to remind our clients that they will go in and out of control throughout their labor, and that both are okay. She also tells us to remind them to eat and drink in early labor in order to avoid an IV and to maintain their energy. If their labor has a slow start, she suggests nipple stimulation (which, she points out, can be done manually, with a breast pump, or a willing mouth), and also urges techniques such as walking, squatting, and drinking lots of water. Castor oil (which can cause diarrhea which releases prostaglandins, thus stimulating labor) is for their midwives to do. Pam makes it clear that never, ever, should a doula make any medical suggestions at any time during a woman's labor.

"Mothers should rest," Pam continues, "even sleep, at the beginning, if they can. When you meet them at the hospital, go find their nurse and introduce yourself to her immediately. A good relationship with the nurse can be crucial. Later, if you do piss off the nurse, acknowledge it." Pam gives us some examples of typical, awkward situations. For instance, the nurse comes in and says it's time to get hooked up to the IV, apparently just because that's her normal routine. Pam instructs us to "Look right at that nurse and, in your nicest voice, you say to her, 'These parents don't want to do an IV unless it is really necessary. What are the range of choices here? I know this is the way you usually do it, and it might even be what we want. But before we decide, can you tell us any other things we might try first? Look, here's the cooler of juice she's been drinking, and she's had a lot.'"

Or, Pam continues, maybe the mom has expressed a desire to avoid drugs, her labor is in full swing, she's making her good loud sounds, and the nurse walks in and asks if she wants her epidural now. "You just say to the nurse, 'They hired me to help them do it without drugs—isn't it in their chart?'" Pam says, oozing sweet naivete. "Always address the nurse first, then turn to the father or partner, and say something like, 'I remember you saying you'd like to try something different.' Give *him* an opening he might otherwise miss." Courtney adds, "You can also say to the parents, 'Would you like a minute alone to talk about this?' and offer to leave with the nurse." That way the nurse is reassured that the doula isn't calling the shots. Pam nods and says, "Whether it is an epidural or some other intervention, back down if it is *your* issue. Don't, if it is the client's issue."

After this, Pam urges, the doula needs to go to the mom and tell her, "You are doing it," not just "You can do it." Suggest to her that she go a little further, "So you know you've gone as far as you can." After all, this is what she hired a doula for. Suggest a change of position. Ask the mother what *she* thinks might help most. Try getting her to go to the bathroom, and ask her to try six more contractions. But then, "if she wants the drugs, don't be an obstructive force between her and her epidural. Sometimes women are angry that they didn't get one."

Courtney agrees with Pam's position on honoring the mother's decision, saying, "Once it's a done deal, be supportive by saying things like, 'When you get the drug, it will be easier for you to let your body do its work. When it wears off, you'll feel the pain again, so when that happens we can go to the shower or try something else, just let me know.' Always help her finish her labor with dignity and pride. Don't make her feel bad. If something negative happens, the doula's reaction is going to influence the mom's ability to deal with it. Don't vilify anyone—not the doctor, and not his or her actions, and not the parents. Embrace whatever happens."

Courtney leads the next part of the class, which focuses on the height of labor. She begins by telling us that even though we may be dealing with people in pain and confusion who have temporarily lost their ability to be nice, doulas should always respond with spontaneity and joy. She says this wryly, not saccharinely, so I imagine she's pretty good at being convincingly upbeat without being an annoying Pollyanna. "Imagine," she says, "that your client is deep into labor now and complaining, or crying, or pleading for help, or maybe she's silent, but it looks rough." Courtney waits to see that we are all picturing this before she continues, "Tell her 'I know it is hard. I know you need help. You go ahead and handle the next contraction however you can. Do more of what you're doing. Freak out if you need to. Then on the next one, I'll offer you something that might help.' On the next contraction, mirror what she is doing. Let her know you're right there. Then say, 'Remember I said I would show you something. This won't help a lot, but it might help a little. I want you to notice your outward breath, each one all the way out.'" Courtney pauses as the class scribbles in their notebooks. "Or you can ask if it is all right to rub her back. But you need to build a bridge by agreeing with her first. Say, 'Yes, it hurts, I know it hurts.' *Then* offer a pain-reduction technique."

Next, we cover how to deal with transition. This is the outrageous, mind-warping time when your cervix is making its final morph from cute little cherry to thrumming basketball hoop, the point when everything my husband, Richard, offered as help was greeted with clenched teeth and a snapped, "Cut that out." I'm sure some women deal with transition gracefully, but panic is pretty common. Some women think they will die. One direct-entry midwife told me that when she has moms who fear death, she tells them that a part of you does have to die so the mother can be born. Transition is more than a medical term. I know that when I went through it, I was pretty sure I was going crazy and that this would be the beginning of a long institutionalization. I remember thinking how sad it was that my baby would be raised without me. Courtney suggests that at this point we should say, "You are safe. You are okay." She urges us not to say, "You'll be done soon," both because that might not be true and because soon is never soon enough. Instead, try, "You're closer, you're getting close."

Courtney reminds us that we need to offer the mother a drink after every contraction and keep an eye out for dehydration. Sweating is a good sign that she's getting enough fluids. Some hospitals still insist that women get their fluids through IVs instead of letting them drink, and some insist that ice chips are the only official fluid. When this is the case, the doula can urge her clients to ask that they be allowed to drink. But if the hospital remains firm, she's limited to feeding ice chips as often as she can.

We're told that when the mother feels like she wants to push, the doula's job is to find the nurse, because if the staff arrive to find her already pushing, they'll be pissed. At this point, you can suggest that she try sitting on the toilet, since women are conditioned to push and release there. If they have an epidural, give them directional information: Push down through your bottom. If the staff take the epidural dose down a bit, warn her that it can really hurt then, and it may still be hard to push. Remind her of the power noises you practiced prenatally. Tell her, "That's a great noise" and follow her lead. If she's making a high-pitched squeal, however, you might want to tell her, "Go lower with me." Imitate her noise and modulate it downward; help them bring their voices lower, into their gut. Remind her that making low noises can help her relax and allow the cervix to open.

Pam reminds us not to forget to encourage the dad at this point, too. Praise his efforts. Tell him, "The way you work together is great." Remember, the partner's main question is often, "How do I help her when she's in pain?" but he needs to know that he also needs to be asking himself, "How do I get used to it? How do I just deal with her being in pain?" Encourage him to take care of himself; he should eat and drink, and yes, go to the bathroom. If, at any time, the partner or another family member is not pleased with you, discuss it outside the mother's room. Apologize, explain, and be concise.

During pushing, the doula should be right by the mother's ear. While the baby is crowning, remind her that she needs to do softer pushes. Right in her ear, or her face, say "Gentle, gentle,

gentle," forcefully but calmly. Remind her that this will help her to not tear. Don't stroke her while she's pushing; a firm, stationary touch is usually better. If the mother does end up with a C-section, tell the mom that the staff are doing what is necessary to keep the baby safe. Go to the dad. Help him find and put on a sterile gown if he is allowed in, but he might not get to be in the operating room with her if it is a crisis.

When the baby is born, gather up your stuff, clean up where possible, and when you see an opening, ask if there's anything you can do for either parent. They might want you to get some food, or make some calls, or they may just want to be alone. Hang around in the background for a while. When it seems to be the right time to leave, make sure everyone knows that you are going, even the nurse, and leave your phone number with your clients. Tell them you'll call to schedule a postpartum visit.

The class takes a break, and Caitlin, one of the students, tells us that she tried to be a volunteer doula at a local hospital, but that without certification she wasn't allowed to physically touch her clients, which, Caitlin rolls her eyes, definitely made the work more challenging. She tells us the story of one birth she attended. The woman had had laser surgery on her cervix, and at one point, when the doctor was checking to see how far she had dilated, he announced to the room brusquely, "She's just a big knot of scar. We've decided to do an epidural." Caitlin shakes her head, remembering, and says, "Talk about the 'royal we.' She didn't want that, but he said she better just do it. It took a little while for the epidural to arrive, and when they checked her right before administering it, she had dilated from three to five centimeters. But the doctor said he still wanted to go ahead with it. She wasn't asking for medication. They were pushing it on her." Caitlin tells us that after she got the epidural and reached the pushing stage, the doctor acted annoyed when the baby wouldn't pass the pubic bone. "He would roll his eyes, sigh, and leave the room. Even the nurse had to call him back. And he got annoyed when she pooped while pushing. They cut an episiotomy, which she hadn't wanted, and used the Mighty Vac. When she reached for the baby as it was born he said, 'No, don't. We've got to dry him off.'"

At this point in the story, Caitlin wells up with tears and says, "They were taking her baby away from her right away, even though Mom and baby seemed to be fine. There seemed to be no real reason—at least they never gave her one. It was so sad." Pam nods and tells us that we'll all see situations like that at some point, but we'll also see wonderful, joyful births as well. As she wraps up her teachings on labor support, Pam says, "Think of the doula as a flight instructor for the mom, who is the pilot, with doctors and nurses as the air traffic controllers. But also remember that the docs often think *they* are the pilots and Mom is the plane."

Pam's comment reminds me of anthropologist Emily Martin's formulation of our culture's most common childbirth analogy. Martin writes:

> Medical imagery juxtaposes two pictures: the uterus as a machine that produces the baby, and the woman as laborer who produces the baby. Perhaps at times the two come together in a consistent form as the woman-laborer whose uterus-machine produces the baby. What role is the doctor given? I think it is clear that he is predominantly seen as the supervisor or foreman of the labor process.[9]

A number of childbirth historians and cultural critics have remarked on the way that the medicalization of childbirth has fostered an understanding of pregnancy and birth as parts of technology, as somehow alienated from social settings and separate from feelings of connectivity. Barbara Katz Rothman writes that "the ideology of technology encourages us to see ourselves as objects, to see people as made up of machines and part of larger machines." She laments the disempowerment of women that occurs when the "institutionalization of childbirth as a medical event" places "doctors in the active role and mothers in the pas-

sive position of patient, recipients of services rather than con-
troller of their own birthing."[10] British birth authority Sheila
Kitzinger sees women influenced by advanced birth technology
thinking of themselves as mere "containers" for fetuses whose
bodies are "inconvenient barriers" to the process of birth.[11] In our
doula class, we are often encouraged to help women reclaim a vision of themselves as social, attached beings, more akin to animals than to machines, connected to one another, to their families,
to their children, and to a long spiritual, as well as physical, history of birth.

Our class includes a lengthy session on postpartum visits and
postpartum depression. Doulas are supposed to review the birth
with the mother, help out around the house, offer breast-feeding
advice, take the baby and/or older children to the park while
Mom gets a bath, or a host of other helpful activities. If your
client is struggling with the blues, some useful strategies include:
telling "bad mommy" stories about the parenting mistakes you
and your friends have made, talking about her favorite part of the
birth, and using solution-focused questions. This last one involves staying with the stress and defeat for ten minutes or so,
then praising what she is doing well, and finally, asking questions
that help her access her inner resources and help create a picture
of a better future. We are encouraged to ask questions such as,
"What have your tried that has worked? How can you do more of
that? What have other people suggested? If a postpartum fairy
magically solved this, what would you do differently first thing in
the morning? What would keep you from doing this?"

Doulas need to be on the lookout for postpartum depression.
"If she's crying every day, she's depressed," says Pam. Although
doulas should definitely talk to new mothers about their difficulties, Pam stresses that we always refer them to trained professionals for further help.

Next, we review how places like the Netherlands do so much
more than the United States to support a safe, comfortable, low-

tech birth environment with high-tech options readily available as backup for difficult or emergency situations. The Dutch have the fewest mothers and babies to be injured or to die in childbirth, episiotomy rates far below ours, and a caesarean section rate of only approximately 5 percent, as opposed to U.S. averages of more than 20 percent.[12] Among the many factors that contribute to these successes, significant ones include the fact that 70 percent of births are attended by midwives, transfers from home to hospital are easily facilitated, national health care covers everyone, and there is no financial incentive to use unnecessary technologies. In addition, malpractice suits are less common, making practitioners more likely to trust the natural process since they don't need to prove in court that they used every available intervention.[13] This last item seems to be evidence of a positive feedback loop; less inclined to sue over problems, practitioners avoid the complications of intervention, thus bettering their birth statistics, which, in turn, encourages the tendency to accept the rare occasions when childbirth does go wrong. Pam urges us, as doulas, to be aware of institutional barriers to positive birth experiences and urges us to both work within the situation we are given and work to improve it.

At the end of the class, Pam reads a story she's written called "If You Give an Elk an Epidural." It is accompanied by a set of funny storyboards that show a mama elk hooked up to bunch of machines and tubes, talking on the phone, and being cheered on during pushing by a cheerleading squad of pompom-bearing mice. Clearly, the implication is that using an epidural is far from "natural." Still, Pam is careful to begin by pointing out times when epidurals are worth the risks, including sheer exhaustion and discouragement, extremely long early labors, when labor is really stuck, if you've tried everything else and you still need help, if you have a caesarean, or induction when the cervix is not ripe.

"Normal pain, normal labor is not a reason for an epidural," she says, "abnormal is."

As Pam reviews the pictures of the anesthetized elk she explains, "An epidural means you get IV fluids, so you have to pee, but you won't know, so you get a catheter. If your blood pressure drops, which it can with an epidural, it can make the baby's heart rate drop. Ten to eleven percent of cases have moderate to severe fetal distress after an epidural. You have to stay in bed, so your pelvis won't be as open as it would if you were walking around, gravity won't be helping bring the baby down, and sometimes the baby won't move into the best position if it needs to rotate. Once sensation is gone, your body will not produce as much oxytocin, so you will need Pitocin, which produces harder and longer contractions. Sometimes this can deny the baby enough oxygen. Often you can't feel enough to push effectively, so they may have to use vacuum extraction or forceps that lead to tears or episiotomies. If you really can't push the baby out, you can end up with a caesarean. Some mothers have subsequent problems with bladder control, headaches, and backaches caused by the epidural. There is often decreased motor activity and responsivity with the baby and sometimes a decreased ability to suck, which can disrupt nursing. Your baby is more likely to be in the nursery because of the chance of a maternal fever caused by the epidural; since the staff can't tell if the fever is from the anesthesia or from an infection, they'll need to do a septic workup on the baby, which can include a spinal tap."

It's a long list of potential problems. Frankly, just being reminded that my baby could get a spinal tap is horrifying enough to make me try biting the bullet for as long as I can.

⌒

The final hours of our training are spent at a local Zen center that offered us their meditation room and eight massage tables. When we arrive, eight hugely pregnant women, whom Pam has solicited, are changing into kimonos in preparation for the pregnancy massage class we are about to take. They alternately lumber and float around the room, their matching loose robes making them look like a fleet of beamy boats bobbing in the large sunny room. I'm jealous; we doulas look like the mortal slaves we are named after in the company of this tribe of ripe goddesses—

that is, until they have to climb up onto the massage tables. Then, what an ungainly galumphing, heaving, and sprawling occurs.

Once they are all up, lying on their sides and panting noticeably, we get to work. My partner's name is Zora. She has a waterfall of auburn hair and is absolutely radiant. She is from Brazil, studied at Juilliard, and is married to a yoga instructor named Shiva. Zora is very patient with my clumsy attempts and even arranges for me to give her a professional visit postpartum—something I need to get my certification.

As the sun sets, the class winds down, and the participating mothers leave. The doulas remain. We are given contact numbers for potential clients and hospitals. We need to attend ten women to become officially certified. Our last assignment of the day is to write in our journals about our "strongest responses" to the course. At first, I decide that the most powerful things I learned were 1) birth is a mental process as well as physical one, 2) in dealing with mothers in labor you must meet them where they are—mirror their behavior and then you can shift that gently, and 3) doulas can make small drops of sympathetic change in a large bucket of less-than-ideal childbirth practices.

As I think further, I realize that the course also intensified my frustration and anger about how limited women's birth choices are in the United States. It seems so difficult to avoid the cascade of technological interventions at the hospital; birth centers are few and far between (there isn't one in my city of half a million people); home birth, while statistically very safe, is often expensive (since insurers are reluctant to cover it) or hard to come by (since some states either actively discourage it or even make it illegal); and doulas, while wonderful, are often an option only for those with disposable income. Despite decades of reform, and although many wonderful authors have written on the subject (including Suzanne Arms, Jessica Mitford, Henci Goer, and Naomi Wolfe), I can't help but feel that while doulas can certainly help, the state of childbirth in the United States still needs major improvement.

Addressing the need for doulas in low-income communities is part of Pam England's mission. She arranges for student doulas to work at a local school for pregnant teens, a drug-rehabilitation program for women (many of them homeless), and at local hospitals on an on-call basis for women who arrive with little or no support. I participate in these programs and find them at once rewarding and challenging, as they don't always allow for important, rapport-building prenatal sessions. There are huge, unanswered needs for birthing women in impoverished or difficult situations, and the few clients I do serve in these communities all request that I not write about their experiences.

I also see some private, self-paying clients as a doula-in-training, including Sharon Levine. Sharon is on bed-rest and needs some prenatal support. She suffers from severe nausea for which she takes a medication that makes her dizzy and exhausted. Sharon went to an Ivy League school, and used to be lawyer, but now works part-time as an archivist so she can spend more time with her little girl, Cara, who is the same age as my son, Max. On my first visit, we discover that she and I are due on exactly the same day. Sharon hesitates after telling me this, then confesses that actually she added two days to the date of her last menstrual period when she and her midwife were figuring out her due date, since last time she went way past her due date and this time she wanted a little buffer before the hospital threatened to induce her. I can't believe it; I've done exactly the same thing. When I tell her, we bond pretty quickly. And in fact, we will end up giving birth on the same day, two days ahead of our official due date.

Sharon had a very traumatic first birth. Cara's shoulder got stuck and her arm was broken during the delivery, and Sharon tore terribly. She tells me that she thinks her nausea may be partly psychosomatic, brought on by the dread of another birth. I nod and tell her I see how this could happen. But I add that whatever the cause, nausea is real and debilitating. I hate the way arguments that morning sickness is all "in the mind" work to make pregnant women feel guilty without giving us any relief.

Sharon is lonely and gets very animated when I come over. We talk about pregnancy, labor, and birth, and then I make her some rice and wash the stack of dirty dishes in her sink. We talk a lot about books and connect over the fact that we both read and loved Jane Lazarre's *The Mother Knot*. Lazarre tells of her trials as the mother of a biracial child and as the wife of a Yale law student. Removed from any intellectual community of her own, unable to find the time and energy to continue her writing, and overwhelmed by the responsibility and boredom of parenting a baby, Lazarre's book recounts her struggle to break the silence of the "good mother," to find a community of women who will tell the truth about their experiences of birth and motherhood, and to understand who she is becoming. It is an intensely honest book, and, in telling the truth of her experience, it is a feminist book as well. Sharon tells me she's never met anyone else who has read it and lends me what she calls her "bible," *The Play Group*, by Nina Barrett. *The Play Group* is another honest, disturbing, funny, and liberating book about women in their first years of motherhood. It chronicles the way we can lose our public voices, the way diapers and feeding take over our lives and our minds, and the choices we feel forced to make. The book resonates with my own bittersweet experience; reading it is both sad and comforting.

I visit Sharon several times over the next few weeks. Each time I bring some new remedy for nausea: crystallized ginger, ginger tea, peppermint tea, red raspberry leaf tea, miso soup, popcorn, rice cakes, and advice to eat more protein, eat more often, get outside, exercise, or go for acupuncture treatments. Often we'll take a very slow walk down her suburban street, Sharon sometimes leaning on me when her dizziness gets bad. Because our babies are due on the same day, I won't be able to help at her birth, but I know how much these simple comforts have already meant, and it feels great to be her doula now.

In the next few weeks, I talk to a number of people about their experiences with doulas. One is David Anderson, whose wife, Laurie, gave birth to their first child ten weeks ago. Laurie has just gone back to her job in city planning, and David is staying home with the baby and going to business school. He comes to visit me lugging their baby, Fiona, in her car seat. He plunks her down on the floor and drops onto my couch. His hair is tousled and he looks exhausted. When I ask how he's doing, he gives me a look that asks, "What do you think?" and says shortly, "Sleep deprived." When I ask David to talk about his experience with Fiona's birth, he sits up a bit and becomes more animated. He tells me they decided to get a doula because neither he nor Laurie had been through the experience of birthing before. "I'd never even seen a birth," he says, "and both of us were feeling insecure about how we, as a couple, would handle the various situations. We'd heard a lot of stories about labors that go on for thirty-six hours. So we thought that if we were in the hospital, and really tired, our doula could help us and be our advocate. She could be clear-headed and help us make any decisions we might face." David makes an analogy between laboring and moving to a new house. "When you move yourself, it's exhausting and really emotional. You're too wrapped up in your stuff, in what's fragile and what's not. But if you invite a friend over to help you, it's just boxes to them, so they move it without a lot of worry. And a professional mover can do that even better and faster. That's the kind of perspective we wanted from the doula."

David and Laurie's doula, Heather, had attended dozens of births, so they felt confident that she would know what to do. And she did. To start with, Laurie went past her due date and was about to be induced, but she was worried about the additional pain a Pitocin induction might bring and the reduced mobility an IV would cause. So Heather helped Laurie find an acupuncturist, encouraged her to take the herb blue cohosh, and recommended that she do nipple stimulation. About a day later, Laurie was in labor but the contractions were very mild. She took some castor oil (in a milkshake), and they quickly picked up.

Once in labor, one way Heather was really beneficial for Laurie, David explains, "was that whenever Laurie showed an inclination toward something, Heather would just jump on it. As soon as Laurie would hesitantly say something like, 'Maybe a bath would be nice?' Heather would say, 'Now's the time for the tub, let's get it going!' She did it so quickly that it never even entered my mind, 'Oh, we should do the tub.' That really worked for us."

Their doula's willingness to take the initiative came into play as soon as they arrived at the hospital. The first time Laurie was checked, her cervix was already at six centimeters. "When Heather heard that," David says, "She just jumped up and said, 'Great! Let's keep this ball rolling. Laurie, get up!' She got Laurie out of bed and they started walking." That allowed David to get their stuff out of the car, and by the time they got back from their walk a half-hour later, Laurie was close to the final phase of her labor. She spent two contractions in the tub, then felt pushy and moved to the floor, where she knelt on all fours on the floor, draped over a birthing ball.

The doula provided massage and counterpressure on Laurie's back. She also squeezed her hips in a way that David couldn't. "I tried, but I've broken both my wrists in the past, so I can't really do that, and it really helped Laurie." Heather also put warm compresses on Laurie's bottom and talked to her, saying things like, "You're doing great. Remember this is for your baby. Relax, go ahead and give in, surrender," Later, Laurie remarked that the things Heather said were extraordinarily helpful and kept her from panicking. "If it had been just me there," David confesses, "I wouldn't have said all those great things. Having a doula was great. It was absolutely worth every penny. In fact, I thought it was a bargain at four hundred bucks. The value of having her there was just incredible."

Yvonne Frank, a woman I met while observing childbirth classes, hired doulas for the births of both her children. We get together and sit in her sunny back yard where she watches her two-year-old play while her infant alternately sleeps and nurses. "I'd never heard of doulas until we took that childbirth class, but it seemed like a good idea, just because of the way they said the doula can be a substitute for an epidural," Yvonne says. "Maybe I've been brainwashed. I was afraid the epidural might cause other problems. Plus, I had the idea that if you take the easy way out, you wind up paying for it somehow." Yvonne chuckles. "And I didn't want to do that."

One of the benefits of having a doula occurred at a prenatal visit during her first pregnancy. "We talked about the things I was afraid of," Yvonne says. "We had a long conversation about my fear that the baby wasn't going to be normal or perfect and that I wasn't going to love it. I hadn't ever said it out loud to anyone. So it was very hard for me, and emotional. I was crying. But she knew what I was talking about and told me some stories about other women she'd worked with who had had similar fears, and she told me about a situation where something like that had actually happened. And that really helped a lot. After that, I just wasn't worried at all. Getting rid of that fear made me feel better, and I think it helped me have an easier birth than I otherwise might have."

Yvonne explains that her first doula, Stephanie, was in charge of helping her husband comfort her. "She did a fabulous job. She looked for what I needed and first tried to get Alan to do it. If that didn't work out, then she would do it. For instance, I liked having really hot water poured on me. Sometimes Alan did it too fast, or not quite how I liked, and so she would do it. Alan never it took it personally; there was a fine relationship between the two of them," Yvonne says. When Alan wanted to get something to eat after several hours, their doula was able to stay with Yvonne. "She talked to me. She really helped me," Yvonne recalls. "And I could tell she was really proud of me. I could tell that I was doing it the way that we had talked about and that we had both hoped for. I felt like we were in the groove."

Yvonne also credits her doula with helping her squat, as she wanted to, during much of her labor. "You know, that opens your hips and gets gravity to help bring the baby down, and that probably wouldn't have happened without our doula," Yvonne says. "She actually held me while I was squatting whenever Alan got tired. And I weighed a lot!" She laughs. "There were times when she said, 'Do four contractions standing up,' and I didn't want to do it because it hurt so bad. But she just totally encouraged me and physically supported me. Afterward, Alan said I did way more than the four contractions she asked for, and that was when my labor progressed the most. I couldn't have done that by myself. There's no way."

After the baby was born, their doula remained and helped advocate for what the couple wanted. "They started to take the baby away immediately," Yvonne recalls. "We didn't want them to take him right away because oftentimes the baby's temperature will go down when they bathe it, and then they need to keep it away from you even longer so it can warm up under the lights. Stephanie reminded us that we didn't have to let them do that. She said, 'That's your choice.' So we didn't let them bathe him; we bathed him the next morning." Yvonne stops talking to pick up her baby, who has just woken up and is chirping and grunting, on the verge of tears. She gets him settled at her breast and says, "Having our doula there was so important. Without her, I just don't think I would've had enough support to get through each stage. I would've given up on trying things, and my labor might not have progressed as quickly. I think I would've suffered, and I think Alan would've lost his nerve, because he was very close to freaking out. It's a very delicate balance in labor and birth, and she kept us on the safe side of that, on the strong side."

With her second child, the baby she's nursing now, Yvonne had another doula. This time, she used Heather, the same doula Laurie had, and like Laurie, Yvonne, too, went past her due date. "I was set to go in to be induced at 1:00 P.M. that day. I called Heather and she asked, 'Is that what you really want?' And I said. 'Yes, I really want the baby.' And she said, 'Well, you know how they induce you, right? They basically put something on your cervix that's synthetic sperm. You can do that yourself. Is Alan there?'" Heather recommended that they have sex and that Yvonne also use a breast pump for nipple stimulation. Yvonne was having contractions by the time of her 1:00 P.M. induction appointment.

At the hospital, Heather did pelvic presses, squeezing Yvonne's hips together. "She was *so* good at that," Yvonne says. "When she squeezed, I almost couldn't feel the contraction. I could feel the pressure, but it didn't hurt, and what she was doing didn't hurt. Oh my God, it was unbelievable. And, she's small and was six months pregnant herself! She did it every single contraction. Once she did that, I wanted her to do it every time, because I knew I could get relief. She showed Alan how to do it, but he couldn't do it right." Yvonne rolls her eyes and laughs. "He tried twice, and I was like, 'No. No. No. *She* has to do it.' I don't think I was very nice about it." Yvonne pulls a face. "But, I guess they understood."

One of the things that both of Yvonne's doulas did was make sure she got enough to eat and drink. They kept a cup with a straw in it next to her mouth, and between every contraction they made her drink the Gatorade she had chosen. "I don't think there was a contraction that went by without a drink," Yvonne says, "I would take a single sip and Heather would say, 'Drink more.' It wasn't like I could do a sissy, cheater sip. And she literally helped put cookies into my mouth, because I couldn't do anything. I was out of it. I was a functioning unconscious person, if that's possible." At one point, when Yvonne emerged from her interior state and started to get a little hysterical, the doula brought out some peppermint oil. "She put some where I could smell it, and I remember thinking, 'Ooooh, that's nice.' It took my mind off what was going on for a little bit." Finally, there was the postpartum visit. "That was *lovely*," Yvonne says emphatically. "She brought a whirlpool footbath, and she gave me a foot massage and fed me strawberries. She brought a whole basket of giant, ripe, cleaned strawberries. We talked about the birth and she told me how great I was. Now, that was a pretty nice feeling," Yvonne says, beaming.

The last person I speak with about her experience with a doula is Nora Carter. Nora has two children; one is nine and the other is one. She says she hired a doula simply because she wanted to be better supported for her second birth than she was during the first. "It was so good to have her help settle some of the things I was worrying about," Nora says, as her one-year-old, Liam, crawls around on the couch between us. "My very biggest fear was of being induced, because I had been before, and it was so awful. I remember looking at the monitor and seeing the contraction coming up, and that was like torture. The anticipation was so bad, the dread. I would see the needle start to rise, and think, 'Oh my God, here it comes again. Oh my God, it's coming!' I didn't want to do that again if I could avoid it, and a doula can help offer alternatives."

Nora had a doctor who she really liked and who was comfortable with the doula. Nora didn't mind that her doctor only showed up when the baby was about to be born, because she had the attention she needed from her doula, Amy. "She was completely focused on me," Nora recalls. "That was her job, and that was what she did. I appreciated that so much, because nobody else really was. I mean, my husband was. But, you know, he has his own stuff he's dealing with, and he's not used to doing this."

When I ask what else the doula did to help her birth experience, Nora thinks for a minute, then laughs to herself before telling me, "Well, one of the best things was her postpartum visit. She brought a tray of sticky buns. I highly recommend every doula bring sticky buns to their clients! It was great!"

Nora's mother had come to stay with her for a week after the baby was born, and her doula was scheduled to do a postpartum visit just after her mother left. "My mom was leaving, and although I didn't exactly have postpartum depression, I was sad and my heart was full with everything I'd been through and been given. I had waited eight years, and now I had this baby. So I was actually happy, not depressed. But I was very emotional. Also, it happened to be Mother's Day." Here Nora tears up and begins to cry as she tells me this story. "My husband gave me a picture of the two boys, taken at the beginning of the week when my baby was one day old. Then my mother left. I felt so full and so sad. So I went up to check on the chickens (Nora lives in a rural community not far from a big city) because I didn't want to cry in front of anyone. I cried all the way up to the chickens, the whole time feeding them, and all the way back. When I got back to the house, Amy, my doula, was there for her visit. And it was wonderful. We just talked and ate sticky buns. I still had that fullness of feeling, but she made me feel so good." Nora smiles and tickles Liam until he squeals.

"I'm really glad we had a doula," she concludes. "I tell people to at least explore the possibility of getting one, and not to see that person as an unrelated bystander who is just an extra body in the room, because that's not what they are at all. When you first meet them, you already have a project in common. By the time you go into labor, you know them and you've worked through important things with them. When people ask me about doulas, I say, 'Explore the possibility.'"

I tell Nora that my favorite line to encourage people to use doulas is doula researcher Dr. John Kennell's statement, "If a doula were a drug, it would be unethical not to use it."

Home Birth

I AWAKE into a still, quiet darkness. The illuminated blue numbers of my clock read 3:34 A.M. Briefly, I wonder why I am suddenly no longer sleeping. I realize the phone may have rung, so I
pick it up. A woman's voice says, "This is it. Megan's contractions
are five minutes apart, and you're invited to the birth." The gift of
this invitation is slow to dawn on me.

I went to sleep only half expecting this call. For weeks, I have
been trying to attend a home birth. However, as I suspected, few
people want to invite a stranger, a writer, to the birth of their
baby, especially when they've already opted to give birth in the
privacy of their own home. But then I met Megan, who is pregnant with her fourth baby and, while not jaded, is more matter-
of-fact about her upcoming birth than most of the pregnant
women I have met so far. At a recent prenatal visit with her midwife, she said that since she had two midwives she wouldn't need
me as a doula, but she would invite me to simply observe. However, she could only invite me if she went into labor at night, because then her kids would be in bed and there would be room for
me in the living room of her family's small trailer. It is night. She
is in labor. I am invited. In a moment, the good fortune of these
facts add up, my slumbering mind comes alive, and I'm off the
phone, into my clothes, and flying down the street in my truck.

Driving down the shadowy, vacant streets of my neighborhood, I check my gas gauge and curse. I'm almost on empty, and Megan lives a good forty miles away in a small, rural town. I pull into the bright, white fluorescence of the nearest gas station and as I pump, I pray with each tick of the meter that she isn't giving birth without me. My heart is racing, and I am as wide awake as I've ever been. The baby-catching adrenaline I've heard about from midwives must have kicked in . . . either that or the gasoline fumes.

According to plan, I stop first at the house of Megan's midwife, Julie Bradshaw, who delivered two of Megan's other children, because Julie knows the maze of winding dirt roads that lead to Megan's trailer. I screech into her driveway and jump out, ready to apologize for taking so long. Julie promptly opens the door and puts her hands on her hips. "Well all right. You get an A+ already!" She looks neither young nor old. Her stocky frame fills the doorway and is balanced by a fluffy mane of blow-dried, mousy brown hair. Her apprentice, Andrea, a young blond woman with a willowy figure, appears behind Julie. She looks slightly bohemian in her music festival T-shirt, black clogs, and blue hospital pants slung low on her narrow hips. Nodding in agreement with Julie, she says, "Great timing." Apparently, I'm not late, but it is too soon to relax, since Megan is still far away and who knows how close her contractions are now. This is her fourth baby, so things could be progressing quickly.

I watch as Julie and Andrea pack a few last things. Julie tells a lot of jokes, yet she exudes a no-nonsense attitude. She used to be a third-generation park ranger, where she fought fires, had emergency medical technician training, and did a lot of paramedic work. It is easy to imagine her cheery toughness serving her well in those jobs. Of her time in the park service she says, "There was no intermediary care. If a Band-Aid didn't fix it, then we had to call out the chopper. That's when I saw some babies born in the back of the ambulance, and I thought there shouldn't be so much panic." In fact, it is hard to imagine Julie panicking. She is cool-headed despite her jocularity. She usually wears hospital-style nurses' scrubs, which is unusual for a home-birth midwife. "I take advantage of the preconceived notion that this looks a little nursey, and that makes you feel safer," she explains. "But I don't wear a white jacket that says 'Now you're in the hospital zone.'" Her specialty as a midwife is attending water births, and later she'll laughingly tell me of various tricks she's used to keep dry during deliveries, including wearing a full-length yellow rain slicker and using duct tape to secure her extra-long rubber gloves to her sleeves. Her slightly wacky earthiness differs sharply from the sensitive, spiritual disposition I had imagined all midwives would share.

A minute later, we take off into the quiet night with me tailing Julie's truck, clearly identifiable by its collage of bumper stickers, the most prominent of which reads, "Water babies rise to the top." As we drive, I find myself chanting, "a baby is coming, a baby is coming," over and over. I am surprised by how pumped I am feeling, given that I've already seen several births at the hospital. Maybe I'm so excited because this birth will be at home, and I'm hoping to catch a glimpse of a different way of birthing, some subtle spiritual shift I haven't seen yet. I think to myself, of course I'm excited, I am on my way to a miracle. Just down the road a woman is bringing a new life onto the planet and, with any luck, I'm going to be there to witness it. Something from nothing. It truly is a miracle every time, no matter that thousands of babies are being born every minute. Pattiann Rogers, a poet and naturalist, writes about the way birth crosses the marvelous with the mundane, saying, "Sex, conception, the beginning of life, the moment when that boundary between the inert and the living is crossed and all the ramifications inherent in that moment—these subjects are a wonder to me, such common, everyday occurrences, and yet so absolutely astonishing every time they happen."[1] On top of the usual astonishment is the fact that the woman I am driving toward, Megan, hasn't left for the hospital and isn't planning on doing so. Like women for millennia before her, she will be attended by an experienced woman who is rushing to her side, rather than rushing herself to an institution in town. My suburban upbringing has limited my experience of this kind of scene to a childhood fascination with *Little House on the Prairie*. So yes, I'm pumped.

Julie is really cruising along now, and I'm having a hard time keeping up with her. As we get off onto a side street, the "Check Engine" warning on my dashboard lights up. I curse and ignore it. Several side streets later we turn down a dirt road that is completely washboarded. My body bumps and shudders over the turbulent pulse of the road. The springs under my seat squeak out a crazy, jolting, rhythm. We're doing what speed we can, vibrating viciously at only twenty-five miles per hour. Choking on the dust raised by Julie's truck in front of me, I reluctantly drop back a bit. The dust and pebbles are white in my headlights, a line of barbed wire stretches forbiddingly alongside me, and beyond there is only blackness. Finally, with a crunch of gravel, we pull up to Megan's steel blue trailer. Several unseen dogs bark wildly in the dark. My stomach is clenched in anticipation of what we will find. Will she be screaming in pain? Will the baby already be there? Will we be too late?

Inside it is quiet. Cozy. There is a single, yellow lamp on next to the couch where Megan lies wrapped in a blanket, resting. Her long blond hair is pulled off her face and hangs loose behind her. Her face is flushed, and she looks pink, pretty, and young. Although she is breathing hard and only smiles weakly when we walk in, it is immediately apparent that we're there with plenty of time to spare.

I meet Megan's husband, Jeff, who is a carpenter, and we chat as Julie and Andrea bustle around bringing in equipment: bags full of towels, blankets, scissors, a thermometer, a hot pad, a suction device, intubators, and finally, a large mover's dolly with an oxygen tank. As she hauls this last item up the steps Julie catches my glance. "If this is all set up, we won't need it." Once everything is inside, Julie sits down and unwraps a condom. At my raised eyebrows, she shows me a handheld Doppler for listening to the baby's heartbeat and then shoves it into the condom. "Voilà. Waterproof." Megan is planning to have her baby in a tub—actually in a bright aqua-colored, kid's blow-up swimming pool that takes up a third of the trailer's living room.

Water births are becoming more and more popular (Julie says two-thirds of her clients opt for an aqueous labor and most remain in the water to deliver), mostly because women love the pain relief the water provides and see no reason to get out when the baby actually arrives. The water's soothing warmth decreases a woman's anxiety and, thus, her perception of pain, allowing to her relax both mentally and physically; it may also stimulate further oxytocin production, which produces both a mellowing effect and more rigorous contractions. The buoyancy provided to a heavy pregnant body, when the water is sufficiently deep, adds to this relief, and the fluid ease with which one can change positions is a great boon to labor and birth. Some studies have also suggested that giving birth in the water may decrease the chance and the severity of perineal tears.[2]

When I first heard about water birth, I confess, it sounded pretty odd. Humans are not exactly water creatures, so how could this be "natural"? Wouldn't the baby inhale water as it was born? As it turns out, the baby does not breathe underwater because it does not truly perceive that it is beyond the barrier of the mother until its nose and mouth are in the air. Some theorize that the first breath is triggered by the air itself; others think it is the change in temperature, so midwives are careful to ensure that the water is warm. Fifteen minutes after we arrive, Megan, wearing only a long T-shirt, hoists her large, unwieldy, pregnant body into the warm water of the pool. Submerged, her contractions seem to ease off a bit. She reports that "They don't pull down so much."

Julie turns to Jeff and asks, "Did you check her?" He has, and estimates that his two thick fingers show her cervix to be dilated four centimeters. "It's pretty soft, and the baby's head was just a little farther in, kind of low." I'm surprised and impressed. This is not information your average expectant father can offer. However, Julie, like many home-birth midwives, regularly delegates various simple health-care procedures to both fathers and mothers-to-be. This is just one manifestation of midwives' belief in emphasizing the normalcy of birth. Overall, delegating tasks to the woman and her family is a small step in their efforts to demystify the care of pregnant women.

Julie listens to the baby's heartbeat with her waterproof Doppler, then gives the thumbs-up sign. Everything in the trailer is very peaceful. I can't help but notice already how different this scene is from the hospital. Nobody talks, and with each contraction Megan simply breathes a little heavier and closes her eyes. In a while, Andrea suggests a trip to bathroom. Out of the water, Megan clearly feels more pain with each contraction. We hear her moan loudly and then vomit. Andrea and Julie move toward the bathroom. Julie snaps on a pair of rubber gloves, since throwing up can sometimes be a sign of the mother entering the last stage of labor. But Megan isn't quite there yet. She gets back in the pool, which Jeff has kept warm by intermittently siphoning the cooling water out the nearest window and adding hot water via a long, yellow, garden hose attached to the kitchen faucet. Julie checks the baby's heartbeat, and we settle back into our places. Jeff moves gently back and forth in a gliding rocker, Julie and Andrea share a floral couch surrounded by family photos, and I sit on a soft, old beige armchair in the corner. The adrenaline of the ride has subsided, and I am feeling pleased and eager with a hint of sleepiness, like a child allowed to stay up past bedtime, feeling privileged to be part of this expectant scene.

The minutes and the contractions pass with a steady sameness. Has it been an hour, or more, when Megan's son, Max, age five and the oldest of her three children, wakes up and wanders sleepily into the room? He climbs into his dad's lap holding his red, stuffed Teletubby doll. He is mildly curious but unconcerned. He's seen this before at the birth of his two younger siblings. A few minutes later Natalie, age two and a half, joins him. She, too, climbs up on Jeff's lap and listens calmly as her mother moans softly through the next set of pains. I've seen children at hospital births, but here their presence seems more integrated, more appropriate; they are, after all, at home. Many hospitals still don't allow siblings to attend births, and where they do, doctors are less likely than midwives to be supportive of this option. But midwives, both at home and in the hospital, are also sensitive to the ways in which children might have difficulty with the situation or can interrupt a labor when the mother is too focused on them, and recommend that families be flexible about their presence.

At 6:30 A.M., the sky is still dark when a friend and neighbor, Sylvia, arrives to take the children. She is clearly curious and stays to watch for a while. Megan begins to groan more insistently, and Jeff and the two midwives move to stools next to the pool. By seven o'clock the sky is beginning to lighten, and Megan is noticeably more out of it. Her face is very flushed, and she says she may need to throw up. Andrea tells her she has a bowl ready and shows it to her, saying, "You're doing great. Keep it up." Julie doesn't say much. Jeff alternately rubs Megan's back and holds her hand. Her contractions are now one minute apart. She says, "I feel nauseous," moans, and starts to move around in the pool. Andrea holds out the bowl and Megan vomits. She vomits again. Three times she heaves into the large stainless-steel bowl Andrea holds out for her. Julie puts a cold washcloth on her neck, gently touches her head, and says quietly, "You know it won't be much longer now." As Andrea goes to empty the bowl, Megan blurts out, "Wait! I'm not sure I'm done," and throws up again as Andrea passes the bowl back just in time. Andrea intones, "It won't be long now. This will pass."

All this action has woken everyone up a bit. Jeff, myself, Max, Natalie, and Sylvia the neighbor are all watching, engrossed. The baby, Benjamin, seventeen months old, toddles into the room and joins the crowd. For a moment it feels like a bit of a spectacle. Max asks Sylvia, "Why can't we go to your house and then go to church?" Sylvia responds, "We can." But she doesn't move. She's transfixed and clearly wants to stay for the birth, even though it is just as clearly time for her to go. I don't blame her; the anticipation is intense. Each moment is fascinating simply because it is a step along the way to a birth, to the arrival of a new person.

Julie seems to sense that Megan's labor is becoming something of an exhibition, and, knowing that performance anxiety is not going to ease her labor any, shoos Sylvia and the kids out of the trailer into the dawning day. There is silence again. Julie gives Megan a homeopathic remedy for nausea called nux vomica. Megan comes out of her trance a bit and says, "Well, that sucked," and we all settle in for the remainder of her labor.

⌒

The chair I'm sitting in is wedged between the pool and a bookcase crowded with an assortment of dictionaries, *The Norton Anthology of Literature,* Walt Whitman's *Leaves of Grass,* Kahlil Gibran, Isaac Asimov, Calvin and Hobbes cartoon books, Grateful Dead books, Dr. Sears's *Parenting and Child Care,* and several Bibles. I flip through their copy of Whitman until I read

> This is the bath of birth, this the merge of small and large, and the outlet again.
>   Be not ashamed women, your privilege encloses the rest, and is the exit of the rest,
>   You are the gates of the body, and you are the gates of the soul.

I linger here and find myself trying to figure out, if, like Megan, I, too, could choose to birth at home. What do I have in common with Megan and Jeff? We may both have an affection for Whitman's life-loving verse, but beyond that, what beliefs about life do we share? Why did they choose to have their baby with a midwife? Why did they decide to have their baby at home? Jeff and Megan are practicing Christians, and I suspect this has a lot to do with their decision. Their religious community and their faith support them in this choice. I wonder, if we are fundamentally very different people, could someone like myself also choose this alternative, or will my more mainstream lifestyle and beliefs stop me? It is quiet in these early morning hours, and we all rest, even doze a little, as Megan continues to labor, her focus internal, her contractions making her moan gently.

It is 8 A.M. The sun shines more brightly, and I can see the line of the horizon out the window, the desert mountains brown and dusty, separated from us by a field full of trailers. Megan drinks some water. Andrea says, "You're doing great." Megan groans and slides her hands along the top of the pool. "It's hard," she says. Andrea responds, "Yeah, but you're doing great."

A few minutes later, Megan complains of feeling dizzy. Julie gives her one whiff of oxygen and asks, "Better?" Megan nods yes. Andrea checks her and says there is a bit of cervix left, but it is really soft and she could push past it. Julie suggests she push with the next contraction, so she does. It clearly hurts. Megan looks like she's going to cry and says, "I'm afraid to push." Julie puts a hand on her shoulder and says firmly, "You send that fear out in the hall. You can do this. You were afraid to push with the last baby, but he got here all right, didn't he?" Megan nods. Reassured, she gives a big push, strains, and groans. Andrea listens to the baby's heartbeat; it is fine. Julie asks, "Do you have rectal pressure? Do you feel like you have to poop?" Megan nods, and Julie says, "Good. Good."

Even as the pressure is literally mounting, Megan suddenly falls asleep. Two minutes later she wakes up, groans loudly, pushes, and turns red. Julie puts one hand on Megan's side and then the other inside her and says, "Push past this point." Now Megan is yelling and moaning, "Oooooh! It hurts. Oh fuck, it hurts." Julie kneels beside the pool saying, "Lots of pressure. The baby's right there. Move your baby." The contractions are coming one right on top of another. Megan cries. "It hurts. I want it to be over. Please God, let it be over." Andrea says, "Try not to fight it." Megan's eyes are closed and she croons out, "Okay. Okay. Okay," and then, "I'm afraid." Julie tells her, "It's okay to be afraid, but your baby's fine and you're fine." Megan seems to relax for a minute.

Julie suggests she can pull on her legs since it might help the baby come out. Megan reaches down and grabs her legs, moans, and cries, "Come out! Come out!" Suddenly, Julie says "It's going to burn. Head's coming out," and then, "Head's out." Megan is shaking, and in the shadowy water of the pool I see a dark, round form between her legs. Her baby's head. Another contraction comes and Jeff says, "Here comes the rest of it." Andrea, too, says, "Here comes your baby." The baby slips silently out into the water. Everyone is quiet as we watch Julie reach into the water and lift her baby to the surface. Tears are running down my face and making watery blue splotches on my note pad. Jeff says quietly, "Praise the Lord."

The baby's face is bluish red, the body white. Megan asks if the baby is okay, but Julie is too busy to answer. She has Andrea pass her the bulb syringe. She quickly squeezes the bulb at the baby's mouth twice, then switches to a more effective DeLee suction device. She pops one part in the baby's mouth, a tube in her own, and sucks hard. Megan is now stroking the baby, saying, "You'll be okay." Andrea listens to the baby with a stethoscope. The wait seems eternal, but when I check my watch, it is actually only a matter of seconds before Andrea says that the baby is breathing, and its heart sounds fine. Julie reports that although the amniotic sac was stained with meconium, which is dangerous to the baby if inhaled, the mucus is all yellow, and that is good. Julie is trained in how to intubate a baby and administer oxygen, should it be necessary, but she doesn't need it today. Jeff sighs, "Thank you, Lord."

The baby lies peacefully on Megan's chest. After five minutes the umbilical cord is still pulsing, meaning that the baby is still getting nourishment from its mother, easing its transition into the world, so it is not cut yet. Fifteen minutes later, Megan says she's crampy, and when Julie tells her it's the placenta coming, Megan says, "That doesn't seem fair. I should be done." Twenty minutes after the birth of their child, Jeff cuts the umbilical cord and only then do we see that it is a girl, Hannah Beth. While her baby nurses with tiny, beautiful, little sucking sounds, Megan births the placenta. Most midwives encourage immediate nursing, as it helps release more oxytocin, which aids uterine contraction, which helps the placenta separate and be expelled, and, thus,

reduces the likelihood of hemorrhage. Julie checks Megan's perineum and tells her she didn't tear.

All this is so different from the births I've seen in hospitals,
where the bustle of activity around the birth moment itself can
seem alarming. In the hospital, when the baby begins to arrive
somebody suddenly yells for a "baby nurse!" who then comes ca-
reening in with her heating table and equipment. In the hospital,
the birth is sometimes attended by the use of the Mighty Vac
electric suction device, or the cutting of an episiotomy, and the
baby's sex is announced almost immediately by a staff member,
not discovered by the parents. And in the hospital, even when the
mother gets to hold her infant at first, they soon whisk the baby
to the cleaning table, usually within five or ten minutes. These
may seem like minor differences, but they strike me forcefully
here at the calm, respectful, and intensely loving arrival of Hannah Beth.

Megan gets out of the pool and climbs onto her big double
bed. It is fully day now with the sun streaming in and Jeff playing
the Jerry Garcia Band on the stereo. Julie checks her perineum
again. Definitely no tears. I am reminded of a study on genital
trauma that found that the highest rates of intact perineums
were among women who give birth at home (the highest rates of
genital trauma were among women delivered by obstetricians in
large urban hospitals).[3] "Yeah," Julie says, "just a bit of rug burn.
It's going to sting when you pee, so we'll leave you a peri bottle."
The peri bottle is like a squeezable sports water bottle to use instead of wiping with abrasive toilet paper. Julie breaks into a story
about a woman whose doctor saw her at the six-week postpartum
visit and asked her, "What did you do, sit on a chain saw?" after *he*
had cut an episiotomy for a forceps delivery. Julie informs Megan
that if the baby refuses to latch on, something might be not quite
right with the lungs, but if they nurse, they're probably okay. The
baby is nursing busily, and Megan is smiling. Finally, Julie tells
Megan that if the baby isn't fine two hours after the birth, then
we'll all go in to the hospital, but she isn't expecting to have to
do that.

Andrea sits on the bed filling out forms and then does a complete baby examination. Hannah Beth is eight pounds, three ounces, and twenty inches long. Andrea puts some olive oil on the baby, then asks if they want the eye goop, an antibiotic ointment to help prevent infection. They say yes, so she puts it in, but not until Hannah Beth's dark, inquisitive eyes have been gazing up at her mother for well over an hour. Jeff makes us all eggs, toast, coffee, and juice. We squeeze around the yellow formica table in the tiny kitchen area of the trailer and eat hungrily. Everyone is tired and happy.

We leave just after eleven o'clock. It is a Sunday morning and a brilliantly sunny southwestern day. Driving down the dusty, gravel road, I see the soft blue-brown of the nearby mountains rise peacefully in the near distance where there was only blackness when we arrived seven hours earlier. The new day has brought a new life, a new baby born safely at home.

⌒

Seeing Megan give birth to Hannah Beth is liberating. It opens the way for a paradigm shift in my thinking about home birth; suddenly everything looks different. Instead of being an unknown entity, something vaguely scary and definitely on the fringe, home birth is now not only imaginable, but a reality—something that has been normalized. Witnessing the competence of the midwives is also hugely reassuring. I find myself thinking that as long as my pregnancy remains trouble-free, I may want to have my baby at home. I know this would mean shelling out more than two thousand dollars because my insurance won't cover home birth, but I think I could manage that. I'm new to this, and not a die-hard convert, so I figure that if anything starts to go wrong, I'll transfer to the hospital without a murmur. Also, if the pain is truly unendurable, I'll transfer and get that epidural. In her book, *Birthing from Within,* Pam England, my doula class teacher, writes that for her second labor she gave herself an outside limit to the number of hours she was willing to be in serious pain. This seems like a reasonable and comforting strategy to me, so I tell myself I can do ten to twelve hours at home; I'm not interested in toughing it out beyond that. I'm not feeling hardcore about the whole home-birth thing. But wouldn't it be nice, I let myself daydream, if everything just went smoothly and I had my baby in the peace and safety of my own home, just like Megan?

8

Choosing

I AM more than half-way through my first trimester and I still haven't chosen a midwife. With my first pregnancy, I was so excited to get started, I had my first clinic visit when I was only about ten days pregnant. This time, I'm feeling more laid-back about the process, but also, I've struggled to find what I really want.

After seeing Megan's home birth, I've been thinking seriously about having my baby at home. Megan's labor and delivery were reassuringly well-managed, and there was something almost inspiring in its normalcy. Most of the midwives I've met have chosen to have their own babies at home. And research has shown time and again that, statistically, home birth for a healthy woman, attended by a qualified individual within a system that allows for hospital backup when necessary, is as safe as or safer than birth in the hospital.[1] I am especially impressed by a recent study from the University of Copenhagen, comparing planned home births backed up by hospital systems and planned hospital births, showed no difference in survival rates between the babies. The home-birth group had fewer medical interventions, fewer babies born in poor condition, fewer maternal lacerations, and fewer inductions, medications, caesarean sections, and forceps- or vacuum-assisted deliveries. There were no maternal deaths in either group.[2]

My background as an academic and a medical doctor's daughter makes me trust statistics more than anything, and yet I still have reservations. Many of the home-birth midwives I've talked to are assisting at only a dozen, or fewer, home births a year. They're not seeing a wide range of births, and that makes me nervous. While I understand that scheduling a solo practice limits the number of women you can see, and that there just isn't a huge demand for home birth, I still want my midwife to have a lot of experience. And while there are one or two home-birth midwives in town who are quite experienced, I didn't really click with them on a personal level, so I'm not enthusiastic about becoming their client. For instance, I have total confidence in Julie's abilities after seeing her at Megan's birth, but I don't feel either an intellectual or an emotional connection with her, and I want that.

As for having a nurse-midwife at the hospital, my on-site observations have left me with mixed feelings. I saw a few very nice births where the woman was well-supported by her midwife, nurse, and family; and even a few births that seemed to have that elusive element of the spiritual that is so appealing to me. But I also saw a lot of births that were tied up in the technological apparatus of the hospital—electronic monitoring read from the nurses' station as opposed to someone listening more intimately to the baby with either a fetascope or a Doppler right on the mother's belly; an IV instead of someone patiently urging the mother to keep drinking; nurses who expressed irritation with mothers who preferred to try nipple stimulation to start their labors instead of Pitocin; and so on.

Also, there's the nagging issue of not getting to choose your midwife when it comes time to give birth. I've realized how important this is to me, and at the hospital, you just cannot guarantee who you'll get. Still, although I would prefer to have my birth attended by the person who did my prenatal exams—someone who knows me, my health history, and my concerns—I think I could live without that if my attending midwife could at least provide a continuing supportive presence during my labor. If nurse-midwives could always sit with women through their labor, if they didn't have anyone else to attend or paperwork to complete at the nurses' station, I could forego my attachment to a particular person. But the certified nurse-midwives at Skyline Hospital, where I've been observing, don't labor-sit very much. If you get lucky, a good nurse will do some of that, but you have to get lucky.

Recently, I went to see one of the certified nurse-midwives who is covered by my insurance company. One of the first things she did was to hand me a pastel-colored, mini diaper bag full of complementary "goodies." When I asked what was in it, she said, "Oh, it has a video, and coupons, and some stuff." I peeked in. It was full of formula. I told her I was planning to breast-feed and didn't need the formula. She suggested I keep it anyway. I declined politely, but later I wished I'd said, "I can't believe you're pushing formula. Yes, there are times when it's necessary, but surely you realize that handing this stuff out sends moms the message that formula is the best way to go. There is so much data out there on how much healthier breast-feeding is for babies and mothers, the American Academy of Pediatrics goes so far as to say that 'breast-feeding ensures the best possible health as well as the best developmental and psychosocial outcomes for the infant.'[3] So aren't you an advocate of breast-feeding? Isn't that part of what midwives do?" I was really shocked. Even so, I might still have considered becoming a client of hers, but she works with only one other midwife and a group of doctors, which means that it's possible neither of the midwives would be on call when I deliver, in which case I would be attended by a doctor I had never seen before, and that's not what I want at all.

I finally go for my first prenatal visit with another certified nurse-midwife who accepts my insurance, Jane Elliott. She used to do home births but now works for a practice that employs a mix of obstetricians and nurse-midwives. Jane is in her forties, trim and stylish, with short, blond hair in a boyish cut, and a bright, attentive manner. She comes across as intelligent and thoughtful. I ask her why there is no birth center in town and she tells me it's an economic issue. "The volume that you have to have to sustain a birth center and not be on call constantly is such that it takes a pretty good population density," she tells me as she starts a chart for me and measures my belly. "The rule of thumb is that in order to pay for yourself you have to deliver ten babies per month per midwife. And a reasonable call schedule is a one-in-four call schedule, so that means your volume has to be forty births a month at a birth center, and we just don't have enough demand here."

When I ask if it was hard for her to switch from doing home births to being in the hospital she nods yes but defends her choice saying, "My main issue was, am I going to be able to translate those midwifery principles to a hospital setting? And I am happy to say yes, I've been able to do that." I ask if it isn't hard for her to really pay attention to mothers in the same way during labor, and she nods again, backpedaling a bit on her initial stand. "Oh yes, that is one of the drawbacks at the hospital. Sometimes I feel so frustrated because I'm so torn, you know. I have the postpartum people who are over there yelling at me because they need to get someone discharged and out the door, and I have to go over and write up a note, examine her, and write the orders. And then somebody is in triage with a bladder infection who I need to check on. And there's this woman laboring, and I know if I can just sit with her that's all she needs, someone just to sit with her the whole time and she'll be fine. If I could do that she'll walk away from that experience with a better birth and a sense of gratification. And that's why we do our work, to be able to empower people in that way. But I can't always do that."

I tell Jane I'm considering a home birth and ask if she could attend me at home and then transfer to the hospital if necessary. She sighs and says that, unfortunately, and despite the midwives' protests, the doctors in her practice have decided not to provide backup to midwives transporting their clients to the hospital. This means that she couldn't attend me if I decided to transfer, and that I would have to be seen by whatever doctor was on call for emergencies at the hospital. Jane pulls a face and says, "And that could mean a doctor who is hostile to home birth." I most certainly don't want that. If I want to do a home birth, I'll have to find someone else. So I am still looking.

I am feeling frustrated and acutely aware of the time slipping by. I am rapidly approaching the window at the end of the first trimester when most prenatal testing is done. I need to find some prenatal care, and I need to find it soon.

⌒

The next midwife I speak to is Sarah Walker-Adams. I have followed her in the hospital for four months and am impressed with her work and manner. Sarah greets me at the door to her house with her three-year-old daughter, Pilar, clinging to her legs. Pilar plays nearby as we settle in to talk.

Sarah speaks in a well-modulated, deliberate way that makes her sound both gentle and purposeful as she tells me about her decision to become a midwife. In her senior year of high school, she wrote a term paper on Renaissance literature, stumbled across a reference to midwives, and became fascinated by the topic. "I ended up writing about midwives, and it changed the course of my life. I decided that was what I wanted to do. I shared my plans with my very best girlfriend and my boyfriend at the time. Both of whom, ironically, were on paths to become physicians. They thought my idea was really . . ." Sarah trails off, then concludes, "bad. No, that's an understatement. They were concerned about my mental health and asked if I was also going to become a witch." She laughs, and says, "Of course, they hadn't read my term paper."

After her friends' response, Sarah decided not to tell her family about her plans. Instead, she merely told them she was going to nursing school; a decision they found baffling, as it didn't seem to fit her previous intellectual and artistic goals. "I knew I wanted the option," Sarah says, "even at just seventeen years old, of being able to do both home births and hospital births, and I'd have to have a nursing degree to do that. So I went to nursing school. But I hated it. It just didn't fit with my idea of feminism at the time. So I quit." She began pursuing other studies and went to work part-time at a local birth center.

The birth center was in a big old house in which the bedrooms had been turned into birthing rooms. Sarah recalls, "It was lovely place. I was twenty-one years old and attending my first day of orientation there. A woman was in labor and the midwife in charge had me sit with her while she saw someone in the clinic. The woman spoke a little bit of English but mostly Spanish, and I speak mostly English and very little Spanish, but we understood each other enough. At one point she went into the bathroom, and as she came out she had this incredible look on her face. Her eyes were wide, and I just knew by looking at her that the baby was coming. She was dressed in just a shirt with nothing on below, so I looked down at her vulva and, sure enough, I could see the baby's head starting to come. We both called for the midwife, but it was a very large house." There was no time to spare, so Sarah says, "I dove down on my knee and caught this little baby as he came flying out. And um," her voice breaks a little as she tells this part of her story. She leans forward, letting her long, dark hair swing in front of her face before she finishes. "I got her back to bed and put the baby up on her belly. The midwife arrived, and I knew right then that I had to go back and finish that last year of nursing school. So I did."

After completing nursing school, Sarah worked briefly as a labor and delivery nurse in a hospital. But she says she didn't last long since she kept "losing" the leather straps that they bound women's hands with in the delivery room. I can't quite believe what I've heard and ask her to clarify when that was. Yes, it was in the mid-eighties that this hospital was still strapping women down during labor. Fortunately, Sarah was able to get a job as a nurse across town at Skyline Hospital, which was just then expanding its midwifery service. While there, she applied to midwifery schools and was accepted to the program at Yale, which she attended. "I chose Yale to legitimize midwifery to my family," she says, laughing. "They still thought that I was . . . ," she breaks off and taps her temple. "Well, let's just say they just didn't understand my passion."

Sarah credits Yale with giving her an excellent education. While there, she learned that they offered a three-year program for students who don't have a nursing degree. "Had I known about that program when I was seventeen years old, I probably would have pursued it; it would've suited my makeup a lot better," she says. She notes that the existence of this program meant that she went to school with a lot of women who were not nurses, and this thoroughly convinced her that one does not need to be a nurse to be a midwife. "I'm really interested in direct-entry midwifery education," she tells me, "and in having paths other than nursing for people drawn to midwifery."

Her one disappointment was that the school did not offer the tender and loving apprentice relationships she was hoping for, relationships like the ones she had witnessed at the birth center. "I expected them to sort of take me under their wing," she says, reaching her arm out widely and curving it back in with exaggerated tenderness, "and I thought they would give me all of these little pearls of wisdom—the treasures they had learned." She shakes her head and smiles at her naivete. "Well, Yale's a very academic place." She did, however, get the opportunity to come back to Skyline for her internship "and those midwives," she says, "*did* take me under their wings, and they did give me their pearls."

Pilar, who has been playing quietly for some time, interrupts us briefly. Sarah bends down and gives her a hug, saying, "You're being really good, sweetheart," and turns to me to explain that her daughter is in "Mommy University this year." Sarah drinks some tea, watches Pilar working hard to get two pieces of a wooden train track to fit together, and says, "Motherhood has transformed my life in ways I just never expected, growing parts of me in my heart that I never knew were there. My first daughter is now eight years old. I had a very magical pregnancy with her. It truly was a transforming experience. Our children grow so fast. They're little and with you for just a few heartbeats and then they're off." Gesturing at my belly because she knows I'm pregnant and that our children will have a similar age split of almost five years, Sarah adds,"Your first will seem even more grown-up when your new baby comes."

Sarah is working part-time so she can be home more with her children. She tells me that she always envisioned herself with a home-birth practice. However, although she has attended friends at home and had both of her children at home, she works in the hospital because the home-birth call schedule is "enormously difficult" to combine with motherhood. "I think one of my biggest challenges as a midwife," she says, "has been to find the balance—to have midwifery in my life as a mother. I love them both. They're my two passions right now, and they both would very much like to be my only passion. And so, finding a way to weave those two together has been challenging. " So she keeps working at the hospital with the thought that when her children are grown, she may turn to home birth.

Sarah and I have been talking for a long time, and Pilar is starting to get restless, so I ask one final question. I ask Sarah what the greatest joy of being a midwife is for her. I ask it mostly as a way to wrap up our interview, so I'm surprised at the intensity of her response. She takes a minute to think, then says, "Well, there is magic that occurs. . . ." Suddenly, her voice breaks and her eyes turn pink and watery, but she keeps speaking, "when a baby comes into the world." Tears slide down her cheeks and she cries quietly for a minute. There is a long pause before she continues, "And almost every day that I work, I get to live in that, and I thank the stars for that every time I think about it." She pauses again to wipe her eyes and grins. "Also, I like working with women. I come from a family of very strong women, and I get to do that every day that I work. I get to be with women during one of the most physically challenging, spiritually altering, and emotional moments of their life. And I love that. I don't know why I love it, but I do."

I am moved by Sarah's heartfelt response. Knowing her attachment to home birth, and that she's caught more than 1,200 babies, I go out on a limb and ask if she would consider doing a home birth for me. I know she's not expecting this, so I preface it by telling her she doesn't need to respond right away, but maybe we can talk about it again when I see her in the clinic next week. She agrees to consider it, and I leave, hoping she will be my midwife.

⌒

Before I see Sarah again, Richard, Max, and I go on a hiking trip to Canon de Chelly on the Navajo Reservation in Arizona. I love to hike. It's one of the reasons I left New York City, where I worked in my twenties. Living there was thrilling but claustrophobic. Living in the immense spaces of the West makes me feel happily insignificant; the landscape provides a constant visual reminder of how temporary we are. I love to get out and feel small, feel lost, feel overwhelmed by nature and what writers like to call "the sublime."

So here I am, trying to do as much hiking as I can before I'm too big to haul my body up a trail and before I am so sleep-deprived by a new baby that I won't want to. The canyon's towering red rock formations rise up against a stunningly deep-blue sky. Autumn has arrived and the cottonwoods are blazing yellow. The hike, down a wisp of a trail cut into the rock face, is a challenge for Max, but also an adventure. He manages to get all the way down the canyon and back up on his own. He is pleased, and so am I, since he's been too big to carry in a backpack for a while now and has spent much of the past year whining whenever we go hiking. Finally, he is actually enjoying himself, playing all along the path. He is so sweet with me these days. I think we both sense that his baby days are drawing to a close. Today, we have what is becoming a ritual, bonding conversation for us: the discussion of baby names. For a girl, I vacillate between wanting something unusual like Iona or Kestrel and old family names like Ella and Marie. Max's current favorites for a girl are Cloudy Dawn and Jamaica.

While we are on the reservation, we visit one of the students from my doula class, Jenny. Her husband is a doctor with the Indian Health Service Hospital here. They have two young children, the youngest born less than a year ago. Jenny, who is outdoorsy, athletic, and a bit of an earth mother, tells us she'd like to take us on the trail she walked when she was in labor, so we hike up to the top of a small mesa behind her government-issue, cinderblock house. The views at dusk are stunning. The Lukachukai Mountains glow pink and blue in the distance, and the enormous bulk of Black Mesa darkens the horizon. We watch the sun set over hundreds of miles of empty desert. The endless expanse of dusty land slowly drowns in the lengthening blue shadows. It is exhilarating. I find both thrill and comfort in the absence of manmade destruction. But the vastness is not entirely benign; it is also a source of threat and fear. What is unseen? How powerfully destructive are the forces of this nature I profess to love? How easily could it break me, even as it holds me high? I know its enormity conceals terrors of its own. The heedless ambush of a flash flood, the unheard attack by animal or man, the killing intensity of the sun at noon. Looking out, I think about my plans for a home birth. I know my romance with the natural world is unrequited. So while I long for a birth as devoid of synthetic interruption as this scene, what potentially brutal realities might mother nature throw my way if I choose to birth on her turf? Of course, having a home birth is not as daring an act as braving the desert wilds, after all; my midwife will be there. Her skills and judgment will be my blanket, my tent, my safety line.

I ask Jenny what it was like to labor up here in this world without end, a space so unbroken by the hand of the modern world. She beams, then laughs as she recalls that it was great until her contractions got really hard and she wasn't sure she was going to make it back down the hill to the little hospital hidden behind a ridge below us. She describes scrambling back at an awkward trot, hoping she wouldn't turn an ankle, her progress impeded every two minutes by waves of pain. As she talks, we descend into the almost completely unilluminated lowlands, what lies ahead unseen. The din and glitter of the electric world barely exist here. Only an impossibly paltry handful of lit buildings, like a lonely constellation in an empty black sky, allows us to retrace her once-heavy steps.

⌒

Our hiking trip thoroughly exhausts me. I'm looking forward to some increased energy in my second trimester. The day after we get back, I drag myself in to follow Sarah Walker-Adams for a full day at her busy clinic. That evening, after a typical round of prenatal and postpartum visits and as she finishes writing up patients' charts in her office, I get up my nerve to ask if she's thought more about being my midwife for a home birth. Yes, she says she has, and she will. This is great news. I'm very excited. I think Sarah is a wonderful person and an extremely skilled midwife. When I suggest a pay schedule, she says, "Actually, it's something I would like to give to you."

"I'm sorry?" I say, confused.

"I would like to do this for free," she says. "One of the things I like about working here at Skyline is that I don't have to consciously mix money and birth; it happens on the side. I would like to offer this to you. I don't want to do this as a moonlighting business; this is just something I would like to do for you. Besides, I'm really flattered that of all the midwives you've met, you asked me to be present for this."

I can hardly believe it. I am so touched and so surprised by Sarah's wonderful offer that I am at first speechless and then embarrassingly inarticulate. She could have charged me $2,000 or more, which I'm sure her family could use. I mumble my thanks and suggest that I could give her a series of gifts in exchange for her work, a sort of barter situation. She nods and tells me about a midwife friend of hers who sometimes gets paid in goats, chickens, and earrings, but basically, she shrugs me off, saying it isn't necessary.

It is night when I leave Sarah's office. The sky is black with a touch of indigo blue on the western horizon. As I turn the corner out of the parking lot, I am suddenly confronted by an enormous moon—full, glowing brightly, and just peeking over the top of the mountains. It is incredible, like a big wafer, or one of those silvery-white pods we used to play with as kids, peeling the brown skin off to reveal a shimmering disk and a few seeds. I'm so stunned by the scene, I worry I'll have an accident as I am already giddy with excitement over Sarah's offer. I pull over and watch the moon rise, thinking how lucky I am. I feel relieved and rejuvenated by Sarah's generosity and also somehow reassured that I am making the right choice to birth at home.

The only remaining hitch in my prenatal care is that my insurance won't cover prenatal testing or hospital visits at Skyline, where Sarah works. I need to work out a backup plan for these. I decide to continue seeing Jane Elliott, the certified nurse-midwife who works at a hospital my insurance does cover, in order to keep up a relationship with her. If I need a hospital, I won't say I'm transporting from home, since the doctors in her practice won't attend transfers; I'll just pretend I was always planning to have my baby with her at her hospital. I ask Jane if this is okay with her and she says yes, as long as I keep seeing her at least every other month and as long as I keep it quiet. She even agrees to be my backup home-birth midwife; she'll assist Sarah at my house, or take over if Sarah is unavailable, when I go into labor. Again, I couldn't be more thrilled. Now I have not one, but two midwives I really like both personally and professionally. The next time I speak to Sarah, I tell her I feel a little sneaky doing this. She tells me to relax; I'm not being sneaky, I'm just keeping all my options open. Yes, it's bending the rules slightly, but it's not breaking them.

Sarah also tells me that if I have a major or very sudden emergency (both very unlikely) we'll just go to the nearest hospital emergency room, which is less than ten minutes away from my house. If it is a major emergency, I'm not going to care who is attending me.

Having chosen my midwives, I immediately schedule some clinic visits, as I'm closing in on the dates when any prenatal testing must be done. Now for another big decision. Amnio or no amnio? I will be thirty-five years old by the time my due date rolls around. I had always assumed I would do amniocentesis, because I don't want a child with Down's syndrome, and I am strongly in favor of a woman's right to decide when it comes to abortion. However, for the next two weeks I struggle and struggle with the decision. I am scared by the risks of the procedure, even though they are low (about 1 in 200 for a miscarriage due to the procedure itself), but I hate to think of losing this baby unnecessarily. Also, I find that it is very, very difficult—agonizing, in fact—to think about aborting my baby even if it does have Down's syndrome.

I am already terribly attached to the idea of my baby. I know it might be better, psychologically, to think of it as a fetus, since there is still the possibility of terminating the pregnancy, but that is an intellectual argument that has little allure right now. To me, not only is this growing life a baby, it is my child, Ella or Emrys. It may be a mistake to think like this, but surely it is also a normal, healthy, loving thing to do. Surely, mothers have been thinking of their unborn as "babies" for millennia. Plus, by the time they can do the amnio, it is possible that I will have felt my baby move—a possibility that fills me with additional longing for my child and dread at the idea of rejecting it.

While I am in the middle of fretting about amniocentesis, at the beginning of my sixteenth week of pregnancy, I go on one last weekend hiking trip, this time with Professor Leah Albers, who has just returned from a year-long sabbatical at Oxford University. As we hike along a narrow mountain switchback, she tells me that in England, most pregnant women do something called an "anomalies screen" at eighteen weeks. This is a high-level ultrasound in which they can tell if the baby has spina bifida, anencephaly, or other neural-tube defects. If I did this, I would catch most of the really huge birth defects that might lead me to decide to terminate the pregnancy, but it wouldn't catch Down's syndrome.

The only other test that is available to me is the alfa-fetoprotein, or AFP, a blood test that is routinely given to help assess the chances of having a baby with spina bifida or Down's syndrome. Unfortunately, it is notorious for giving a huge number of false positives. In other words, it often says you are at a high risk for a problem, when, in fact, your baby is fine. But it also has a significant false-negative rate, meaning you think the baby's fine, but it's not. The standard obstetrical textbook reports that it has a "positive predictive value of only 2 to 6 percent. Thus, the majority of women with elevated levels do not have a fetus with a neural-tube defect."[4] At the same time, it misses as many as 40 percent of Down's cases for women my age.[5] This seems practically useless to me and also seems guaranteed to either make me worry unnecessarily or be falsely reassured.

In trying to balance all this out, I look at the statistics: 80 percent of Down's syndrome babies are actually born to women who are younger than age 35, but the risk does increase for women over 35. I have a 1 in 350 chance of having a baby with Down's and a 1 in 200 chance of having any genetic defect. This means I am more than 99 percent likely *not* to have these problems. Still confused, I call all my female friends and discover that most of them either did or were likely to do amniocentesis, and also that many of them had had the notorious falsely positive AFP and swore they wouldn't do that test again because it upset them so much.

My friend Addie, who is thirty-seven and pregnant now, is considering doing chorionic villi sampling (CVS), usually a riskier procedure than amniocentesis (unless you live in a big city where there is a practice that does this frequently), but one that can be performed several weeks earlier, which might help make an abortion a little easier to handle, should there be a problem. Several friends confess to making their decisions based on an emotional rather than a statistical basis. My friend Mareth did not do amniocentesis with her first, because she was only thirty-two, but she too isn't sure what she'll do with her next pregnancy, and says she hates to even think about it. She's leaning away from it just because she hates big needles, but she also doesn't like the idea of aborting an imperfect child. She is a professor and tells me that she recently read an article written by a woman with spina bifida. This is a wake-up call; I didn't even know you could have spina bifida and live. I don't feel like I'm getting any closer to a decision, so I call home.

My father answers the phone. I begin by telling him that the test I'm thinking of doing, the high-level ultrasound, won't catch Down's syndrome, and though my chances are slim, I have to accept that I might have a disabled child. He says, "Well, I don't know if you know anyone with Down's, but I see quite a few patients who have it, and they are, for the most part, loving members of their families. They are often cheerful, and while they make life more complicated, they bring their families a lot of happiness. Even as adults, they can demonstrate a loving, childlike affection that is wonderful to be around." I am so grateful and relieved to have this little extra picture to add to my mosaic. Before he hangs up, my father adds, "You know, trying to balance the risk of miscarriage from the procedure with the risk of a defect is comparing apples and oranges. You might as well trust your gut."

In a lot of my discussions and reading about prenatal testing, I'm disturbed by what feels like an undercurrent of intolerance. So often it seems to be accepted, almost without question, that, of course, you would abort a child with Down's syndrome or any other serious handicap simply because they would be too hard to deal with. I am somewhat sympathetic to this on the extreme end of the spectrum. Yes, a severe disability could make my child's life and the life of our family very, very difficult. But some disabilities, while offering us challenges, and certainly making our lives more complicated, well, can I really say that that life is not worth living? If we, as a society, all abort less-than-perfect individuals, won't we become even more intolerant of difference? Already, we are so isolated from it; "they" are in separate classes, if not separate schools, and are rarely visible in the workplace. I wonder, what do we lose when we choose to eliminate certain disabilities? What part of our humanity, our ability to be caring and compassionate, gets shut down forever?

This week, I have my first prenatal visit at home with Sarah. It is so sweet. She measures my belly while I lie on my own bed, I pee on a stick to test my urine, then we talk in my kitchen and drink tea. I tell her I'm struggling with my decision about whether or not to have an amnio. Sarah shakes her head sympathetically and says, "At your age, that's a tough call. I wouldn't say it was necessary, but you need to decide for yourself if you want to know if there's a problem with your baby. And you need to know what you would do with that knowledge." She sighs and says, "It's so hard to know what's right. All I can tell you is that I will absolutely support you in either decision." After she leaves, I call my hospital-based midwife, Jane, to tell her I'm thinking about skipping the amnio and just having an ultrasound. When I question her about whether I could still get an abortion if I wanted one, she hesitates a bit. Well, I ask, what's the story? She tells me that yes, I can terminate the pregnancy, but it wouldn't be a surgical procedure. In this city, after nineteen weeks, I would have to be induced in the labor and delivery ward and give birth to my fetus/baby/child. It would be born and then would die almost immediately. I cry just thinking about it. Jane tells me I can see the genetic counselor in three days and make my final decision about testing then.

That evening I open my mail. There is a letter from Addie that begins by saying she has sad news. This is never good, but it is especially scary coming from Addie, whose last letter that began this way told me she had cancer. I am crying before I even know what has happened. I force myself to read on. She is no longer pregnant. An ultrasound has revealed that her fetus has stopped developing. It is a huge loss. I am crushed with disappointment and so sad for her and for myself. I had already counted on our joint pregnancies, on having children the same age. Foolish, I angrily tell myself now. You know you can't count on these things. It was too soon to feel confident.

Two months later, my friend Elena, who is also pregnant,

writes to tell me that she's felt the first "flutters" of her baby. She writes that every time she thinks about her baby, she feels unconditional happiness, pure joy, and yet, there's a part of her that "refuses to believe that things could be okay. I remind myself that many people have many babies, but it still seems too miraculous and fragile." A few weeks after this letter, well into her second trimester, she calls to say she is spotting, and a day later I get a tearful call from her husband, telling me that Elena's pregnancy is also over. It turned out to be an ectopic, or tubal pregnancy, meaning that the baby implanted in a fallopian tube instead of in the uterus. Her tube ruptured, leaving her in agony and in danger of bleeding to death. She's at the hospital now and is doing alright, but one of her tubes is gone, which will make it harder for her to get pregnant again, and the baby, of course, is dead. They named him Angel and had a small ceremony to mark his loss. They will try again, but the truth is that they are devastated. Not long after, yet another friend calls to announce her pregnancy (we're all in our mid-thirties and trying to beat the biological clock), and although I'm glad, my response is muted. I know I should be jubilant for her, but all I can think is that I'm not counting on either of us having our babies.

I grow so aware of the ways that in pregnancy, birth, infancy, and even childhood, it always feels too soon to be sure, too soon to be safe from all the threats that lie in wait. Defects, disease, and death in all its forms hover just beyond the joy of it all. My issues with prenatal testing have already made me acutely aware of the way I swing between being defined by my pregnancy and wanting to distance myself from it, just in case. . . . Just in case the technology available to me tells me I shouldn't have this baby, just in case I miscarry. It all seems so tentative, so precarious.

Two days after I get Addie's letter, the day before my appointment with the genetic counselor, I feel my baby move. It is a surprising squiggle of comfort and love, a single flutter, an opening to the infinite. It is thrilling. Suddenly, I am in love and fierce in my protection. My baby could die at any moment, but I won't do anything to hurt it. I know I could not abort now, so I won't do the amnio. I'll take my chances. If the baby has Down's, well, it will change my life, but maybe not for the worse.

That night I dream of carrying two children, one on my hip and one in my arms, to the edge of a raging river at night. The chest-high water, brown with mud, swirls menacingly. I need to get across. Without thinking, I plunge into the water and start walking. Somehow I make it safely to the other side. I wake up feeling calmer than I have in weeks. I do the ultrasound and everything looks fine, but the Down's question remains and will continue to haunt me throughout my pregnancy, as will all the other shadowy threats to the life I carry within me.

PART THREE

Second Trimester

9

Challenges

THE sky is unusually gray and dark. It is cold. Most of the trees have lost their leaves. A few of the cottonwoods in the valley are still a bright lemon yellow, but many have turned a deep gold, and some are already crisped and brown. In the distance, the mountains are a dark, humped blanket of navy blue with a fringe of snow on the rocky crest. The telephone wires are full of birds, and everywhere crows are cawing. It is late fall and late afternoon. I notice that the clock on my cassette recorder needs to be set back an hour, since daylight savings time has ended. I am driving through a suburb that used to be a rural town. Colossal new houses are being built on dusty, old farm roads. Some people have horses; a few remaining long-time residents have goats and chickens. On the radio, Bruce Springsteen sings the lonely hope of the individual, the perfect somber-but-happy-that-way groove for this dusky day. Despite the bleakness of the weather, life feels good. I am in my second trimester and feel the ebb of nausea and the returning flow of energy. I am on my way to be a doula at a home birth, another one attended by midwife Julie Bradshaw, who took me to my first home birth at Megan's house.

Julie's current client, Melanie, felt her first contractions before dawn this morning. At 2 P.M., she called Julie to say that her contractions were "getting pretty rough" and that it was probably time for Julie to come. Melanie and her husband, Bill, have decided to labor and birth at his mother's house, which is roomier and slightly closer to the hospital than their own home. The house is new and feels like a hotel. There are huge stately carved wooden columns in the entryway, a cavernous fireplace, and, in the room where Melanie is laboring, pale beige wool carpet and a view of the mountains through a gracious picture window.

When I arrive, Julie, who is wearing teal-colored scrubs with little red hearts printed all over them, is setting up her equipment in a corner. A friend of Melanie's and several relatives are milling around the house. Bill is leaning over the edge of a blow-up pool, pouring water down Melanie's back from a green Tupperware bowl. She wears a soaking wet, oversized T-shirt. Tribal synth music plays softly in the background, and there is a large, milk-colored crystal lying in the bottom of the pool.

Bill has long, dark-brown hair and a small, athletic build, as does Melanie. Melanie is very pretty, slight, and has delicate hands. When I first met them at a prenatal exam, Julie made Bill put on a homemade device of hers she calls "the empathy belly," a smock with big weights sewn into pockets on the stomach. Julie told him, "We're going to put you through your paces. Take it home. Wear it all day. Pick things up off the floor and roll over in bed without waking your partner, because, after all, you're just pregnant and 'he' has to go to work tomorrow." They had an easy, joking rapport. So I am not surprised now, when Julie puts gel into a condom to waterproof her Doppler and says to Bill with a leer, "You and I are going to go out in the hall now." Bill grins and jokes right back at her, "I thought you looked a little nervous." Julie gives a big belly laugh.

In the pool, Melanie gets a contraction. As it rises, she leans into the tub wall, squeezing its sides. Julie checks the baby's heartbeat; it's fine. She holds Melanie's hand for the next contraction, commenting, "It seems like they're actually getting shorter," and looks through her collection of treatments for something to speed up the labor. She gives Melanie a tincture of something called B&B labor extract. It contains blue cohosh root, black cohosh root, blue vervain leaf, skullcap leaf, and lobelia leaf. When I ask her about its effectiveness, she says, "Sometimes B&B kicks them right in; sometimes it takes a few days." Julie offers Melanie a grape, saying, "Grapes are good to eat in labor. They're wet, they're quick, and they're gone before the next contraction." Melanie eats a single grape, then gets another contraction. "Oh, oh, ay, yi," she says, pounding the side of the pool lightly. She's complaining but not a lot. Between contractions she sits up and seems just like her usual self.

Andrea, Julie's apprentice, arrives and asks Melanie if she has been peeing regularly. Melanie says, "Sort of," and Andrea says, "Well, go when you get a chance." Andrea asks if she wants to be checked. Melanie doesn't, but Julie interrupts to say that there's some question as to whether the baby may be face up. If it is, they could work with her position to help the baby turn. Julie adds that she's glad Andrea is here, because she has long fingers and Melanie is very sensitive to being checked. Andrea puts on a glove, puts some olive oil on it, and puts her hand in. Melanie winces. Julie says, quietly, "Breathe it out," as Melanie cries out "Ow, ow, ow!" She pants loudly and cries out again. Andrea sits back and says she's two centimeters dilated. Melanie looks shocked. "Only two?"

"Yes," Andrea says, "but your cervix is really thin, almost 100 percent effaced. Baby's nice and low, zero station, maybe minus one, nice and low."

Two centimeters is not good news for someone who has been laboring for almost twelve hours. Melanie asks the midwives if there's anything else they can do to help. Julie gives Melanie a homeopathic remedy called gelsinium, which can help with what the midwives refer to as a "rigid os," which is Latin for "mouth" or "opening," in this case, the cervix. Melanie looks tired. I ask her if she'd like something to eat. Pasta, maybe? No. My doula training kicks in and instead of backing off politely, I persist. How about some rice? "Oh, maybe," Melanie says. Bill goes to start the rice, while I stay with Melanie through a long, double contraction. I pour water on her belly and try out some of the mantras I learned in doula class. "Breathe the baby out, down and out. Ride the wave to the shore. It always hits the shore." After the next contraction, Andrea says she sees some more mucus in the water, which she checks for meconium. Andrea looks with a flashlight, as it is now dusk and quite dim in the room. There is no sign of meconium staining.

Melanie switches her position so she's in more of a squat. Both Julie and Andrea praise the position, and Julie tells her that if she goes to pee, out of the tub, there will be more pressure and that might help her open, though it will hurt. Melanie says "Okay" and gets out of tub, but after a short, painful trip to the bathroom, she's soon back in the pool. She sits back and has Bill hold both of her hands and pull her arms out straight while she's contracting. Bill says, "Pull back harder. Pretend you're water-skiing. Yeah." He smiles. "Look at her ski!" Melanie eats a spoonful of rice. Another contraction comes, and when it passes, she eats another spoonful of rice. After a few rounds like this, Melanie gets out of the tub, briefly, walks around the house for a few minutes, and then goes back to the tub.

At 6:10 P.M., Melanie asks if she can take some more herbs to get her labor going stronger. Julie says, "Time for a pow-wow," and she and Andrea go into the hall to discuss what to do—maybe quiet down her contractions with calcium, or keep trying to speed them up with herbs like blue and black cohosh. Julie says, "We've seen women go for hours and hours with no progress. Sometimes they have to get completely exhausted before they'll relax. And sometimes when I leave them alone, they can give up performance anxiety and cry and fuss in a way they wouldn't in front of me. So far, this is a typical first birth." Julie eats some grapes, and between mouthfuls, she says, "Second-time moms remember birth on a cellular level. A second-time baby is going to trigger the expulsive mechanism and come down farther, and the average second-time mom remembers how to push. Most important, the second time around, the body is more likely to overpower the mind; you use less energy worrying." They decide to check Melanie's cervix again, because she may not need anything if she's progressed to six or seven centimeters.

Andrea checks her; she's made a little progress, but not much. Melanie's friend and Bill's family have been hovering over her through most of her labor, and now Julie and Andrea ask them to come out in the hall, away from Melanie, where the midwives suggest that the onlookers change what they're doing. Andrea says, "You are acting overconcerned and anxious, and you're making her nervous. No more telling her, 'You poor baby,' no more, 'Oh God, it looks hard.' Just say, 'You're doing great.'"

Julie adds, "She's fine. She's well within range of what's normal, but she may be feeling some fear, especially since we just let her know she hasn't progressed much. We need to let her know she's doing great. And she may need some time to just be alone with Bill and cry and say, 'Oh no, I can't do it,' and then let go." The family, who have seemed nervous and uptight, are a little grumpy at being told how to behave, but they agree to back off.

Julie and Andrea give Melanie more blue and black cohosh. Watching them prepare these concoctions, I am reminded of an account I read of Lewis and Clark meeting Sacagawea when she was pregnant. When she went into labor, they were impressed that her husband gave her some water with a crushed rattlesnake rattle in it in order to speed things up, and she delivered very soon after. But Julie and Andrea don't just use herbs and age-old remedies, they also employ some modern, Western technologies. For instance, they give Melanie an IV for fluids, something direct-entry midwives in this state are licensed to do, which can really help when a mom is tired and possibly dehydrated, and later they'll give her some oxygen.

It is about 8 P.M.; Melanie has moved to the bed with Bill lying next to her and Andrea and Julie sitting nearby. When Melanie moans, Julie moans along with a loose jaw and a low sound, and Melanie shifts her tone slightly to match Julie's. Julie says, "That's good," and gives her something to drink. Melanie sounds more weepy than before; at one point she clenches her fists in front of her and whispers, "No more." Her contractions are coming very regularly but most only last forty seconds. In a very small voice she says, "Oh, it hurts so much."

Bill asks, "How's my baby feeling?"

"Icky."

"You're the most beautiful thing in the world," Bill says.

Melanie just moans.

"I know," Bill says, "but you are."

Melanie really is extraordinarily beautiful, with long, wavy black hair, almost in ringlets, an arched thin nose, her face not at all puffy from pregnancy, high cheekbones, a rosy glow, big eyes that sparkle, and a full lower lip. She is exhausted, so Julie gives her a few whiffs of oxygen, which revive her a little.

It is approaching midnight. Melanie is moaning, "Oh no, oh, oh, oh. Please come baby, you're hurting me." Despite my second-trimester surge of energy, I am now so sleepy, I don't know if I can continue to stay up. I go into the living room and lie down. Julie joins me and writes up a hospital transport form, telling me, "I guess this falls in the category of playing games. Sometimes just filling out the transport form is all it takes to turn things around." The next time Andrea checks Melanie's cervix, there's good news. "You've made a lot of progress. You're so close."

It is 2 A.M. and Julie has been checking the baby's heart tones regularly all night. Now it is time to listen again. She turns on the Doppler. Nothing. Silence and slight static. Nobody talks, and the tension in the room rises a little as Julie tries several different positions. She can't find any heart tones and gets visibly antsy. Melanie is back in the pool; Julie asks her to stand up out of the water. She takes the waterproofing condom off the Doppler and listens again. There it is, a strong and steady beat. The baby is fine. Relief. Andrea says, "We need to talk about checking you again." Melanie moans. She really hates it. Julie gently pursues, "We'll wait until after the next one." The contraction ends, and Julie says, "Okay. I'm going to check you now."

"Now?" Melanie asks in a panicky voice.

"Yes."

Julie puts her hand in and says, "You are eight to nine centimeters." Everyone is pleased.

Just before 3 A.M., all the friends and relatives finally leave. I go back to the couch, thinking I'll nap for twenty minutes. Bill comes and puts a blanket on me as I'm drifting off, and I end up sleeping for two hours. When I wake up, it is 5 A.M.—morning, but not yet dawn. I awake with a start, angry that they haven't woken me for the birth. But there is still no baby. Julie tells me Melanie is fully dilated. I think to myself that I could not have gone on this long. Finally, as the sun rises to a pale, steel-blue dawn, Melanie begins to push.

After a few pushes, she says, "I feel like I'm going to poop." Julie says, "Yup. Push right past it, and if some little turds come out, we'll clean 'em up. They're taking up valuable space for the baby's head." Melanie says, "I don't think I can do it." She gets a funny look on her face and says, "Ooops. I think I pooped." Julie nods and uses a little scoop to get it out of the pool, saying, "No problem. I got it." Several more contractions and pushes. No sign of the baby.

"Time to move to the bed and allyoop her," Julie says.

"No, I can't," Melanie says.

"You can. You have to." Julie says, motioning Andrea to help pull Melanie out of the pool.

They manage to get her into bed and on her back with her feet on Julie's shoulders and Andrea and Bill each holding a knee.

Julie says, "Don't you dare push me off this bed. Don't push in your legs; push my fingers out. More power. Now. This is the time. It's going to feel like your butt's flying apart, but you have to do it anyway." To Bill she says, "We're going to use her femur like a fulcrum."

"I don't know if I can do this," Melanie says.

"Well, if you can't, we can go to the hospital. I don't say that to be mean, but you've been working a long time. You may not have the energy to do this," Julie says. Things feel tense and a little scary in the room. Melanie has passed some bloody fluid, and the room smells a little rank, almost sweetish. Andrea says, "You've got to do more. You've got a lot of strength left in you. You can do it. More, more." The next time Julie checks the baby's heartrate, it is slow and then fast. She says, "Oh boy, I don't like this with the low heartrate." She checks it again, and this time it is fine, but Julie's clearly worried and says, "I want your baby out. We may need to get the baby out. I don't know if you can do this. You've worked so hard."

Melanie says, "I don't want to go to the hospital." She bears down hard. "Okay, let's do it." But the next push doesn't change anything.

"We can do one last try on the toilet," Julie says.

"What happens if we go to the hospital?" Melanie asks.

"Well, they might do an episiotomy and forceps, or vacuum, but you may also be prepped for a C-section if the baby is too big to fit. And that baby has not changed position. We don't know if the baby's too big. While you go to the toilet and push, I'm going to call the hospital."

I go to the living room with Julie. As I look out the window at the gray sky and the cluster of sparrows at the feeder, I find myself praying that this baby will be born soon and well. Bill and his mother come into the living room. They are near tears, they are so worried. Julie fills out the remainder of the transfer form she had started working on earlier and calls the hospital. Bad news— the doctor on call is a hostile one—the same one I saw threaten and complete a C-section not long ago, the one who had made a midwife cry. Julie shrugs, goes back to Melanie, and says, "We're going to the hospital."

Julie's official diagnosis for the hospital is possible CPD (cephalopelvic disproportion), or a head too big for the pelvis, and maternal exhaustion. Melanie has been in labor for more than twenty-four hours. We drive to the hospital in a convoy of vehicles. I am in my own, and I am worried; it's very hard not to think of my own plans for a home birth. What would I be feeling now, if it were me? I am almost certain I would have gone in earlier; I don't have Melanie's total aversion to hospitals, and I definitely don't have her strength and determination to stay at home.

I remind myself that although this is nerve-racking, it isn't a real emergency. The last heart tones on the baby were good, and although Melanie is really tired, she has made steady, albeit slow, progress. There were no problems until the pushing turned out to be somewhat ineffective, and then Julie decided to transport. Still, I find myself deciding right then that I definitely want to set myself a time limit for staying at home. I don't want to transfer because of exhaustion.

When we get to the hospital, I find Melanie sitting in a wheelchair and Julie arguing with a nurse. Despite the fact that she called ahead, they are not expecting us at O.B. triage. Julie explains that she called and was given the green light to come, but the nurse just shrugs her shoulders and says, "There are no beds. She'll have to go someplace else. Or she can wait. If you want to do that, she needs to fill out all the forms," and holds out a stack of papers. Clearly struggling to stay calm, Julie says, "I am very concerned about this baby. We've been at this since yesterday. She's been pushing for an hour and a half." Bill starts to fill out the insurance forms, and Melanie groans. "These contractions are really hurting. They're pushing, pushing all the time." The nurse looks at her, apparently for the first time, and says, "I think she sounds like she's pushy." Julie rolls her eyes and says, "I *told* you, she has already been pushing!"

Finally, another nurse takes us down the hall to Labor and Delivery, where I catch a glimpse of the difficult doctor we were expecting to see. He is in his civilian clothes and is clearly leaving. We are greeted by another doctor, Dr. Olsen, who introduces himself with a smile and briskly gets Melanie onto a bed in a makeshift room behind a curtain. The first nurse reappears, pushes past Bill, and protests, "They can't bring her here. You can't see her here." Dr. Olsen ignores her as he explains to Melanie and Julie that he wants to get the baby on the monitor immediately. He does so, and reports, with a big grin, that the baby is fine and from what he can see it looks like they can proceed with a vaginal delivery—if that is what Melanie wants. She nods. The doctor turns back to the nurse, who is still fuming a few feet away. "I'll take her from here," he says politely but firmly, and escorts Melanie down the hall on a gurney to a delivery room.

A new nurse appears with scrubs for Julie, Bill, and Andrea so they can go in with Melanie. She apologizes that she can't get me in, too. It is about 9:30 A.M.. At 9:50 A.M., I hear a baby cry and get excited, but it is not Melanie's. A half-hour later, Andrea comes out, and, smiling, tells us that Melanie had a baby boy and that they are both fine. "The doctor was so nice," she says. At one point he said to his attending students that normally this would be the time to cut an episiotomy, but why bother, since the tissue was swollen, and, besides, the baby's heart tones were still fine. So she got no episiotomy, only a tiny tear, no vacuum extraction, no forceps, not even an IV (at one point a nurse asked if they needed one and the doctor said no).

It has been a long day and a half, and for Melanie it is still not over. She has a retained placenta. Afterward, she tells me, "They gave me some drugs after the baby was born, so they could go up and do a manual extraction, but then it came out on its own. I was so glad. After that long labor, I didn't want anybody putting anything in there." Ten minutes later, Bill walks down the hallway holding a tiny bundle of blankets wrapped around one very cone-headed baby with piercingly alert, dark eyes.

A few days later, at a postpartum visit, I get a chance to talk to Julie and Melanie. Melanie holds her sleeping baby as she reminisces about the birth and tells me that, "In the car, on the way there, I suddenly felt the baby pushing. Before that, I had to make myself push. By the time I got to the hospital, the baby was down there, ready to come."

Julie shakes her head and says, "I'm thinking about just driving people around then checking them again and going back home!" She pauses, then adds, "It turns out we could have had the same outcome at home, but with your exhaustion, it was just too risky. You did work hard for a very long time, Melanie. You were incredible; so strong. Although, at one point when Andrea asked if you would like to pray, you did say, 'I want the drug god!'"

They both laugh.

"Your strength really touched all of us who were present," Julie adds.

Melanie smiles, looking proud. "It was a true initiation into motherhood," she says. "I found I had the ability to let go of my personal self for someone else. I feel I gained a strength way, way inside myself—for someone else. It was worth it. To bring another life into the world, you have to give up part of yourself. I had no choice. I couldn't give up. I had to get him out. And I just didn't want drugs. I am very, very stubborn. I wanted to experience it fully without drugs. I've always taken the hard way," she says, snuggling her face down onto her son's tiny head. "For me, it really was an initiation."

I am drained after Melanie's birth, both by the endurance test of staying awake for most of twenty-four hours and by the emotional roller coaster of transporting to the hospital. I remind myself that nothing went wrong, and, in fact, this worked as the system should. She stayed home until there was a true need for the hospital, Julie acted prudently in deciding to transport, Melanie did not arrive with an emergency, and the hospital didn't even have to use any equipment or technology. Nonetheless, Melanie's birth reminds me that every choice has its down side, especially in a system that is not set up to optimize the potential of home birth, a system that doesn't have ready and habitual hospital backup. Home birth needs to be a fully integrated part of the spectrum of available birth options for it to become more viable for more people and, thus, to become the valuable part of our culture it could be.

I remind myself that when home birth is legal and attended by a trained practitioner, study after study has shown it to be safe.[1] And I remind myself that I want my decision about where to birth to be based on statistical evidence as well as my emotional needs. I decide to see what some of the midwives have to say to my specific fears about home birth.

I go to see Nancy Elder, one of the certified nurse-midwives I followed at the hospital, and tell her about a friend of mine who once told me, "You know, I know someone who had a home birth, and she's not my friend anymore because of this." I was taken aback and asked my friend what she meant. "I think it was really irresponsible," she said, "to have a home birth when she could have been in a hospital. What we're talking about here is that it could have been brain damage for that child." The woman was attended by a midwife, she did not live very far from a hospital, and both she and the baby had been fine. But my friend was still appalled. My response was to tell her, hesitantly, because I did not want to offend her and risk losing her friendship, that it was my understanding that home births are really pretty safe and that if you have any complications you generally have time to get to a hospital. I also told her that midwives are trained in neonatal resuscitation and that they have basically the same equipment that the hospital would use, except maybe a warming table. She shot back, "Well, what if the cord is around the baby's neck?" I smiled and relaxed a bit; this was an easy one. Roughly 20 percent of all babies are born with the cord around their neck, and either you disentangle the cord as the baby emerges, or, if it is really tight, you can clamp and cut it as the baby is being born. A tight cord doesn't take any major piece of equipment or any skill that a good midwife wouldn't have. I realized that my friend's viscerally negative reaction to home birth was probably not based on some piece of knowledge or information that I had overlooked, but rather on ungrounded fears.

Nancy, who is not a home-birth midwife and who had told me earlier that she was very proud of her nursing background, listens to my story, nods, and tells me that she's read that there has been little to no improvement in the neurological health of newborns as a result of the medicalization of birth. She adds that brain damage can occur for multiple reasons. "It can happen in utero, it can happen during labor, it can happen during birth, it can happen after birth, or it can happen in the person's infancy. It's very difficult to pinpoint. But most cases occur during the prenatal period. There are, however, some risks at birth if the baby is out of hospital and the midwife is not well versed in neonatal resuscitation." Nancy points out that this is where having legal and licensed midwives (as we do in our state) is a great help, because those midwives will be fully trained in neonatal resuscitation. "Also," she adds, "if there's real sticky meconium, that can be a concern since the baby may have already sucked it into his lungs. But, that's a call the midwives can usually make early enough. I think if you see meconium coming, that might be a reason to transfer." Later, when I talk to my midwife, Sarah, she concurs, telling me that some midwives might not transfer at that point, but she would, and if I want to stay home beyond that point, then she might not be the midwife for me. I have no problem with going to the hospital if we need it, so, of course, I agree.

Nancy, meanwhile, tells me, "There are some risks in hospital as well as out of hospital. So I think your perception is totally right. Home births are safe, and I think they're safe because the woman's ability to birth is protected instead of controlled. This is where home birth actually surpasses hospital birthing, and that's a pretty subtle thing for people who don't know or believe in this sort of energetic experience of crisis. Birth is a crisis, and when people gather around women who are in the middle of this crisis with love and openness and protection in their heart instead of the fear that they might get sued, or fear that if they don't get this kid delivered in two hours she's going to get a C-section, or fear that the nurse isn't going to like the way they're handling this, then it tends to work out better."

I am surprised at the way Nancy's response ranged from technical concerns about resuscitation to a more nuanced take on birth as an "energetic experience of crisis." Her words resonate with me, as I have recently read a passage by the French writer Michel Leiris that said:

There are moments which may be called crises and these are the only ones that count in life. Such are the moments when what is exterior seems abruptly to respond to the appeal which we make to it from the interior, when the outer world opens so as to establish between itself and our hearts a sudden communication.[2]

Leiris was actually talking about art, but it seems to me that his words beautifully capture the moment in birth when that which is literally interior to oneself, the baby, becomes part of the exterior world, and how the moment of birth makes visible the communication between our hearts and the world. I tell Nancy this and she says, "Wow. Yeah, I think birth mirrors that perfectly, and the question is, how best can a woman be supported when she's in that place, that crisis, when she's going through that door? You know, birth is one of the milestones of human beings' existence. Quite frankly, women who have the nature to be courageous and not follow the mainstream are probably better supported in an out-of-hospital birthing situation, provided they have knowledgeable caregivers."

Unfortunately, the barriers to getting knowledgeable home-birth caregivers in the United States can be steep. Not only does direct-entry midwifery still face legal challenges in more than a half-dozen states, but where it is legal, midwives face both cultural and economic stumbling blocks. On the cultural side, midwives have to overcome general misconceptions about home birth fostered, in part, by the medical model. One economic challenge to midwifery is insurance. Malpractice insurance is both extremely expensive and hard to find. One midwife told me that the only plan she was eligible for did not have the liability limits HMOs require. "They were looking for one million to three million," she said, "but because this is our first time ever to get malpractice insurance, the company said they would only give us a $300,000 limit for the first year. Then, depending on what our results are, we could get increased to the typical one to three million. So we're appealing to the HMOs." The difficulty in obtaining malpractice insurance contributes to patient insurers being unwilling to cover midwifery services. In a few states, Medicaid covers direct-entry midwifery, but usually at an abysmally low rate, often only half of their regular fee. Most women who want a home birth have to pay for it themselves, usually at the rate of around $2,500 for prenatals, birth, and postpartum visits. If you have hospital insurance that can get you through the process for one tenth the cost, home birth can be a hard option to justify.

Another deterrent to home birth is the fact that in many places, including one of the largest cities in my state, doctors refuse to provide hospital backup to midwives. One midwife told me she knew a doctor who used to hand out bumper stickers that said, "Home Delivery Is for Pizza." While the doctors often cite the difficulty of attending emergency transports as the reason for their refusal, most midwives are quick to point out that doctors are also protecting their territory, keeping the pool of patients to themselves, no matter what their personal beliefs about the efficacy of midwifery. This has long been so. In *Brought to Bed: Childbearing in America, 1750–1950,* Judith Leavitt quotes a 1912 letter to the editor of the *Journal of the American Medical Association* (*JAMA*) written by a doctor who, commenting on the problems associated with medical intervention in childbirth said, "Perhaps the best way to manage normal labor is to let it alone, but you cannot hold down a job and do that."[3]

I am so glad that I am able to have my prenatal exams at home with Sarah; I look forward to each one. She comes over and we usually drink a cup of tea and talk about what's happening in our lives. She asks me how I am and tells me I look radiant. I know she doesn't mean it this way, but I can't help thinking that "radiant" is just how *Charlotte's Web* described Wilbur, the pig; and it's true, I, too, am feeling fat, pink, and a bit vapid.

Sarah strikes me as both a romantic and a perfectionist. She tells me her daughters are learning to play the harp and that she herself is in a harp circle. She wears elegant dresses, dangling earrings, and her long hair swings loose below her shoulders. She always looks immaculate and arrives precisely on time. When she describes her life it sounds well ordered and full of music, dance, and learning. Mostly when she comes over, she is quiet and simply listens to me. Sometimes I'll tell her about a dream I've had, like the time I dreamt I was lying in bed, looked down, and found the baby was being born, still in the bag of water. Sometimes I'll tell her that I'm still scared about going into labor, frightened by the prospect of the pain, and then angry at myself because I know this fear might actually increase the pain or make my labor longer. Sometimes she comments, reassuring me; sometimes she just listens. She'll do the basic exam, take my blood pressure, record my weight (which soars as my belly begins to blossom outward), listen to the baby, and so on.

Throughout my pregnancy, Sarah keeps a detailed record of everything she does and observes. Her handwriting is delicate and legible, always in a fine, blue cursive. She notes the day she tells me how to make a raw potato poultice for hemorrhoids; how far along I am in gathering home-birth supplies (plastic sheets, heavy-duty sanitary pads, a pile of receiving blankets); the position of the baby; when I'm feeling tired; when I'm feeling good (one entry reads "Looking beautiful, doing great!"); the gradual dilation of my cervix toward the end; and her consultation with a doctor about my case and his opinion that, yes, I'm a good candidate for a home birth.

I deeply appreciate my midwife's loving attention, and as the weeks pass, I find myself growing more confident in her judgment and expertise. Despite the slightly nerve-racking experience of witnessing Melanie's transport to the hospital, I discover that I am also growing more confident in my decision to take control of my birth by avoiding the hospital if I can, while remaining willing to accept its services should I need them.

10

"With Women"

U m, hi, It's Nima. So, um, I think I'm in labor. Can you come over? I don't think I'll have the baby for a while, but maybe you could come soon anyway?"

Nima Eisner is on the phone. She has agreed to let me write about her birth in exchange for my services as a doula. She sounds more lonely than nervous, but I don't want to miss her birth and I am her doula—my job is to support her—so I agree to come over right away, even though she may not be in active labor. I get Richard to take care of Max, make a stop to buy grapes and watermelon, and head over to Nima's place.

Her apartment is small with wall-to-wall carpeting, low ceilings, and toddler toys cluttering the living room. Nima meets me at the door. She has pale brown skin, glasses, and long, kinky black hair twisted into a bun under a white kerchief. A few curls escape by the side of her broad face. As I walk in the door, I am immediately hugged around the legs by her two-year-old son, Kerem. He has a soft floating cloud of curly black hair and coffee-colored skin. He is incredibly cute, despite the fact that he has a bad cold, which has turned his nose into a streaming snot machine. He wears a T-shirt and a diaper. A blow-up pool is inflated in the middle of the room for Nima to labor in, but there is no water in it yet.

Nima is mellow, almost beatific, and smiling. Every ten minutes or so she gets a painful contraction, but they are short and still far apart. She sits curled up on the couch, and with each contraction she'll close her eyes and sway gently to the Lauryn Hill CD that's playing. The music is smooth, rhythmic, insistent, and, at times, intense. Every now and then, Nima will get onto all fours and rock back and forth. She moans gently and doesn't want much attention, saying, "I'm okay," every time I ask her how she's doing. After an hour or so, Nima's husband, Hasan Bradley, arrives home from his job at a local music store. Hasan has a shaved head and the tracing of a beard. He is short, has very black skin, and has a contained energy. He is a musician who used to tour with a well-known ska band. He's also a martial arts expert. At times, he moves around the apartment with a lilt that combines dancing with bobbing and weaving. He is very physical with Kerem, often mock fighting with him. Hasan says he is more anxious with this birth. He's not sure why, maybe because now he knows how much it can hurt. He does seem a little nervous, talking rapidly and sometimes abruptly leaving the room.

We hang out all afternoon, chatting and playing with Kerem. He draws all over my notebook, climbs in my lap, and shows me his toys. The television is on with the sound turned down low—soap operas and kids' shows. Nima tells me about her first birth at a maternity center with midwives in New York City, where they used to live. She says it was disappointing, because there was not enough focus on her. Hasan chimes in, "It was false. They gave one impression at first, and then it was something else entirely. When we got there, the midwife on call was someone we had never met. She wasn't sensitive to our family. She kept saying that Nima should be quiet because she wouldn't be able to hear what the midwife was saying. They broke her water without asking and without even saying what was happening. They said we could wait to cut the cord, but they cut it right away." He shakes his head in disbelief. "So we said, next time, at home."

Nima and Hasan have chosen Anne Healy-Kerr and her partner, Claire Hamilton, to be their midwives. Anne is young, maybe in her late twenties. She has a clean-scrubbed beauty with long, shiny, golden-brown hair, clear skin, an open face with a distinctive aquiline nose, and big, light eyes you can see way into. We got together to talk in the midwives' small, pleasant office.

I ask Anne how she became interested in midwifery. "From the time I was a little girl, I was curious about birth," she says. "That got translated into 'Oh, you want to be an obstetrician,' because that's all that anyone that I grew up around knew about. So I grew up thinking I wanted to be an obstetrician."

Anne earned good grades in high school and went to a prestigious college that had a high success rate of getting people into med school. While she was there, suffering through physics and organic chemistry classes that she hated, she happened to take an anthropology class titled "Sex and Culture," for which she was required to read Suzanne Arms's book *Immaculate Deception*. "When I read that book," Anne says, "something just clicked. I just knew that American birth practices were really bizarre and strange, so her saying that we need to reclaim natural birthing made so much sense. That was the first time I ever heard the word *midwife* in a contemporary context, and I realized that what I really wanted to be was a midwife."

A number of the midwives I've met reported that same sense of "something clicking," of recognizing their calling through a sudden and deep realization. Some found it through experience, but many, like Anne, were introduced to midwifery through books, most often through Ina May Gaskin's powerful work, *Spiritual Midwifery*. I remember Liz Donahue, one of the Skyline Hospital midwives, telling me that she read *Spiritual Midwifery* in high school and decided on her career right then. Gaskin's book is a collection of fascinating birth stories and instructive essays on midwifery that grew out of her work as a midwife in a Tennessee commune known as The Farm. For Gaskin and that community, childbirth is a physiologically normal and spiritually transformative process. *Spiritual Midwifery* was written in the

1970s, so the wonderful photographs of parents and their children tend to feature lots of long hair, and the stories are salted with a groovy, hippie vocabulary (contractions are "rushes," and the birthing parents spend a lot of time "smooching," "making out," and generally getting "tantric"). Despite its dated look, it is a phenomenally timeless book, brimming with vivid and immediate portraits of people and their positive experiences with natural childbirth.

After Anne had her "ah-ha" moment about midwifery, she did an internship at a birthing center in Pittsburgh staffed by certified nurse-midwives, where she says the midwives "were wonderful and were very committed to natural birth and to empowering women. But they had a lot of negative ideas about direct-entry midwives that they passed on to me—that direct-entry midwives learn through correspondence classes, and they sew people up with fishing line, and they will attend triplets, at home, in a bathtub. Things like that that." Anne laughs. "I guess there's some degree of truth to that. There's probably a midwife out there who meets that definition, but it really isn't indicative of direct-entry midwifery in the whole country. So of course, I thought I was going to be a nurse-midwife."

Anne chose the midwifery program at Yale (where my midwife, Sarah, also studied), because it doesn't require a nursing degree and its prestige was in keeping with her academic background. But then, during the next school year, something inspired her to write to Ina May Gaskin and ask if she could visit The Farm for a summer internship.

"I didn't hear from her, and didn't hear, and then, finally, I got a letter back that said, 'Tell me when you're coming.' That's all. Just one line," Anne says. So Anne wrote back, drove to Tennessee, and stayed on The Farm for a summer. "And Ina May, her life and her work, convinced me that *that's* the kind of midwife I wanted to be. It really was an amazing experience. It was a real blessing to be able to go there. There was no going back after that; I couldn't go to Yale after that."

Also, Ina May had pointed out that if Anne did the program at

Yale as a working-class young adult, she was unlikely to get out without at least $60,000 of debt. "I would be forced to work in hospitals to pay that off," Anne says, "because no home-birth practice can pay off that type of debt." So Anne finished her undergraduate degree and moved to a state with licensed midwifery where she could get an apprenticeship. "I had no idea how difficult that would be. I really thought that I could come here, sign up, and someone would take me on as an apprentice." She pauses, then adds, "It was more of a twisting path." She called every midwife in town the day she arrived, and nobody wanted an apprentice. She started studying herbalism, and shortly afterward got pregnant and had her first child at home with a licensed midwife. "After that, the path opened up to me. All of a sudden I had an apprenticeship."

Anne was a single mother at the time. When I ask how she juggled all her responsibilities, she holds her head in her hands briefly, then says, "I was just thinking this morning, how did I ever do all that? I had a list of people who said I could call them in the middle of the night if I got called to a birth, and I would just go down the list at two o'clock in the morning and think 'Which one should I pick?' People were very accommodating, but when I look back, I think if a young woman came to me and said 'I'm a single mom, is it possible to do an apprenticeship?' I wouldn't believe it was possible. Even though for me, it magically worked out." Anne finished her apprenticeship in two years and then became a licensed midwife.

As part of the licensing process, she attended births with every home-birth midwife in town and spent some time observing certified nurse-midwives in the hospital. "That was more traumatic than helpful," she says. "The midwives there were very supportive and accommodating, but it was *so* different from home-birth midwifery." Anne recalls how she would sit in the lounge with the midwives, discussing the patients, "and the moms were just a name on a list, not someone you already knew." When they finished getting updated on the patients' status, they would all go sit at the nurses' station. "For the most part," she says, "you just went into the room when someone wanted to be checked or someone needed medication, and then you'd go in to catch the baby. Now I know why nurse-midwives get called "mini-docs" or "med-wives" or "L.O.B.s for Lay-O.B.s." It was so foreign to the midwifery I knew. I don't consider that midwifery. The word *midwife* comes from *mid wif,* which means 'with woman'; it doesn't mean run in and catch the baby."

Anne is touching on a sore point among midwives—the divisions that exist between nurse-midwives and direct-entry midwives. Anne says that she sees their separate histories as the primary stumbling block to better communication within the profession. "From the point of view of a direct-entry midwife," she explains, "there's a perception that the history of nurse-midwifery comes out of trying to pacify the existing system. Nurse-midwives have worked within the system, so they feel that they have played by the rules and should be rewarded for that, whereas direct-entry midwifery came out of a more radical, 'We're going to do what we want to do, whether or not it's legal.' Mothers saying, 'I know I can birth my baby by myself.' It came out of a very different place of grassroots activism. Direct-entry midwives have consistently refused to follow the rules, whereas nurse-midwives have played by the rules and worked to change the rules when they were not in their favor. And nurse-midwives have made incredible progress both in changing the medical system and in being recognized as a profession. But many people would say that nurse midwives still have to practice in very compromising situations because of the rules. And many of them are not really happy with the restrictions that are placed on their practices."

Liz Donahue at Skyline Hospital once told me something similar. She put it this way: "Physicians are less threatened by midwives who are nurses, because they think they can keep us under their thumbs much easier. This is exactly the political reason why licensed midwives aren't comfortable with nurse-midwifery, because it puts you in a subservient position on some level." She acknowledged the struggles of direct-entry, or licensed, midwives, saying, "Being a licensed midwife is definitely more of a battle than being a certified nurse-midwife."

Anne tells me that her personal experience with certified nurse-midwives has run the gamut. Many obviously enjoy helping her out and are supportive of women's choices. "They really want to help women who are willing to take this radical step in our culture and have their babies at home." But others are more critical of her work. "Some see that they were good girls, that they studied very hard, that they went to school—which was a less than happy experience—that they jumped through all these hoops to get their degree, and that everyone else should, too. Kind of the classic, virgin-whore dichotomy of one woman who is having sex for money and a place to live is a wife and in another situation she's a prostitute. It just depends on whether or not you play by the rules." Anne gives me a mischievous grin, then turns serious again, "Also, because they practice within the medical model, they sometimes practice medicine more than they practice midwifery." She shakes her head. "There is so much tension between those two paradigms."

After a brief pause, Anne chastises herself gently, saying, "But people like me need to stop thinking in terms of those stereotypes I just named. A lot of the certified nurse-midwives are really great women whose hearts are into being there for the mothers, but they can't always do it in that system. People like me need to go out and talk to nurse-midwives and appreciate them for what they have done for women. Again and again, nurse-midwifery care has been shown to be superior to obstetrical care," Anne says. She sighs and carefully tucks her long hair behind her ears. "There's so much animosity between the hospital practitioners and home-birth practitioners, and I'm certainly guilty of divisiveness as much as anybody else. I'd like to see more unity among all midwives. I would like there to come a time when there's one type of midwife."

What's really sad, Anne says, returning to her observations of midwives in the hospital, is that those births were so much better than what a lot of women in obstetrical practices are getting. "The moms come out with these stories," she says, "like, 'Oh my birth was so great. They let me walk around.' And I mean who's in charge here? Look at where the power is in that sentence. '*They let* me use the bathroom.' '*They let* me hold my baby.' But to the women, that was a wonderful birth experience, because in their last one maybe they got cut with no one asking their permission, or they weren't allowed out of bed, or they had to be catheterized, or their baby was taken away immediately. For me, it's hard. I know in one part of my heart that that's progress, but I'm also kind of sickened by how little progress that is, and I'm sad that women put up with it."

The experience of observing hospital births seemed "really fragmented and bizarre" to Anne. "I hate coming across so negatively," she continues, "but so many times when I go to a hospital birth I feel like a passive witness to violence, and its a very hard thing to see. I can't imagine why women would want that." She concedes that the hospital is necessary for some women and thinks we live at the ideal time for giving birth when it comes to having access to technology, should we need it. "But," she emphasizes, "we don't *have* to access it if we don't need it."

As for her own practice, she says she doesn't often have to transport her clients to the hospital, and almost never for an emergency. "Going to the hospital in the event of an emergency," she says, "is just very, very rare." Most of the women in her practice who have to be transported are women who do so for "failure to progress," as excessively slow labors are called. Also, Anne notes, they are usually women who have decided on home birth late in their pregnancies. "The women who have already been in the medical system have a much, much higher transfer rate. Virtually all of our transports are those women." She and her partner tend to transfer first-time moms a little more often, but even that is a lot less likely if they started their care with the midwives. "I think part of that is because we have such incredible rapport with them," Anne says. "They trust us. When we say, 'You can do it,' they believe it. Women who have been in the system where the whole message is 'You might *not* be able to do it' have a much harder time. They have faith in that paradigm of birth. The essential paradigm shift has not happened. They still have faith in that complication-minded belief system, rather than knowing they can trust themselves and that birth is safe and happens on its own. Often they place too much power on us to get the baby out."

When she does have to transport to the hospital, Anne says, "At that point, I tell women that part of being strong is knowing when to ask for help. That's an important lesson for many people, myself included. So if we're going to go into that system, we're going to go in thankfully and graciously, and take what it has to offer." She breaks off, looks at me and cocks her head to the side, and bites her lip for a second. "But it's certainly harder to view birth as empowerment with the transports." And for Anne, that's what midwifery is all about, "having the chance to help women empower themselves and the opportunity to bring babies into the world without violence."

I ask her if she has any theories about why there is such a dichotomy in women's birth choices in the United States. Why is there such a divide between the medical model and home birth, with only a handful of places offering something in the middle of what could be a broad and continuous spectrum of options? And why aren't women pushing for those options? She responds eagerly, clearly invigorated by the opportunity to explore and articulate her ideas about the culture of childbirth. "Ohhhh. It's such a multifaceted problem," she says. "I think what it gets down to is that we live in a culture that represses women's sexuality, and men's as well. We live in a culture that does everything it can to keep women from being sexually powerful, and birth is the climax of women's sexuality. It doesn't get much more powerful than that," she adds. "But from the time we're little girls we're taught to do what we're told. We're taught that doctor knows best, or daddy knows best, or someone else knows best."

Anne brings up the comments of prominent midwifery advocate and former officer of the World Health Organization Dr.

Marsden Wagner, whom we both heard speak recently. "He said that when a woman is birthing in her own space naturally, it is frighteningly powerful to people who live in a culture where we do everything we can to repress that," she recalls. "There is so much truth to his statement. If you take that away from a woman, if you make her believe that her power to give birth is in the hands of someone else, that it's not her power, you've got her for life. She's going to come in every time she's got menstrual cramps, or every time her kid has the sniffles, and you own her power. I don't know what all can be done to help women reclaim that. I'm doing it one family at a time."

⌒

One family Anne is helping is Nima and Hasan's. Back at their apartment, it is now around 5:30 P.M.. Nima's labor still hasn't picked up much. She has been lying around most of the afternoon, so I suggest we take a walk. She gets a contraction and says she doesn't want to go. I shift into assertive doula mode and after the contraction passes, I say, "Now is the time. Let's just go get the mail. It isn't far." So we walk slowly across the lawn of the apartment complex, Nima moving like a ship in weeds. Several times she gets down on her hands and knees right in the grass, moans a bit, then gets up and keeps walking. She has three or four contractions like this on the way to the mailboxes. She's still calm and even laughs a bit. But on the way back, I notice that the contractions are closer together, and she's not smiling anymore.

When we get back, I urge her to go to the toilet. She does, and immediately has a huge contraction. For the first time today, she yells loudly, and Kerem, frightened, suddenly jumps up on my back while I squat next to his mother. I hold him while she has three big, strong contractions very close together. All three make her yell. Clearly, her labor has taken off. She says, "Ughhh. They hurt here."

"Yes, but that's good," I say and ask, "Are you ready to have the baby?"

"Yes."

"Good. Let's do one more on the toilet then. These are good strong contractions, just like you need. Now we're getting somewhere."

After another big, painful contraction, I get a bit nervous that her labor might suddenly be quite far along, and ask if I can call the midwives. Nima just nods. It is 5:55 P.M. when I call Claire Hamilton, Anne's partner who is on first call, and leave a message. I decide to page her. Two minutes later I haven't had any response. I'm too antsy to wait, so I call Anne, who says she'll try Claire again and then come. Claire calls back two minutes later and asks if I think she has time to eat dinner. I hesitate for a moment, and she says, "Never mind, I'll be right over."

I move Nima to the pool, which Hasan has filled with warm water. Her contractions are still hard there, but not quite as intense as they were on the toilet. Still, Nima continues to yell loudly through these contractions. There is a knock on the door. It is a young woman, a neighbor, who has heard Nima and has come to check on her. When she leaves, Hasan says, "Whoah. She lives upstairs, way on the other side of the building." We all laugh, even Nima.

Around 6:15 P.M., both midwives and their apprentice, Leah, arrive. Claire's T-shirt says "Midwives Hold the Future." Anne wears loose beige linen pants, a dusk-blue T-shirt, and silver earrings shaped like goddesses with their arms raised, each one holding a moon. Her honey-colored hair swings loose around her shoulders. They begin to unpack. Claire sets up the oxygen tank while Anne listens with a Doppler and reports that the baby is fine. Kerem is fascinated by the oxygen tank, so to distract him, Anne makes him a balloon out of a rubber glove, draws a face on it, and tosses it to him; to me she jokes, "Bet you didn't know that chicken balloons are the heart of home birth."

As Claire attends to Nima, Anne finishes unloading their equipment and tells me that they have more and more clients who use water in labor or even to birth in. "The water provides really nice counterpressure when the baby is coming out," she says, "and it takes the edge off that burning sensation of crowning. Plus, you're less likely to get a tear in the water. Although," she shrugs, "sometimes a tear is inevitable." One thing they like to do at water births is to encourage the mothers to catch their own babies. "I see far fewer tears when women have their own hands there," Anne says. "With my first baby, I counted on my midwife to provide perineal support and then I tore through my anus. With my second baby, I didn't want anyone touching me. If I was going to tear, I was going to know who was responsible for it. Having my hands there just completed the circuit. I knew not to push too hard, I could feel myself stretching, and I knew how to ease my baby out. Even with first-time moms, I've really seen that they seem to be able to hold that stretch much more patiently and let themselves stretch around the head while they're crowning if they have their hands there. Plus," she adds, lifting her head high and grinning, "there's nothing more empowering than catching your own baby."

Suddenly, Nima gets a contraction and yells so loud my ears chime. She squeals and moans. We all move in closer. Anne asks if she's peeing in the tub. She doesn't think so, so Anne suggests a trip to the toilet. But right then another really intense contraction comes, followed right away by another one. Hasan is holding her left hand, the midwives are facing her, and I have somehow ended up with one hand wedged between Nima's back and the side of the pool and the other one holding her right hand. My wedged hand is starting to get pins and needles, so I slowly try to pull it out. Nima barks, "Whoever that is, don't you move that hand. I need it." I stay right where I am.

With the next contraction, Nima closes her eyes and grunts. I realize she is probably pushing, and I must have been the last to notice, because I now see that the midwives have rubber gloves on. A moment later, the baby is being born into the water. I crane my head around Nima's shoulder and catch a glimpse of his head and body squeezing out. The umbilical cord is wrapped twice around the neck and once around the shoulder. As the body emerges, Anne loops some cord off with one hand and rolls the baby over and over to untangle him, lifting him out of the water at the same time. It is just after 7 P.M., about an hour and a half after Nima's contractions finally got really hard, and a little less than an hour since the midwives arrived.

Within a minute the baby is crying. It's a boy. He lies on Nima's breast as Hasan rubs the baby's feet at Claire's suggestion. The baby wiggles his fingers. He opens and closes his eyes, then slowly opens them again. "She did it!" says Hasan and sings a little song to himself. Nima is smiling and stroking the baby. "It was shorter than with Kerem," she says. "I am so glad it's over. It's over. That wasn't so bad. Ah. It's over." She scoots the baby up closer to her face and says, "Look at his eyes—so big!" Around fifteen minutes after the birth, the cord is cut. Ten minutes after that, the baby latches on to Nima's breast and nurses. Nima bleeds a little with the birth of the placenta, and Anne says, "I want to keep an eye on that bleeding," so Nima gets out of the pool and into bed.

The midwives estimate that Nima passed close to 500 ccs of blood. "It doesn't overly concern us yet," says Anne. Nima's belly is firm and her uterus feels small, but she is still bleeding a bit. "Maybe we're missing something," says Anne, looking a bit concerned. They massage her belly to keep the uterus contracting, at which Nima lets out a large "Ow!" Then they urge her to pee, which she does. Claire checks her for tears and wipes her with a clean, warm cloth. Nima, the midwives, and the two children are all on the couple's large air mattress, and every time somebody moves, everybody else moves up and down; it is like being on a bobbing raft.

"Your bleeding is minimal now, and you are completely intact," Claire says. "It doesn't even look like you had a baby! Plus, that is the best postpartum pelvic tone I've ever seen!" Nima grins and says, "My mom taught me to do Kegels when I was a kid so I would never be incontinent. Maybe they're paying off now." Kegel exercises (named after Dr. Arnold Kegel, who popularized them) involve squeezing and releasing the muscle that surrounds the birth canal, the same squeezing motion you use to stop the flow of urine. Women with good muscle tone around the vagina tend to suffer less damage to it during childbirth, less incontinence afterward, and are more likely to feel pleasure during intercourse.

Kerem gets in the bed and cuddles into Nima while the baby nurses. Hasan sits next to them and says, "This time was so much better than the first. First, with the prenatals, we always got all our questions answered. They listened to us, and they respected our choices. Now, with the birth, it was no stress. No hassle." He beams, nods, and says, "Home birth. This is the way to do it." Nima says, "It was so nice without the math. The first time, there was so much math, so many numbers. Check the baby's heartrate, check the dilation, check the length of the contraction. Figure out how many hours left by how many centimeters still to go. This time was so much nicer."

I ask Claire if they even checked her cervix, since I don't remember them doing it. Claire says, "We both tried, but she didn't really give us a chance, and that's okay with us. I mean, why check her cervix? We could hear the baby was fine, we could see she was contracting. Some people do it just because they feel they have to do something." Anne adds, "Yeah, the baby will come whether we check or not, and most moms hate being checked." Laughing, she says, "Imagine if you did all that checking for a mother cat giving birth. She'd kill you!"

Anne says that her job as a midwife is to have complete confidence in the woman's ability to give birth and to instill and reinforce that confidence in her. "Because I can't have her baby for her," she says. "I wish I could—I'm good at having babies, you know. I wouldn't mind taking a turn every once in a while. But all I can really do is believe in her and tell her, 'Your body knew how to grow the baby, your body knows how to get the baby out.' The medical model is based on the belief that 'your body might not really know how to grow the baby, let's check. And your body probably will do all right during labor, but let's check you and monitor you the whole time anyway just in case your body kills your baby.'"

At 9 P.M., Nima passes another clot. Anne gives her some

shepherd's purse, an oxytocic herb, to help keep the uterus clamped and stop the clotting. Nima pees again, then gets back into bed saying, "Come here, pumpkin," to the baby, and nurses again. At 9:30, there is yet another big clot, and Nima reports that she feels a little dizzy. Claire and Anne are paying close attention. They look concerned. After giving her a whiff of oxygen and a vigorous massage, the midwives discuss whether to administer methergine or Pitocin. They choose methergine, a tablet and a shot, and Anne sets up an IV "just in case," as she says to me. She tells Nima that if this doesn't clear up in a few minutes she's going to have to call the ambulance. To her apprentice she says, "Be ready to call 911," and gives her the address where we are. Anne asks me to keep talking to Nima to make sure she's "really here." I hold Nima's hand and talk to her about baby names. She's still feeling a bit faint, so the midwives go ahead and give her the IV with fluids and now some Pitocin and continue massaging her belly.

In a few minutes, Nima is noticeably more alert and says she feels fine now. Her bleeding has stopped, and everybody seems a little calmer. Any crisis has been averted. But the midwives stay for quite some time after, longer than usual, to keep an eye on her. The Pitocin seems to have done its job; she doesn't bleed any more in the next two hours. Anne estimates that altogether Nima lost close to 1,000 ccs of blood. At the midwives' request, I go out to buy some iron pills at a nearby pharmacy and bring them back.

This was my second home birth with a slightly scary moment. I am nervous about hemorrhaging myself. But once again, I saw the situation handled professionally and prudently. The midwives were ready to transfer if they had to, but they were able to employ the same resources the hospital would have in the same situation—oxygen, fundal massage, an IV, and Pitocin. I am enormously reassured by the midwives' actions. I recall Seattle midwife Heike Doyle, who usually attends births at home or at a birth center, telling me of the first time she attended a birth at a hospital with a doctor observing. She said, "For about 15 years, the physicians had seen us bring our transfers in, and they had seen that we made appropriate consultations and appropriate transfers. The first birth I actually did at the hospital ended up with shoulder dystocia (where the shoulder gets stuck coming out), a frayed cord, and hemorrhage. We turned the mother on her hands and knees so the dystocia was handled quite easily, and we managed the other problems as well. The doctor watching was blown away. He said, 'You really know what you're doing!' And he was so interested in our techniques. He asked us, well, what do you do for this or that, other birth issues. It was gratifying to have our skills acknowledged."

As Anne packs to leave, she tells me that she's been to two births in the last few days and is feeling worn out. "I'm so tired, and I haven't seen my family in so long," she says. "To me, the challenges of being a midwife are having time for the other important relationships in my life. Many times I feel really compromised and I'm not able to give my children what they really need because I have to give to my clients." She pauses, then says, "The other challenge is the challenge of being an activist all the time. The challenge of bucking the system by your very existence and the challenge of knowing a truth that the culture doesn't recognize."

I ask Anne why this is so. As she loads her bag into the back of her car, with its bumper stickers that read "Birth at Home Naturally" and "Peace on Earth Begins with Birth: Support a Midwife," she shakes her head and says, "We're up against this huge machine that is promoting the medical model of birth. I would like to see all women who are even considering having children have access to true and accurate information about their choices. I would like to see all the choices presented truthfully as legitimate options for women."

PART FOUR

Third Trimester

Reaching the Summit:
A Birth Center Fights for Families

Over the past few months, whenever I have mentioned how frustrated I am at women's lack of birthing options (Why is there no birth center in my city? Why don't home-birth midwives have better hospital backup? Why won't insurance companies cover home birth? Etc., etc.), someone has said to me, "You should go visit Elizabeth Gilmore's birth center in Taos. They offer home birth, birth-center birth, and doctor-attended hospital birth all in the same practice." They usually add something like, "She's amazing."

Elizabeth Gilmore is, indeed, rare among midwives. In a reversal of the usual hierarchy wherein a group of doctors might decide to hire some midwives (to please their patients and save the practice money), Gilmore runs a midwifery practice that decided to hire some doctors (to care for patients who need them or who feel more comfortable with them, to provide backup, and to protect the midwives' social and legal standing). The doctors Gilmore hired are Board-certified obstetricians who are unusually committed to the midwifery model of care. A husband and wife team, the new doctors had one of their own children with the direct-entry midwives on The Farm in Tennessee (the setting for Ina May Gaskin's *Spiritual Midwifery*), and the other at home.

In shaking up the usual dynamic of medical care, the Northern New Mexico Women's Health and Birth Center has fundamentally altered standard maternal health services, offering families an exceptionally wide range of woman-centered care. They now help deliver two-thirds of the babies born in Taos County.

So in my eighth month of pregnancy, reduced to wearing only long, floppy dresses that hide both my enormous belly and the tops of my unsightly knee socks (maternity tights are either strangulating or have to be yanked up every few minutes), I drive several hours to Taos, New Mexico. The town lies at the foot of the Sangre de Cristo Mountains. It is made up of a mix of Native Americans, Hispanic families who have lived here for generations since before this was part of the United States, Anglo hippies, tourists who come for the stunning scenery and excellent skiing, restaurant owners and workers, artists, and others. I have an enormous fondness for this place. I worked here one summer as a seventeen-year-old from the overcast snowbelt of rural New York and was immediately (and forever) dazzled by the southwestern landscape. When I arrive today, it is cold, and although it is early spring, winter hovers in the wings, ready for a comeback. The sky is a swirling, slate-colored sea of clouds. Tufts of white mist creep down the face of the pine-covered mountains. It is snowing at the higher elevations, and the hazy foothills look like a scene from a Chinese painting. The valley floor is pale brown and dusty green-gray with sage. My feet are cold as I get out of the car at a gas station to ask for directions.

The pumps are crowded with Mercedes Benz SUVs and other fancy tanks. No doubt they belong either to Los Angeles folks in town for the annual film festival or to some of Taos's wealthy landowners who have come to live in what is, nonetheless, still one of the poorest regions of the nation. A few beat-up compact cars and pick-ups signal the presence of locals. Inside the gas station, just beyond the prewrapped burritos, decorative covers for cell phones are for sale next to little green foam boxes containing "One Dozen Canadian Night Crawlers by Bait Master." I ask for directions to the birth center. The guy behind the counter just shrugs, but two people in line start talking at the same time, telling me the way.

The birth center is perfectly located next door to the hospital and on the edge of an open field with spectacular views of Taos Mountain. It is big, new, and beautiful. A long, covered *portal* in front leads into a central waiting room between the midwives' wing and the doctors' wing. The hallways are painted just the right shade of warm, buttery yellow, and the walls are hung with huge bulletin boards blanketed by a papery patchwork of dozens and dozens of snapshots of new babies and mothers. Behind the receptionist's desk, a collection of thank you notes from new mothers surround a sticker that reads, "Women of Earth, Take Back Your Birth."

Elizabeth Gilmore comes out to meet me. She is middle-aged with shoulder-length, graying, wavy blonde hair pulled back on the sides by little combs. She wears a white blouse, a wide navy blue skirt, a tooled-leather belt with a horse on the buckle, and short, brown lace-up granny boots with white ankle-high lace-topped socks. I've seen her a half-dozen times this year, and she's always wearing an almost identical outfit. It looks very 1980s, which I suspect was probably the last time she bothered to up-date her wardrobe. She has better things to do: working as a midwife, administrating a busy birth center, running a college for student midwives, lobbying local politicians on maternal and child health issues, campaigning to get businesses to support family-friendly practices, and making time for her own family. Now, she graciously takes time out to show me around the birth center.

⌢

The practice just moved into this new building recently; before they were located in a little place called the Birth Cottage. "I've been in town for a long time," says Elizabeth as we walk down a hallway, "and I've been at births helping mothers with their deliveries here since 1977." We step into a gracious, high-ceilinged, combination kitchen/living room. The kitchen area has pale wooden cabinets and sand-colored tile on the floor; the living room walls are hung with a collection of large, clay pieces in the shape of a woman and a baby who flies a kite on its umbilical cord. A small note says the art was made by Elizabeth. Through a pair of wooden doors are two separate birthing rooms, each with their own bathroom. The birthing rooms have a homey atmosphere—windows with gingham curtains, a double bed with a headboard carved with flowers, bedside lamps, a rocking chair, a birthing stool, and framed prints of Southwest and Native American scenes. Tiled into a corner of the room is an enormous, deep, oval bathtub.

The center cost more than $800,000, and it shows. When I ask how she afforded it, Elizabeth says that they still owe a lot of money, but they've managed to raise funds from foundations and individuals. She's delivered so many babies over the twenty-some years she's been here that she knows a lot of people in town; at a single fund-raising lunch they raised more than $100,000. Still, she adds, "I would never have done the new birth center, except that these new doctors told me they wouldn't come unless I did it."

Elizabeth tells me that the impetus for getting the doctors on board, after years of practicing without them, was that there was a very hostile obstetrician in town. "I was concerned," she says, "because the C-section rate was between 35 and 54 percent in town, our low-birth-weight rate was very high, and when we had to send people to his practice, sometimes he would pay very little attention to them." She tells of one client who was diagnosed with placenta previa, a condition where the placenta lies close to, or covering, the entrance of the cervix. This obstetrician scheduled her for a C-section, even though she had many weeks to go in her pregnancy and placentas have been known to migrate. The woman decided to get a second opinion by going to another city, and that doctor was willing to wait until closer to her due date to decide whether she needed a C-section. The placenta shifted, and she delivered vaginally.

Elizabeth says this is just one of many examples she could give. "I was concerned that we weren't getting good enough care," she says, "and that our mothers and babies were in jeopardy in this community. His priorities seemed to be elsewhere." She pauses. "And he hated us," she says. "He absolutely hated us. He told me he was going to take my license, shut down my center, buy it, call it Doc's Gun Shop, and I would be working for him." I raise my eyebrows, and Elizabeth nods and grimaces. "Every time we did a birth, he felt it was money out of his pocket. He did handle some emergencies rather nicely; he wasn't a completely destructive person. But he wasn't proactively *for* women and children."

Just as things with the local obstetrician were getting difficult, Elizabeth says, "As if by universal design, three sets of doctors came looking to work here. *They* approached *me*. I never had to approach them. And one of the sets of doctors was Heidi Rinehart and Rudy Fedrizzi, who came to be with us."

Elizabeth takes me over to the doctors' wing and introduces me to them. Dr. Fedrizzi is a balding man with glasses dressed in a colorful sweater. Dr. Rinehart is a slim, petite woman. I ask if the doctors attend births at both the center and the hospital. She tells me yes, and although they do see more clients at the hospital, she always encourages moms to consider the birth center, saying, "It has so many advantages: intimacy, flexibility, privacy, and the woman is the center of what is happening—not the staff, not the equipment, not the routine—the woman. Also, we have some women who live far from the hospital, and if something did come up in their labor, it would be hard to reach the hospital from home."

When I ask if she encourages home birth as well, she says, "Absolutely. Statistics show that both birth-center births and home births are safe, and probably safer, for women who are healthy and having healthy pregnancies. But you need to have a feeling of safety and security, privacy and support. And different people will define that safety and security differently. I had one child at a birth center where hundreds and hundreds of women had given birth naturally. It gave me confidence. I had my other child at home. With me, what made me feel safe was feeling like

I didn't have to worry about behaving properly. I wasn't going to be judged for being too loud, I was going to have continuous support and encouragement, and I wasn't going to have technology pushed on me that I didn't need. But," she adds, "we feel very strongly that the safest place for healthy woman to give birth is the place she feels the safest."

Dr. Rinehart explains that some women aren't confident that they can give birth without pain medication or that their bodies can give birth safely, and they feel safer in the hospital. "They have a belief that the staff, or facilities, or the equipment will help them," she says. "And if they believe it, it can be true for them. But in a healthy woman, medical technology does not improve on her physiology, and those medical technologies can introduce side effects and risks of their own." Still, she says, there are situations when a woman is not healthy or has complications that make the hospital safer. "Then, I think the most important thing is to have a doula. She doesn't take the place of a partner or husband; she is additional support who is calm, confident, and loving throughout the labor."

I ask Dr. Rinehart if there's anything else she wants to comment on. She pauses then, looking a little impish, says, "At the birth center they do the laundry. At home it was nice not to have to go anywhere, but the laundry was a pain!"

⌒

Elizabeth takes me down the hall to see her next client of the day. In the clinic rooms, the exam tables are not the usual, narrow metal and vinyl items, but custom-built, adjustable, wooden beds. Over this bed hangs a handmade mobile made of twigs fabric hearts, moons, and stars. Elizabeth washes her hands and introduces me to one of her students, Callie, who will be joining us, and her client, Mimi.

Mimi is in her mid-thirties and is a curator at a local museum. She is wearing black leggings, black boots, a lime-green sweater, and cat-eye glasses. Her mother is visiting from New York City and has joined her for this appointment. Elizabeth shows Mimi how to use the calendar wheel to figure out her due date and how far along she is. Together, they look at a book of week-by-week, life-size pictures of a baby in a womb. Mimi is sixteen weeks pregnant and pores over the picture of a sixteen-week-old fetus. Elizabeth pulls out a homemade doll that lies swathed in netting (meant to represent the amniotic sac, or bag of waters) and a knitted, wool uterus complete with cervix. "That's where the contractions are," Elizabeth says, pointing, "and they really hurt."

Elizabeth hands Mimi her chart, an unusual gesture in a medical office in the United States, where charts are often closely controlled by doctors and can, thus, become a symbol for their control of the patient's body. Elizabeth's act is a deliberate part of this practice's efforts to put control of women's bodies back in women's hands. In Europe, many practices have their clients keep their own charts.

Now, Elizabeth asks if anyone explained why and how they take blood pressure readings. Mimi says yes, they did that the last time. Elizabeth takes her blood pressure and says, "If your husband comes the next time, he can do this part." Next comes the urine test, which clients at the birth center do themselves using a little paper testing strip. When Mimi goes to the bathroom to do this, Elizabeth tells me, "We try to get them to do as much as possible so they have an actual grasp of how they're doing. The more moms and their partners and families participate, the easier it is for them to take good care of themselves."

While Mimi is out of the room, I look around at the birth art covering the walls. One large color photo shows a woman who has just given birth. Her long, blond hair is piled loosely on her head and she stands naked in a pool of water, emerging like Venus from the waves, her baby, all pink, cradled in her arms, still joined by the umbilical cord, which loops and twines up the mother's body. There are three images of Native American women and their babies and a bright picture, painted by Elizabeth, that shows a birthing woman attended by a midwife and two angels. A poster full of women's faces reads, "Many Strong and Beautiful Women."

I comment on what a welcoming atmosphere this is. It feels homey, but, I point out, like a rather wealthy person's home. Everything is so clean, pretty, and artfully chosen. Elizabeth nods proudly, and tells me she wants women to feel good here. "What I'd like us to do is start treating mothers as if they were as valuable as an expensive Arabian mare. As if every mother were worth at least $500,000, and her foal was going to be worth $700,000. Do you know how they treat an Arabian mare? She's worth a lot of money. She gets fed special food, and she gets washed, groomed, and massaged every day. She's taken swimming every day, and if they're on the road, she has a special swimming tank." I must look incredulous, because Elizabeth says, "I'm not kidding you. And when their foals are born, boy those little foals are kept right with their mothers. They're allowed to do anything. They're petted, gentled, and loved. Tons of money is spent, and nobody bats an eye. Horses are great examples because they produce nothing. You can't even eat them; they are a purely luxury item. But we don't treat women and children as if they're worth one penny," a little anger creeps into Elizabeth's normally cheerful voice.

"So often," she says, "I think there's a part of our society that doesn't like mothers and babies. They're a pain in the neck. The kids are crying. They're messy and noisy. Kids get sick. It's not nice and neat. They disrupt the workplace." She ticks off each item on her fingers. "In Taos, between 52 and 54 percent of our mothers are single mothers who are really isolated and have to do everything themselves. And if they're getting state assistance, they are even more despised. People ask, 'Why are we paying her to have more babies?'" Elizabeth shakes her head. "Mothers can't get abortions because it goes against God, but if they have babies, it goes against society. So they are put into a corner and told to shut up and deal with it themselves, because nobody else wants to, and I don't think it's right." She pauses, "That may be an exaggeration," she concedes, "but it has enough elements of what's really happening."

When Mimi returns from the bathroom, Elizabeth says, "Now

climb up here," patting the bed, "and we'll see if we can hear the baby and measure to the top of your uterus." She pulls out a soft tape measure and says, "It measures about 15½ centimeters. Can't get better than that, since we're looking for about a centimeter per week of pregnancy."

Callie, the student midwife, puts the Doppler on Mimi's small belly. At first she doesn't hear anything but static, and in the crackling silence Mimi asks in a small voice, "Is there a possibility the baby isn't alive?"

"Well, it is possible," Elizabeth says gently, "but not probable. Usually that would cause bleeding or fever." Suddenly the Doppler crackles and throbs with the sound of the baby's furiously pumping heart. Everybody smiles, and Mimi's mother digs in her purse for a tissue to wipe away her tears. As Mimi sits up, Callie gives her a big hug, congratulates her, and invites her to join a creative mom's group the center sponsors. I feel a twinge of jealousy. I want to join their cool club.

"Let me show you the results of your bloodwork," Elizabeth says. Then, going through the chart, asks, "Have you ever been pregnant before?"

Mimi says "Ummm. I had an abortion, so I guess, yes. But no children."

Elizabeth nods and asks, "Any complications? Didn't need a transfusion?"

Mimi says no, and Elizabeth continues down the list she's reading, "Have you ever been hospitalized?" No. "It says here you didn't want the AFP." Mimi shakes her head no. "Okay, declined."

Mimi complains about some achiness. Elizabeth gestures for her student to answer this question. Callie says they recommend calcium-magnesium, but not to take it with the prenatal vitamins because the iron will make a soap with the calcium, and then you just pass it. She tells Mimi that calcium-rich foods include spinach, broccoli, chlorophyll, tahini, and almonds.

Elizabeth spends the next few minutes chatting with Mimi, explaining that her feelings of sexuality may be decreased in the beginning and that this is quite normal. She tells Mimi that she may experience worries and fears, saying, "The truth is, it is best to talk about your fears. It helps them to go away, otherwise you may also feel lonely." As Elizabeth wraps up the visit by telling her to make an appointment for four weeks from now, Mimi's mother smiles and says, "Oh, you are so lucky. It is so much nicer than when I had mine."

Elizabeth's next client is thirty-four weeks pregnant, as am I. Because our due dates are so close, I really connect with this exam. Monica, the client, is twenty-three years old and wears black, corduroy overalls and a black-and-white striped T-shirt. Elizabeth shows her the calendar wheel and calculates that the baby probably weighs around four pounds now. She shows her how long the baby is with a tape measure. Then, out comes the book of babies week-by-week. The thirty-four-week baby looks so big to me. I notice that Monica and I are both stroking our bellies as we gaze at the picture.

Monica and Elizabeth take turns listening to the baby with a special, oversized stethoscope called a fetascope. In keeping with their commitment to a minimal use of technology, the midwives in this practice don't always use the fetascope's modern cousin, the electronic Doppler. There are some lingering concerns about the long-term effects of exposure to the ultrasound waves it uses, but also the fetascope keeps the midwives in a more direct and quiet contact with the mother, one of the hallmarks of this practice. Elizabeth says, "Little baby sounds wonderful. Heart around 150 beats per minute."

Elizabeth runs down a list of questions: "Religion?" Catholic. "How many hours a week do you work?" Twenty hours as an administrative assistant. "Any problems with sexuality?" No. "How's your back?" Sore after sitting for a while. "What do you do for it?" Stretch, get rubbed. "Constipated? Diarrhea?" Borderline constipated, but she's trying to drink more water. "Have you ever had herpes?" No. "Will you have this baby at home or at the center?"

Monica pauses, purses her lips for a few seconds, then says, "Well, I was going to do the hospital, but last week I got to see the rooms at the birth center. They're so nice. Now I think I want to do it here."

"Whatever feels best for you," Elizabeth says. "If you choose the center, the midwives will be there for you. We will make suggestions and tell you the truth—even if you have an emergency. Say the baby's heartrate is going down. We'll tell you what is happening. And if we think you should go to the hospital, we'll say so and then ask if that's okay. With us, you can be very direct. Sometimes being too polite can slow things down. With us you can walk, wear your own clothes, go outside, get in the bath, move around. Birth-center births have been shown to be safe.[1] But the choice needs to be yours."

Monica nods and says, "I want to do it here, if I can."

As Callie does the physical exam, Elizabeth turns to me and says, "We try to get people to look at the birth center, look at the hospital, and consider their home, and have them think about where are they going to feel—in their heart—the best. We hesitate to encourage anyone to give birth in a place that doesn't instinctively come to them."

I ask if most of the clients get home birth presented to them as an option and comment that even the suggestion alone, coming from a health professional, seems to help normalize home birth as an option. Elizabeth looks almost surprised and says, "Oh yes, everybody gets told about it. I just take it for granted. Of course you get to have your baby at home, or at the center, or hospital. And I will point out to you the statistics that show that if you have a home birth, you have the home court advantage and you're likely to have fewer problems. So if you're one of those people who is comfortable at home, you should definitely stay home if there's any way to pull it off. Although, people who go for home birth usually do so from an emotional point of view. They don't usually say, 'Oh, well I know it is safer, so I'm going to stay home.' They usually say, 'I want to have my baby at home!'" Elizabeth pounds her hand on her thigh, mimicking their enthusiasm, and laughs.

After writing in Monica's chart for a moment, Elizabeth turns back to her and talks briefly about the psychological side of labor and birth, telling her, "We encourage people to start thinking positively about the birth at this point. See the baby coming out. See it coming up to your chest after it is born. We find this can really help. Sometimes people find themselves crying, isolated, and cranky at this point in their pregnancies. We suggest you talk about your feelings and your ideas about birth, not just think positive. Allow yourself to ask, even, are you and the baby going to live? To be all right? Nobody knows for sure, and everybody worries about this. We, the midwives, are your advisors. Call if you're worrying about anything, even if it is just a feeling. Call if you have bleeding but also just if you're worried. Don't be shy." Monica nods and says okay.

Elizabeth reminds Monica that she should be doing fetal kick counts to monitor the baby's activity. She tells her to do them after dinner for about an hour for several days. If there is some change, she is to call the center. I am plunged into fear, as I haven't felt my own baby move all day, and yesterday I barely got any kicks after dinner. Throughout my pregnancy, this baby has been so much quieter than the first. Maybe because I know more about the fragility of babies now, I often worry that this quietness is a sign of trouble. I resolve to call my midwife as soon as I return home, and in fact, I end up going in to the hospital the next week to do a nonstress test, which confirms that my baby is fine. Why I don't just ask Elizabeth to listen to my baby now to give me some reassurance, I don't know.

Monica tells Elizabeth she has some trouble with congestion, and I listen carefully for the response because I, too, have a horrible stuffy, runny nose. In fact, I have a sinus infection, which I'll manage to hang on to for a month. It makes me feel cruddy all the time, thickens the usual fog of pregnancy into an impenetrable barrier, and ends up defining much of my late pregnancy. My midwife Sarah suggested a number of things, including certain over-the-counter drugs and a concoction of honey, lemon, and pepper, which, with a powerful whiff, does help clear my passages temporarily. Now, Elizabeth recommends a little steamer you can buy at the herb store. "You can put echinacea and golden seal in it," she says, "or you can use a hot compress on the cheeks with grated ginger in the water. Make sure to drink lots of water before bed, too."

As Monica gets ready to go, Elizabeth reminds her to draw a map to her house on the back of the chart "So we can come see you after the baby's born." They say good-bye and Elizabeth heads down the hall to pick up the next client's chart. At the front desk, she quickly fills out some paperwork for a lab test, picks up an HIV test form for a client, then returns to tidy up the exam room. Before her next appointment arrives, she takes a phone call in her office. It is from a woman who gave birth recently and is calling to thank Elizabeth for her help. Elizabeth chats animatedly for a few minutes.

When she gets off the phone, she says, "You know, the greatest joy about being a midwife is getting to be with people when they realize how strong and wonderful they really are. I guess you could say it is mothering the joy that mothers get. When people feel competent and confident, they take good care of themselves and their families." Elizabeth speaks with passion and conviction when she adds, "I've been given the gift of being able to truly enjoy the strength and happiness of others. And I know that that is what heals the world."

She pauses for a moment, then says, "About that sense of competence . . . I think that's one problem with the overuse of epidurals, that by numbing women in childbirth, they don't have the opportunity to grow in their self-confidence. They think they are wussies, that they aren't able to deal with the pain. What they don't realize is that they probably could. Of course, there are times when the pain is abnormal, and we really do need to give women pain relief. It's not across the board that we shouldn't be doing these things. What we're talking about is using technology judiciously, in a way that enhances health rather than in a way that detracts from health."

The phone rings again. This time it is the front desk getting back to her on a question she'd had about a client's insurance situation. Hanging up, she groans and says, "The challenges of this profession are that I'm not really a businesswoman. I have great vision, and on some levels I have great leadership ability, but I am *not* a businesswoman." She shakes her head. "I don't really have a lot of savvy about things like billing and managing an organization. So the challenge has been to find people to help me who do have those skills and then give them the authority to work and to help me. I have been fortunate in getting good people."

I'm surprised to hear that she thinks of the business aspects as her greatest challenge and not the battles she's had with doctors who wanted to shut her down. I suggest that they might be more of a challenge, and she laughs and says, "Oh, I consider those to be minor challenges." It's time for the next appointment, so we head back to the exam rooms.

The next prenatal exam is for Arianne, a beautiful, stylish woman in her late thirties with curly, blonde, slightly dreadlocked hair. She wears a long, brown sheepskin coat, chocolate-colored velvet pants, and some hip-looking jewelry. Arianne is thirty weeks pregnant and planning a home birth. When Elizabeth comments on how fit she looks, she says, "I'm a textile designer, and I get a lot of exercise loading and unloading my truck. Plus, I work in my garden, and I walk three or four miles a day." I feel like a slug. I'm lucky if I can haul my body across the pool twice, and sometimes I'll actually walk to the curb to get my paper, but most days I'll make my son, Max, do it. I resolve to go for a hike later this afternoon. If I'm not napping.

Elizabeth explains what blood pressure is and how it is measured as she takes Arianne's, which is fabulously low. Arianne says, "Thanks for that explanation; nobody ever put it quite like that before. I sure appreciate how informative you all are." Arianne compares the diet chart she's been keeping on herself with the ideal the center has printed up. She needs to drink more water, eat more protein, and should cut down on sugary foods. Callie says it's too bad it's still a little early in the season for good watermelons, because they can provide lots of water and vitamin

C and can satisfy sugar cravings without giving you the fat most sugary foods have. Arianne complains of some digestive tightness, saying, "Sometimes I feel like I'm having a backward fart." Elizabeth chuckles and tells her she could try taking chlorophyll; one tablespoon three times a day can sometimes help keep you clear.

Arianne is in the creative moms group Callie mentioned earlier, and now she tells Elizabeth how great it is. "I have a friend who wants to henna my belly. Wouldn't that be neat?" she says. She seems very happy and is all smiles. She tells Elizabeth and Callie that she thinks she's going to go into labor early, before her due date. Elizabeth says, "Yes, hmmm, well, we're ready," laughing softly. Then she tells Arianne that she would really like to paint a picture of her in her garden while she's still pregnant, so Arianne draws her a map to her house. Elizabeth and Callie both hug and kiss Arianne good-bye.

⌒

After cleaning up the room again, Elizabeth goes down the hall to throw a load of laundry in the washing machine and ducks into her cluttered office. Behind her desk is a sign that reads, "Pregnancy Is Safe, Let's Make It Special." We sit for a few minutes, and I tell Elizabeth that in the course of my research for this book I have often found myself angry and at times depressed at the way women are treated in labor and birth in this country and at the political and social obstacles to improving the situation. At times, it has been hard to remain hopeful. Here she is, struggling for year after year, and yet she seems to have an exceptionally positive attitude. How does she do it?

"Well, I grew up in Mexico City," Elizabeth says. "There, I saw many children die of polio, diphtheria, and tetanus. My mother almost died of tetanus, my little brother had polio, and my mother had to take care of him around the clock. So I saw that life is very short, and that has been a tremendous gift for me; it has made me really strong and passionate. It made me see that one person can make a difference. For instance, when you love somebody and you tell them, it makes a difference. People are going to suffer anyway in life, all of us. And for me, when I'm able to tell somebody that I'm sad, or I'm able to share somebody else's pain, well you know what, I understand, and I feel a little better. It's that simple."

Elizabeth often speaks in a high, almost girlish voice that belies her strength and determination, but the more she talks, the more commanding her voice becomes. Now, her tone has modulated to a more serious register. She says, "I've noticed about myself that it's not so much that I'm skilled or whatever; I'm just willing to be there. And that's true for the political work, too. Because I come from Mexico I'm very, very, very patient. It's the land of mañana, and that's true here, too. I don't freak out because something didn't happen instantly. I am extremely patient, and I'm persistent. I know I probably have more persistence than somebody who opposes me, and I've had plenty of people oppose me. There have been times when I, or my practice, have been reported because the medical community felt that we didn't handle something correctly. And I've thought, well, conceivably, they could close us down, if the state agrees with them. They could take away our license. But the state *didn't* agree with them," she says brightly, "and so our license *didn't* get taken away." She sounds victorious and raises her arms lightly in the air.

"Usually, people who are blocking efforts don't have as much energy as I have," she says. I believe it; following Elizabeth around proves to be challenging work. "So instead of getting uptight about, oh my God this person's going to block my effort, I just persist," she says. "I know what I'm doing is right, and I love what I do. I love the women and families I work with. So I do the things I know are going to make a difference. I do see myself as an activist, but not in the classical sense of 'This is wrong, so we've got to fix it,'" she shakes her fist and speaks loudly. "I'm more of an activist who says, 'This is right, so let's do more of this.' You get further if you focus on things you know will work. And I'm willing to take even very small steps. I figure if I'm still alive it's a total triumph," she laughs. "With each breath I have another opportunity and nothing is stuck. Like I said, they're going to have to kill me to stop me, and by then I'll have gotten everything done anyway." Her energy, enthusiasm, and faith are enormously contagious. We both smile broadly as she finishes this little speech, sitting in the middle of the birthing center she helped create, looking out at the site where she plans to build a "labor garden" for the mothers she loves.

Before I leave, I ask Elizabeth about her goals as a midwife, and she responds, "I want Taos to be known as the best place to have a baby and raise a family." From what I've seen here, it is easy to imagine that Elizabeth doesn't have far to go. But she tells me that there is still so much work to be done. For instance, even though the Birth Center's C-section rate is down around 15 percent, it is still up near 35 percent for the town, and the low-birth-weight rate is still quite high. When I ask why we should care about these statistics, Elizabeth shoots back at me, "A C-section mom is twice as likely to die, and low-birth-weight babies have a much, much higher death rate in the first year." In fact, low-birth-weight is the single factor most closely associated with infant death, and some sources find that the maternal death rate is at least four times higher with a caesarean.[2]

In order to make birth safer for her community, Elizabeth is looking at standards required by a number of national and international organizations, including the Coalition for the Improving of Maternity Services, the Safe Motherhood Initiative of the World Health Organization, and the Baby Friendly Hospitals standards set by UNICEF. "We are a small enough town that we can work to make Taos a safer place," she says, "and we realized that most of the things that are required have to do with a cultural shift from the norm where you try to engage in what is known as 'outcome-based practices' rather than continue with what is known as 'the standard of care.'"

Elizabeth explains, "If somebody's going to sue me and I don't have a fetal-monitor tracing, they'll say I wasn't up to the standard of care, even though fetal monitors have not been proven to help mothers and babies. Reliance on fetal monitors may even cause

C-sections, because a lot of people don't really know how to interpret the tracings in concert with the actual clinical findings of what's going on with the mother and baby. Sometimes people just go to the fetal monitor, and if it looks bad, then it's time to have a C-section."

Another habitual practice that is cultural, and not based on the best outcomes, is planning our birth dates, Elizabeth continues. "There's a lot of elective induction. We ask the doctor to induce us on March 7 because we want to do it then. Or the doctor wants to be somewhere." The number of induced births doubled between 1989 and 1997, going from 9 to 18 percent, a fact that also concerns some doctors. Dr. Fredric Frigoletto, of Massachusetts General Hospital, says, "Most often, women are tired of being pregnant at the end of their pregnancy. It's always a bit of a challenge to convince them they just have to hang on because it's better for them and their baby."[3] Elizabeth tells me that once induction becomes a habit, it dies hard. "In order for it to change," she says, "people would really have to understand that elective induction is one of the causes of low-birth-weight, and, like I said, a low birth weight baby really does have a much, much higher chance of dying in its first year." Elizabeth insists that, as a nation, we need to be asking some basic, logical questions. "Why don't we care that mothers and babies are dying at greater rates in the United States than in so many other places? If we know that outcome-based care does reduce maternal and infant mortality, can we talk about why we refuse to go there? Do we care about mothers and babies?"

Elizabeth is confident that change will come, slowly but surely, through education, saying that it isn't a matter of opinion vs. science but of making the data known. "I mean, obviously, the science isn't improving across the board," she says. "In 1989, our maternal mortality rate in the United States was around eight deaths per hundred thousand; it has actually risen to ten per hundred thousand! Some people would argue that we're counting it better, but in any case, we haven't improved. Not only have we not improved, but nobody's objecting. Maybe they don't know.

Maybe they don't know that, statistically, you should go have your baby in Japan or Spain if you want a better outcome." Elizabeth raises her eyebrows. "Working to improve birth has to be a campaign," she says, "and that's what I'm doing. I'm practically going door to door. We're talking on the radio, and we hope to have interviews in newspapers and on television stations. We're also talking to local businesses about what they're doing to support families."

In fact, that evening, when I return to the place I am staying and flip on the television, the first thing I see is Elizabeth in action. She is on a local cable channel talking to the Town Council. I'm stunned by her omnipresence and impressed by this additional evidence of her commitment not only to birthing mothers but to the social and political continuum of birth to family. She refuses any compartmentalizing or atomizing trends, repeatedly asserting the importance of a healthy and empowering birth on a healthy and empowered family. She tells the council about her "campaign" to "Honor Taos Families," by providing safe birthing and improved family life to their town and says, "I'm asking the council members if they will be willing to support this initiative. I want to energize the community to increase harmony and well-being."

There is a pause as the council members speak quietly among themselves, then one steps forward and says, "I think this is wonderful. I'm all for it." Another adds, "This effort on your part to support the family in the community is very important. I think the council has taken to heart that it takes a community to raise a child. Anything we can do to show other members of our society that we are *all* of value is a good thing. The council applauds you and very strongly supports your efforts." They move the motion, second it, and all vote yes. The chair pronounces their support of maternal-child health "Duly done."

The next morning, I return to the center and meet one of the four midwives who work with Elizabeth. Her name is Joan Norris.

Joan has chin-length gray hair and a serious, centered demeanor. She looks very familiar to me, but it takes me a few minutes to realize that I had met her several years earlier in Chiapas, Mexico.

In Chiapas, Joan was a liaison between a group of Lacandon Mayans and the clinics, hospitals, and doctors they sometimes came to the city to see. Despite the fact that the Mexican doctors didn't treat them well, many Indian women wanted a hospital birth. Traditionally, Lacandon women have their babies at home, but they do not have midwives; instead they have their babies with their husbands or maybe a sister. "For years," Joan says, "I felt so inadequate and guilty, because I thought I should be helping those women stay in their villages to birth. But they didn't feel safe there, and now I know that you can't do it at home if you don't feel safe. Women should have whatever birth they want. I'm not against hospital birth. I feel like women are pressured to have perfect births, and any variation on that makes them feel bad. I really try to emphasize the importance of a healthy baby and mom, and that wherever you have it is okay. We guilt-trip ourselves so much, especially the ones who transfer from home or birth center to hospital. That's not right."

During the early part of her stay in Chiapas, Joan says she was "consumed with having a family. I tried, and tried, and tried. I used Clomid, and I had a baby." She pauses and looks away. "But it died when it was four days old." For two more years, she kept trying with the Clomid, but it never worked again. So when she had the opportunity to care for a five-year-old Mayan boy who was being so severely abused that the people in his village begged her not to bring him back there, she adopted him. Two years later, she and her husband adopted his older brother. "Adopting filled my need for a family," she says.

When her youngest son, who, unlike his older brother, didn't want to return to traditional Mayan life, needed schooling he couldn't get in Chiapas, Joan and her family moved to Taos, a town with a similar mix of Native peoples, Spanish-speakers, and Anglos. "I always felt I would leave Mexico," Joan says, "because

I knew there was something else I had to do. I had no idea that I would have this amazing opportunity to become a midwife. It just fell from the sky like a miracle or a dream where things are just handed to you. For instance, there was a long waiting list for the midwifery school here, but they took me right away because they wanted a mature student. And then, when I finished my training, a job unexpectedly opened up here. I'm so lucky." She now works at the birth center full-time, which means five twenty-four-hour shifts every two weeks.

"I love being a midwife," she says. "I'm sure my becoming one had something to do with the fact that I lost a child. I'm still so sad that I lost my baby, and I have a lot of grief, but that is an impetus for working with women and babies, although I rarely mention my baby's death to anyone. But I was always passionate about birth. I went to friends' births as often as I could. While I was raising my sons, I was a family-oriented person. I could only concentrate on one thing at a time, so it worked out perfectly that this is a later career for me, even though it is still a challenge to balance it with my home life. It can consume your whole life, and you have to learn to say no. The hours are challenging. It is hard for me to stay awake, so I try to take naps. But I've read that you have to make up every hour of sleep you miss!" Joan laughs at the impossibility of this suggestion. "Also, it is emotionally draining. You're with women, and their problems, and their family, and you bond with them and experience their suffering. It is hard to let go of that and say, 'What's for dinner?'"

When I ask Joan to describe the joys of being a midwife, she says, "Being able to share that sacred passage, having people confide in you, and enabling women to feel stronger. Although I'm not really enabling; I'm listening and having a dialogue, but the enabling comes from them. I learn so much from them, too. I think it's a great spiritual practice to be a midwife. I feel really humbled by it."

One of the center's students, Kiersten, arrives. She is in her twenties and wears green overalls and funky work boots. She,

Joan, and I pile into her car and drive to the home of Jill, whose thirty-six-week prenatal exam is scheduled to take place at her house, because she is planning a home birth.

Jill's place is down a tree-lined, bumpy, dirt road. Kiersten checks the address and says it is NDCBU 231, a rural post office designation. Kiersten remarks that the mail carriers say it stands for "No Dogs Can Bite Us." Actually, stray dogs bark at us all the way down the road.

Jill lives in an apartment that is part of a larger house. It is small but very pretty with smooth pinkish-white plaster walls, terra-cotta tile floors, a wood burning stove, and lots of light. Jill is an artist, and she has filled the rooms with her work—textile pieces with geometric patterns and hangings made of brass bells and beads. Rows of brightly colored Christmas-tree balls hang from the beams above the brushes, paints, and paper that crowd her work table in the living room. In the corners of the room and along shelves are baskets, candles, feathers, and a drum. Everything is very neatly arranged. A copy of Ina May Gaskin's *Spiritual Midwifery* lies on a countertop.

Jill looks like she's in her early thirties. She has long, blond hair and wears a black skirt and a beige, linen blouse unbuttoned to reveal a black jog bra and a large, firm, and very sunburned belly. "I was only out for ten minutes!" she says defensively as Joan and Kiersten wince at the expanse of bright pink skin.

The midwives have brought in their supplies in a large, orange plastic toolbox; it looks like the kind of jumbo first-aid kit paramedics carry. As they start to unpack a few things, they ask Jill how she's feeling.

Jill says, "Okay, but have you ever heard of women in the ninth month not being able to drink hot tea?"

"Is that what's happening to you?" Joan asks.

"Yeah. It makes me throw up."

Joan ascertains that Jill is able to eat a little at a time, and says she isn't too concerned as long as Jill is able to eat some and is drinking sufficient fluids. If tea makes her sick, she should just skip it. Kiersten hands Jill a test stick for her urine, which Jill takes to the bathroom. When she comes back, she reads the results off to the midwives, noting that, in fact, she is a little dehydrated.

"I'll drink more," she promises them.

As Joan measures Jill's belly and takes her blood pressure, all three of them chat about baby names; Jill wants something unusual but her partner wants something mainstream. When her exam is done, she takes us to see the bedroom where she hopes to birth. "The bed is a little high," Jill says, and it is. Kiersten says, "Oh that's okay. It's good to lean over." Joan asks if she has lots of baby blankets, saying, "We go through them quickly when the baby's first born and we're wiping him off. Oh, and do you have an infant carseat yet?"

Jill's partner, Jonathan, and her six-year-old daughter, Willow, arrive and we go back into the living room so they can review emergency procedures. "If the baby comes early," Kiersten says, "call us. But if it comes first, just catch it, and dry it with a towel, and keep it really warm—warmer than you think it might need. Keep the baby with Jill." She explains that emergencies during labor and birth usually emerge slowly. If they need to transfer to the hospital, they'll probably have some time to decide and then do it.

Jill asks, "If the cord is wrapped around the neck, it's no big deal?"

"No," Kiersten says. "You just slip it over the head. If it is really tight, you just clamp it first. But if you call us as soon as you go into labor, we'll more than likely be here in time to take care of everything." True cord complications are rare, and midwives are well trained in how to handle them.

Jill says that the last time she gave birth she bled for a long time.

"Really? How long?" Joan says, some concern in her voice.

"Two weeks."

Joan smiles and relaxes. She and Kiersten both say, "That's not that long." Jill's answer reveals that she is talking about the normal postpartum blood flow, called lochia, that is similar to a menstrual period, not about a dangerous hemorrhage right after the birth that would have concerned Joan and Kiersten.

Kiersten asks if Jill wants to do a Group B Strep (GBS) test. One in four women carry GBS bacteria, which is considered normal "flora" (a.k.a. germs); their newborns can be exposed in the birth canal. About 50 percent of those babies will get colonized but not sick. Only 1 percent of the colonized ones will get sick, but those babies can get very sick and can die. The Centers for Disease Control (CDC) has said that in order to prevent most incidents of GBS illness in newborns, women should be tested and those with Group B Strep get IV antibiotics in labor, but they also say that close to 70 percent of those cases can be prevented without testing any women and giving IV antibiotics only to those women who give birth before thirty-seven weeks, with membranes ruptured more than eighteen hours, or with a fever during labor.[4]

Joan tells Jill, "If you do it and are positive, we administer antibiotics at home and keep a hep lock in. If you are positive, or haven't taken the test, you have to be in active labor in eighteen hours, and we can't wait until twenty-four hours. But it doesn't rule you out for home birth. If we transfer, we inform the doctors. The main things we can't do are breech births and twins."

Jonathan says, "It's so rare. But you could do the test, and even if you're positive you could decline the treatment." He shakes his head and shrugs his shoulders. "Whatever you think," he says to Jill.

"Ooooh. I don't know," Jill says. "Hmmmm. Welllll . . . I guess I could do it," she pauses, then, having reached a decision, jumps up. "Okay. I'll do it now." She takes the kit to the bathroom.

As the visit wraps up, Jill does some insurance paperwork and comments, "I didn't do this much paperwork when I had Willow with the midwives back at the old center. I never even brought in my Medicaid card."

"That doesn't surprise me," Joan says. "That's why the birth center went broke. We're still broke." She chuckles a little grimly. In fact, Elizabeth tells me later that she calculates that the birth center has donated more than $875,000 worth of care to families who couldn't afford it in the last three years alone. Elizabeth herself only began making a salary just recently, after twenty years as a midwife.

Jill says, "Well, you guys are great." We've been with Jill for about an hour by the time we leave. When we return to the birth center, Joan telephones Maria, an immigrant client from Mexico, who had called in this morning feeling like she was in labor. Now she says her contractions have gone away. Joan says she'll let me know if anything changes, and I go back to the house where I'm staying.

I'm spending the night at a house some friends are remodeling. It is basically a construction site; sawdust covers the floors, saw horses and piles of lumber fill the main rooms, and the bedroom door is draped with plastic. I plug in the portable radiator I brought with me, unplug a large yellow rack of industrial lights, and grope toward my pallet, ready to crash for the night. The normal fatigue of pregnancy is now exacerbated by the fact that I rarely sleep through the night anymore. This is pretty common in late pregnancy, due in part to the fact that rolling over in one's sleep is akin to a whale beaching itself—sure to wake you up. But there is also the frequent need to relieve one's squeezed bladder, and a heightened sense of anticipation and nervousness as birth approaches. Some people say that the changes in one's hormone levels also disrupt sleep. Friends tell me it's nature's way of preparing you for sleepless nights with an infant, but I don't buy that. Wouldn't it be more adaptive to be well-rested before your baby arrives? At any rate, I am bone-tired as I lie down. In the dark, my cell phone rings. I trip over a box of tiles trying to find the phone. It is Joan. Her client Maria just called; she's in labor and will meet us at the birth center.

I struggle back into my clothes and drive fast, gravel flying. I'm so excited. I might actually get to see a birth-center birth. As soon as I get there, a little old lady with neatly coiffed gray hair and a heavy Hispanic accent comes trotting across the parking lot toward me, yelling, "Quick! She wants to push. She's pushing!" It is night in the countryside, and all is pitch black except for the headlight beams of the battered pick-up truck from which she's just emerged. I climb slowly out of my car, stalling. "Hurry! Hurry! She's pushing!" this tiny grandmother yells at me.

As I come around the front of my car, I see a young woman in the truck holding onto a tall man in a baseball cap. She is moaning and, yes, grunting in that pushy way. I don't want to blurt out that I'm not a midwife, since that might unnerve them. So I stall, slowly pulling out my bag from the back of the car, praying that Joan will arrive momentarily. I remember Kiersten telling Jill and Jonathan that if the baby arrives early, the main thing to do is to keep it warm. "Keep it warm," I mutter to myself as I take the first step toward the truck and Maria.

Suddenly there is a loud crunch of gravel as Joan's truck bounces up the driveway. Kiersten pulls in right behind her. I sigh and call out, "I'm not the midwife, but here she is now." Joan unlocks the birth center door, and we all bundle Maria inside. She is leaning heavily on her husband, Ricardo, and a friend she has brought along. She has long, chestnut hair, big eyes, and a trace of cloasma (the mask of pregnancy) across her nose and cheeks, making her look a bit like a heavily freckled little girl. Barely able to walk, she manages to get onto a bed. Maria speaks only Spanish, and now she cries out, "Ya viene!" ("It's coming already!") Joan strokes her shoulder and reassures her, saying, "No problema. Todo esta bien. Descansa. Poco a poco." ("No problem. Everything's fine. Rest. Little by little.") Quickly, Kiersten gets Maria's blood-soaked underpants off. Between her legs is a small dark head.

Maria blows, pants, and cries out, "Ahorita!" ("Now!") Joan says, "Tu vas a ver tu bebe." ("You're going to see your baby.") Suddenly, in one swift, watery movement, the baby slides out and Kiersten catches it. The baby is a bit blue, but cries. Joan says to Kiersten, "Really massage her." I look at my watch and estimate we've been in the birth center for under two minutes. Ricardo says, in Spanish, "It's a girl!" Maria smiles, and says "Ay! Mi amor!" A minute later, the baby is crying a high-pitched, repeated, "Wah! Wah!" She poops some dark, green-black meconium on Maria's thigh. Joan wipes it up nonchalantly, then covers the baby with a few receiving blankets. She places a tube emitting oxygen near the baby's face. "She just needs a little," Joan says. Five minutes later, Kiersten reports that the umbilical cord has stopped pulsing and gets permission to clamp and cut it.

Another student, Wendi, arrives, says "Wow" when she sees how far along things are, and asks if she can do anything. She is in her twenties. She wears Levis, a white T-shirt, a thong necklace, and has long hair tied in a tight knot at the base of her neck. On her wrist is a thin bracelet-like tattoo. All three midwives sport beepers at their hips. Joan tells her to listen to the baby with a stethoscope. Wendi listens and says the baby sounds fine.

Ricardo, the dad, sits in a rocking chair, sighs, shakes his head, takes off his baseball cap, and runs his fingers through his thick, short, black hair. The grandmother and their friend sit nearby, exclaiming over how fast it went. "I told her, 'Don't have it in the truck!'" the grandmother laughs.

There's no sign of the placenta yet, so Joan puts some gentle pressure on the cord and asks, "Tiene dolor?" ("Does it hurt?") A minute later, Maria pushes out her placenta, her baby still buried in blankets on her chest. Maria is slumped down in the bed, her head only slightly raised. She looks dazed, and she's bleeding a little. Joan says, "I want to lift her up a bit," then checks her bleeding and says, "It's okay; it's not much." Joan asks Maria if she's alright, she replies, "Si," and shrugs as if to say, "No big deal." But Joan is watching her carefully, and says, "Tiene ojos de vidrio, pero no?"("You look a little glassy-eyed, but, no?") Maria reassures her again that she is okay.

Joan reaches over and shifts the baby to the breast, where she immediately starts to nurse. Maria looks puzzled and tells Joan that she doesn't have any milk. Joan reminds her about the colostrum she's producing and how good it is for the baby. "Ah, si, si, colostro," Maria says. Some mothers in Mexico don't start nursing until after the milk comes in, ignoring the yellowish fluid called colostrum that breasts produce first. But here, the midwives want the baby to get the benefits colostrum provides. It is high in protein and in white blood cells and antibodies that help ward off pathogens. Colostrum is also an excellent natural laxative that clears the baby of its first stool, meconium, and can, thus, help prevent the most common form of jaundice, known as physiologic jaundice, by preventing resorption of bile products, thus lowering the bilirubin concentration.[5]

Joan wheels a bright light up to the bed and checks Maria for tears, saying, "Just a few skid marks." But now she comments on Maria's bleeding again, saying she's lost about a cup or so. To the students she says, "Can you give me some meth?" They get a syringe of methergine ready. Joan pushes on Maria's belly, saying, "She was boggy, but when I massaged it, it went firm." To me, she says, "We use Pitocin to help the uterus clamp down if the placenta hasn't come out and methergine if it has. Because the baby came so fast, it is a bit of a shock to the uterus." In Spanish, she explains to Maria what is happening and gives her the shot.

Meanwhile, one of the overhead cabinet doors across the room from the bed has fallen off its hinge after one of the students went to get some supplies. Now, it dangles menacingly. Ricardo goes to his truck to get some tools to fix it. For the next few minutes he works hard; he looks happy to be busy and useful.

Kiersten takes the baby's temperature. It is ninety-four degrees, way too low. They are using a digital thermometer. Joan says, "Take it again. No, wait. Let me see the thermometer." She takes Kiersten's temperature and it reads 93.2. Wendi's is 94. They cluck and shake their heads. Kiersten finds another thermometer. The baby's temperature is fine, a tiny bit low, but fine. Kiersten shakes the thermometer down, and it flies out of her hand, breaking and leaving a bright trail of mercury droplets. As Kiersten cleans up, Joan changes the sheets on the bed and chats with Maria, praising her nursing. Maria complains of being hot, so Joan fans her with a Japanese hand fan, gives her some water, and puts a cold washcloth on her forehead. Meanwhile, Wendi takes the baby's temperature again. The baby suddenly jerks, sending the thermometer flying. It shatters on the floor. Joan says, "What is up with the thermometers tonight? That is the third one we've used!"

Joan massages Maria's belly, and she twitches. "I know, it hurts," Joan says. She lifts the sheet and takes a peek between Maria's legs, then says to the students, "I think we might give another methergine for the bleeding." So Maria gets a second shot of methergine. Two minutes later, Maria says she needs to vomit. They get a her a bowl just in time; Maria heaves violently. Joan comforts her and rubs her back. In a few minutes, she and Wendi go to changing the waterproof pads underneath her and find more blood. Joan says, "It might have been the effort of throwing up that made all that blood come out, but we may need to run an IV."

Joan massages Maria again, and although she is very firm, still more blood comes out. Maria says she feels a little drunk, and Joan immediately tells the students to run an IV. They get it in, and Joan says, first to the students, and then to Maria, in Spanish, "We need to stop the bleeding. I'm going to put my hand inside." A moment later, she is swiftly reaching her hand and arm way into Maria's vagina. "Ay! No!" Maria yells, and tries to push Joan's hand away. Joan manually removes several large clots, saying, "That's better." She explains that if the clots stay around the cervix, they can keep it from closing down. As she washes up, Joan says to me, "That was not fun. When you do that, you have to be so determined. If you hesitate, you are lost."

A few minutes later, Maria is much better and the bleeding has completely stopped. Her baby is nursing again, and Maria is resting comfortably. The students do the newborn exam and go to the kitchen to complete the charts. They note that because Maria is from Mexico, she has no Social Security number and no Medicaid, putting her into the "self-pay" category. Since she doesn't have the money for this, she will get a "grant" from the center. They get money from the Department of Public Health for five Mexican mothers per year. "But we take more," says Joan. "We usually see about twelve immigrant Mexican women a year. We take whoever comes."

In the birthing room, everything is quiet. The family rests

silently. Joan takes the baby's temperature again. After being a little low all evening, now it is a bit high. Joan worries out loud that
perhaps the thermometer was too close to the heating pad they
have tucked into the bed with Maria and the baby. So she shakes
the thermometer down to try again and catches it on the edge of
the bedside lamp as she does so. It breaks. There is silence for a
second, and then everyone groans. This is the fourth thermometer they've used tonight, and the third to break. I think to myself
it's a good thing we're in what may well be the best-equipped
birth center in the country. They're down to the last thermometer. Fortunately, it makes it through the night.

⌒

The next morning, Kiersten says "It's too bad you didn't get to see
a *real* birth-center birth." When I look confused, she says, "One
where we get to pull out all the stops, where we do lots of breathing with the woman, use the bathtub, different positions, the
birthing ball, homeopathic remedies, and massage, and walk in
the sage brush." I see what she means, but I know that I did, in
fact, see a "real birth-center birth." Although Maria's labor was
practically over before she arrived, she still received many of the
benefits of a birth center. She was attended with joy and respect;
the atmosphere was homey and welcoming; her family was included in the event; her bleeding was handled efficiently, professionally, and without any sense of panic; her baby was with her
throughout the night; and she will receive plenty of caring post-
natal attention, including home visits.

As Kiersten and I chat, Elizabeth arrives to start another busy
day and launches into one of the impromptu speeches she is
prone to giving. Either she is very savvy about being around jour-
nalists, or she's just used to taking every opportunity to speak
about her passion. I suspect a bit of both. Now, she says, "Good
for you, getting to see the birth, and good for Maria, getting it
done. You know, we should act like mothers have climbed Mt.
Everest. Look how those climbers are treated! Everyone knows

they did it; it's announced in the media. People ask, 'How was it? What would you do differently? What advice do you have?' Most moms just have to deal, and yet they've pulled off these amazing feats. We don't acknowledge them after they've reached the summit. We really should interview them as if they had climbed Everest. We need to let the world know about the scope of their feat." Elizabeth is grinning now. She's on a roll and she knows it. "Mothers put their lives on the line for their babies," she says. "Moms are responsible for the life of the planet."

Childbirth 101

*They are fruit
and transport:
ripening melons,
prairie schooners journeying
under full sail*

> —Kathleen Norris
> from "Advent"

CHING-ching-ching, cha-ching-ching. Cymbals chiming, a supple belly dancer sways across the floor with veils streaming, hips gyrating, and her muscular bare belly pumping in and out. Behind her is a sorry-looking conga line of pregnant moms and their partners struggling to release their inner groove from the constraints of their Dockers and stretch-top maternity pants. Some of the women do a decent imitation, but it has to be said that most of us are quite stiff, and let's face it, the men are downright wooden. They seem to be moving only their arms and shoulders; everything below the waist is pretty locked in. At first, we are all so self-conscious and absorbed in trying to do it right that we barely notice our effect as a group. After a minute or two, it slowly dawns on us how hysterical we look and we start to smile, then giggle, and laugh. This helps; everyone loosens up a notch. Our childbirth class teacher, Pam England (the former midwife who taught my doula training class), says, "Yeah! You're getting it.

Loose! Loose! Open your hips, open your pelvis, open the way for your baby! Breathe! Throw a squat in there! Good!"

As my due date fast approaches, it's time for childbirth classes. I tell everybody that since this is my second time around, I'm only doing them for my husband, who needs more refreshing than I do. But that's not strictly true. I love these classes. I love the opportunity to meet other pregnant parents, and I love the groovy activities a certain kind of class offers. Going to the midwife-lead childbirth class I've signed Richard and myself up for is kind of like getting to go to kindergarten again. We work with clay (making squat, little focal objects or birth totems). We draw pictures (of our babies and of our images of labor). We play with dolls and stuffed animals. We practice making wild animal noises. And we belly dance.

As the belly dancing winds down, Pam leaves the room and returns dressed as the goddess Innana. She wears a crown, several gaudy necklaces, a fringed shawl, a flowing skirt, and holds a makeshift scepter. As we watch, she acts out the story of Innana's descent into the underworld, the tomb and womb of the earth, where she plants the seeds of life by giving up her own. Along the way, Innana encountered seven gates and seven guards. At each barrier she had to give up something to cross over. Pam dramatically enacts the shedding of her crown, her jewels, her cloak, and her skirt, finally entering the underworld naked and shorn of glory. The final price is her life. Innana dies, only to be resurrected by the waters of life. Pam puts on quite a show, and although it seems pretty goofy at first, everyone is entranced. She explains to us how labor and childbirth mirror the descent of Innana, requiring us to give up our preconceived ideas about what it will be like, requiring us to shed some of our former independence, requiring us to give something of ourselves so the new life can be born, and requiring us to surrender to the process.

As she speaks of surrender, her assistant comes in with several basins of ice water. Everybody groans. We've done this before, so we know what's coming. Pain. With the image of Innana to hold onto, we get ready to plunge our hands into the icy water. Two minutes of ice water hurts, but it is nothing compared to a hard contraction. Still, when learning pain-coping techniques, it's better than nothing. Pam is pretty straight with us about labor pain. At the very first class, the first statement we heard was, "Childbirth hurts like hell. I'm not going to kid you about it. This class is about managing the pain." While this sounded pretty cut and dried, Pam's teaching methods, clearly, are not.

Her dramatization reminds us of what should be obvious, that in exchange for the pain of childbirth, we hope to gain the life of a healthy baby, but also that the process itself can be one of transformation, the first of many steps to becoming a parent. Pam doesn't mention that pain and initiation have been intertwined for millennia, yet I know it is true and feel excited and strengthened by the way she has tied us, a very ordinary group of suburban, pregnant parents, to the mythic aspects of birth. Before we start, Pam asks if anyone is already in any pain, physical or emotional. One guy blurts out, "Yes, emotional," then blushes deep red when Pam asks him what that emotion is. She reassures him that he doesn't have to explain it or tell his whole story. "Fear," he says, "it's fear." Pam applauds his honesty and asks us all to look into our fear. Then she suggests that while we are dealing with the ice, we allow ourselves to go into the pain and not try to avoid it. "Soften around the pain," she says. "Begin now."

It is quiet in the room. A few people fidget, but most close their eyes and sit very still, breathing heavily. When the time is up and we pull our reddened hands out of the ice, one woman comments that this technique is "less busy, less involved," than some others we've done. Someone else says the pain kept moving and she had to keep refocusing. Pam nods and says, "Labor pain shifts like that."

Next, we practice a technique called nonfocused awareness. It is a meditation practice in which you allow your mind to wander and simply follow it, gently urging it to take in more than just the crushing pain in your abdomen. You notice the sounds, the light in the room, the color of the floor, the smells around you; notice each thing, positive or negative, and then move on. The idea is to shift your focus away from your pain, but also to maintain a state where no one thing, particularly a negative thing like a beeping fetal monitor or your dread of the next contraction, can tighten its grip on you. Some women prefer to go deep into themselves during labor, but for some, this simple technique gives them a way to distract themselves, even if it's just for part of a contraction.

As we hold our burning, throbbing hands in the ice water, and notice the sounds of the cars outside, people breathing, and the fan whirring, Pam suddenly leaps up and turns on a bright, overhead light. Then she rushes out calling, "Bring her down here! Baby nurse in 303!" She rushes back in, switches the light off again, fiddles with an imaginary monitor, says, "Beep! Beep! Beep!" and asks one couple if they're ready for their epidural yet. Her simulated hospital distractions clearly knock some people for a loop, but some just close their eyes, and one guy starts chanting out loud, "I hear Pam beeping, I see my feet, I smell the candle, I see Pam's skirt, it's blue, I hear the fan . . ." When the minute is over, everybody rubs their hands and listens to Pam's admonitions to be ready for distractions, acknowledge them, and refocus.

After a short break, Pam pulls out a model of a pelvis, joking, "Now I'm going to take off my perineum, which I only do in public!" Holding the fake pelvis in front of her, she shows how squatting opens the birth canal. She demonstrates several vertical birth positions we might like to try, but tells us that if we give birth in an upright position, we shouldn't push much after the head is out, as it can increase tearing. She tells us it's good to have lots of position ideas, but not to get too attached to any one. She says that French birth educator Michel Odent convinced her that women need to choose their own positions during labor. While mothers need to know the value of upright positions, which have gravity on their side, the position of the baby will help dictate to the mother what is most comfortable and probably most effective. Pam also tells us not to feel pressured to push before we feel the need; sometimes there is a lull between reaching full cervical dilation and the expulsive reflex. One woman asks if it is true that when the head is in the birth canal you feel like you have a bowling ball in your bowels. Pam says it is possible. She also says it's fine to push out of your rectum. "And if you poop, well they've all seen it before. No biggie."

Pam asks us to take out the stuffed animals we've been instructed to bring to class. She has a doll, which she tucks under her shirt, indicating we should do likewise with our cuddlies. One woman has a fuzzy red Elmo, one has a wart hog, and one has a small frog. Everybody looks a little embarrassed. Pam says, "Okay, it's time to practice some pushing noises. Some of you may not have made sounds like this for a long time, and now is a good time to lose some of your inhibitions. All right, let's pretend we're mama gorillas pushing our baby out into the world. Hard pushes first, then baby pushes when you're crowning." She takes a deep breath, scrunches up her face, and makes a ferocious, growling "Oooooooggghh!" We all try our best, but she acts disgusted with our pathetic attempts. "Come on," she says, "get mad and tough. Be gorillas!" People get louder. One couple, Ian and Laura, pretend to reach the crowning stage. They look completely involved. He's holding her shoulder, saying, "Slowly, slowly, slowly, there's more coming, just a little push and our baby will be here. Gently." Another man looks at the wart hog emerging from his wife and reports, "Houston. We have a problem." Everyone laughs.

We talk about the crowning phase for a while. Pam tells us it's okay to use warm washclothes on the perineum, but not up by the clitoris, which will be outrageously sensitive. She explains that generally it is better to tear a little than get an episiotomy, as cutting can increase the tear and doesn't always heal as well. She tells us that her one-hundred-year-old midwifery book says to "sopple the perineum with goose fat." Pam says, "You know at Thanksgiving how some people disappear into the kitchen? Well, now you know what they were doing. Yup," she nods knowingly, "soppling with goose fat, uh huh."

We finish off the class by watching a video of birth in the squatting position. While we watch, some parents laugh nervously and some sigh. Several worry out loud about the babies' pointed heads until someone says it's normal. As one woman births an enormous placenta, Laura says, "Wow." Afterward one woman comments that the births looked good but somehow unreal. Everybody nods, and finally someone realizes that the video had been set to music, and all sounds of grunting, groaning, crying, or other expressions of pain had been conveniently edited out.

⌒

At the next session, Pam introduces us to "birth art," a specialty of her classes. In her book, *Birthing from Within,* Pam writes that "language has its limits," when it comes to understanding and expressing our deepest fears and desires, and that "Dreams, reverie, and art all carry messages from the unconscious," which can be brought to the fore and put to use by birthing mothers.[1] We begin by drawing pictures of a "womb with a view," an image of what our baby looks like now. "Your drawings, like your labor, don't have to be perfect. Just try your best," Pam advises.

I draw a large, messy, pastel picture of a baby who is head down and has its face turned away, since I'm terrified my baby, who is still face up, isn't going to get into this optimal birth position. At my next prenatal exam with Sarah, she recommends exposing my belly to the sun, since the baby, who is developed enough to notice this, might try to turn away. I do it the very next day, sitting in a chair with my dress yanked up to my neck and no underwear on, since I've blown the elastic on my last pair. Sure enough, the meter guy arrives at just that moment. I whip my dress back down, and although I won't know for a week, my baby does actually turn, probably out of embarrassment for me.

Our next assignment is to draw a landscape of our labor. It is not meant to be a literal picture of where we will be, but a metaphor. One woman draws a beautiful, chambered nautilus and speaks eloquently of her passage out the spiral, from chamber to chamber. I don't know what to draw, so I make a long snaking line down the middle of my paper. It turns into a river, full of rapids, that flows through a narrow opening into a wide, calm, tree-lined lake. I find myself explaining that the river starts off the edge of the page because I expect to be plunged into my labor. One minute I'll just be me, the next minute I'll be in the middle of something stronger than myself, but I know the river will reach the lake and all will be well. The one problem I have is that the entrance to the lake seems too open, too easy. There is no representation of the pushing stage, so I add an awkward log jam licked by flames to show the ring of fire. But I'm not satisfied. Somehow this part doesn't look right.

Finished with the pictures, we split into two groups—men and women. The women sit in a circle on the floor and are given little lumps of clay. We are told to think about images of opening and then make an object. We squish out a variety of flowers, donuts, and doors, but just as we finish, we are instructed to destroy them as a symbolic way of not getting too attached to a single image, one that might not work for us in labor. Meanwhile, the guys have been getting a lesson in foot massage and each has prepared a basin of warm water filled with bath oils and floating rose petals. When they come in with this gift for their partners, they are beaming. One woman gets a little teary, the rest say things like, "Oh, YES!" and "At last!"

Since it is assumed that fathers will participate during labor, teaching men to be supportive of their pregnant partner is a nice feature of this class. But this class doesn't emphasize the "coach" model that is so prevalent today in the United States. As one father said a little ruefully, "This class is very mother-centered." A number of midwives I spoke with expressed ambivalence about the pressure couples now feel to include the dad every step of the way. Some feel that not all fathers are appropriate birth partners and that some women might be better off without them and better off with a female support person.

In her book, *Telling Bodies, Performing Birth,* scholar Della Pollock comments that "the husband-coached model may also strengthen men's conventional role within marriage," giving men "a kind of imperial control they didn't have in the waiting room." She is concerned that it "broadens their scope of involvement both *in* and *over* women's lives—such that one woman I talked with described her husband as a 'savior' and another mourned what amounted to his cruel detachment . . . one simply dismissed her husband as useless, several felt weakened by what seemed their husband's greater, if well-intentioned, allegiance to the medical staff."[2] She does acknowledge that other women felt "a deepened sense of closeness and partnership" with their partners, and, no doubt, this is what most women are hoping for. As with so many other aspects of birth, surely the ideal is a wider range of choices and less pressure to conform to a single standard of how and with whom to labor and birth.

At any rate, I am glad to have my man learning a few good tricks, like giving the ultimate foot bath. The woman next to me has varicose veins that are so bad it looks like someone's been beating her feet and ankles. She sighs as the warm water envelopes them. I, too, plunge my puffy, swollen feet into the deliciously scented water. I could have opted to take the childbirth classes offered at the hospital where I've continued to see my backup nurse-midwife in case I need to go there to birth, but it is unlikely it would have included this experience.

Hospital childbirth classes tend to focus more on the physiological stages of labor and on hospital procedures. As Pollock writes, "hospital-based 'prepared childbirth' classes" are often "devoted to reducing stress and thus both pain and panic by familiarizing students with all the tests and procedures they might encounter in the hospital setting—including genetic testing, ultrasound diagnosis, internal and external monitoring, episiotomy, induction, epidural, and caesarean section." Although this *can* help parents avoid being set up for disappointment by the disjuncture between the values of many independent childbirth classes and antithetical hospital policies—for instance, when a class encourages parents to avoid interventions, but the hospital has a hard-and-fast policy that all patients in labor must be on an IV—taking a hospital-based class can also mean a limited and limiting experience. Pollock contends that because these classes are "sponsored by hospitals or obstetric groups they enculturate students in scientific and institutional norms. They give anxious parents enough knowledge to feel 'in the know,' but usually only enough to feel indebted to physician recommendations. In general, they preempt opposition by positioning students *inside* the hospital culture."[2]

I think how glad I am to be here, as Pam reminds the men to keep massaging, since they may think they're done in a matter of moments. She dims the lights, and we get our feet bathed and rubbed for fifteen, long, blissful minutes.

Too soon for me, class is over and we're on our own with our impending births. I'm not sure if any class can fully prepare you for the reality of labor and birth. In fact, a *Parents* magazine poll of 25,000 readers recently showed that only 16 percent of mothers who had taken classes found them "very helpful," and 30 percent found them "useless"![4] Still, a good class can give you important information and some helpful pointers. Reading books, which I did obsessively the first time around, can also give you a lot of great information, although one midwife I spoke with warned against books that put too much emphasis on possible problems. Those kinds of books, she says, "are handed out like candy in doctors offices. I'd get rid of them. Women who turn to those books end up worrying a lot and can actually end up manifesting those problems." Even if the books you read serve you well, they can't give you one thing a good childbirth class can provide, and that is community. The childbirth class I took for Max, in North Carolina, continued to meet as a play group for years afterward. And, as was the case with Pam's, some classes can give you ideas about how to approach childbirth that will change the way you approach the rest of your life as well.

"*So,*" my friend Greta asks me one day, "Do you want a baby shower or something more funky, like a mother blessing?" Fresh out of my very funky childbirth classes, I decide I'm ready to go the alternative route, having had a fairly traditional shower the first time around. Greta organizes two events, a belly casting to be done by herself and a friend (they are both artists), and a mother blessing to which my closest friends will each bring a bead to string on a bracelet I will wear during labor to remind me of their loving support.

The belly casting takes place in Greta's kitchen, with its floor of black-and-white squares and light streaming in from the window over the sink. She's made fancy snacks and tea, so even though it's just the three of us, it feels like a party. The casting process itself involves putting strips of plaster bandages all over my naked breasts and stomach, letting it harden, then pulling it off—a permanent, sculptural reminder of my rounded shape, my baby's nine-month house. I sit on the edge of a stool while they swaddle me, since the last woman they did this for fainted after standing up for twenty minutes. When it is done, it is a beautiful white egg-and-teardrop-shaped dome. It is enormous. At this point in my pregnancy I've started telling people I think I might not be carrying a baby; it feels more like a giant, swimming manatee. After a bath that Greta has sweetly decorated with rose petals and candles, I take my belly cast home and make Richard try it on. As soon as he is encased, I ask him to tie his shoes. He bends, gets stuck half-way, laughs, and says, "Okay, okay, I'll put your shoes on from now on." This makes me happy. I don't really need it, but I'm not about to tell him so.

The mother blessing takes place ten days before my due date on the banks of a nearby river on a windy, spring day. Three of my closest friends, Greta, Judy, and Elizabeth, are there, as is Sarah, my midwife. When I arrive, Greta happily crowns me with a wreath of tiny white flowers and miniature red roses; long, delicate pink and white ribbons stream down my back. I am surprised and pretty thrilled to be the oversized center of attention. Greta spreads a blanket for us to sit on near the riverbank, and we go around the circle; each woman gives me the beads she has chosen, lights a candle, and offers a few words of support and blessing. It is pretty amazing, and I find I'm grinning so hard my cheeks hurt.

Judy's beads include an amber one "to calm scattered energy," and a blue one "because it's pretty!" Greta gives a beautiful opal and three wishes: that the love that surrounds me today might fill my childbirth with empowering feelings of self-worth, that I might find the energy I need during my demanding labor of love, and that the creative powers within me grant a beautiful and loving birth experience. Elizabeth presents a bead made of two leaping dolphins ("wise, watery, and fun!"). She asks that I be blessed with a brave heart (to birth my baby with welcoming strength); strong loving arms (to hold and nurture this longed-for gift); a wide, sweeping imagination (to let my child find its own way); and a true gentle spirit (to accept what is difficult and to find the loving answers hidden close by).

Finally, Sarah gives me four beads. First, a rotund, silver earth mother who resembles the *Venus of Willendorf*. "She is one of the oldest spiritual symbols in human times," Sarah says, "honoring the beauty, strength, and power of the feminine forces. May the hand of the lady be upon your shoulder as you journey through your labor." Second is a tiny silver Celtic knot, which, Sarah explains, "shows endless oneness, connectedness, and cycles. May you feel your place among all sisters, in all of time, in all of life. A dream ending is but a magic beginning." I'm touched by this as I have, in fact, begun to grow sad about the end of my pregnancy (despite the discomfort that comes with having gained what feels like an elephantine fifty pounds). So this reminder of the beginning that awaits me is especially welcome.

The third bead is a square cross, a Native American representation of the four directions. Sarah says that the most important direction in motherhood is within. "May you follow your heart and trust your wisdom, and may you feel the arms of all other influences holding you safe on your way," she says. Finally, there is a cluster of tiny moonstones, the crystal for childbirth. "They are said to bring harmony down to the depths of the subconscious," Sarah explains, "that conflicting forces become one energy: bringing forth/letting go, fear/bliss, alone/universal, pain/peace, transformation/oneself, working/relaxing, contracting/opening, screaming/singing, finale/encore, ending/birthing. Oh, I could go on and on!" Sarah says, pushing back her long hair as it blows across her face, "but I'll end by saying, I am honored to be with you."

Well, needless to say, there are lots of smiles and quite a few tears. This is it. This is the spiritual experience I craved all along. In a way, it doesn't matter what happens with my birth now that I've had this. I waddle the long mile or two back to the parking lot, elated. That night, I start contracting, but after two hours of labor and a flurry of activity and excitement as we get ready for the baby, it fades away, only a hint of what's to come.

An Earth Day Birthday

IN April, my son Max's school celebrates Earth Day. It is one of the biggest school events of the year, complete with a parade through the neighborhood led by police on horseback and a crew of African drummers. The kids decorate their little red wagons with flowers and streamers, and papier-màché globes. After the parade come songs and skits celebrating the earth, followed by a huge potluck feast. I wouldn't miss it for the world.

So, wearing a shockingly dowdy, hand-me-down dress that I can barely button over my belly, I saunter out with the rest of the families. As I lumber along, I think, good, maybe all this walking will help start my labor. All along the parade route people joke with me, saying things like "Whoa! Don't have that baby here!" and "Hey! You're bursting your buttons, ha! ha! ha!" I'm going to blame my grouchiness on hormones, but I don't find this very funny. One woman walks with me for a while and, hearing I am just two days short of my due date, says, "You're going to have that baby today." I say, "Yeah, yeah. I hope so." And she says, "No, really. Positive thinking. Tell yourself, 'I'm going to have this baby today.'" Somebody else had told me that if you start to feel some contractions, and you've been having short bursts of contractions on and off as I have, you should visualize your labor kicking in. "Visualize the contractions coming on and staying," she had said.

"Just stay with it and 'think contraction,' basically." Everybody has these great, crazy theories, but today I figure, oh what the hell, it can't hurt. Okay. I'm having this baby TODAY.

When I reach the schoolyard, I collapse into one of the swings. It feels great. If you are in late pregnancy anywhere near a playground, I highly recommend going for a swing. The counterpressure of the U-shaped leather seat, the soothing motion, the way your hips move as you pump your legs, and the little gravity-free moments at the top of the arc are all heavenly. Almost as heavenly as the two-hour nap I take when I get home, only to be awakened by what is quite clearly a contraction.

With a start, I realize that, with any luck, I will be giving birth to my baby here at home some time very soon. I have no bag to pack, no decision to make about when to leave for the hospital. I am a world away from where I was when I first thought about where I would birth my baby. I feel excited to be at home and confident in my choice, assured that my midwife will provide the support and skills I need here and that the hospital and all its services is available as a backup, should I need it.

It is 2:30 P.M. I call my doula, Maia, and Sarah, my midwife, just to let them know that this might be the day, but I'll call them back later. Sarah is half-expecting the call; at last week's prenatal exam, she discovered that I was already several centimeters dilated. Now, I duck my head into my husband, Richard's, home office and tell him, "I think I'm going to have this baby today." He says, "Ooooh. Then I'm taking a nap." I call a friend who is going to take care of Max, should we need it, and leave a message on her machine.

Putting on my beaded labor bracelet, I am reminded of a pilgrim's sign; one of those shells or medals a traveler is given to wear when making a journey to a sacred place. Properly adorned, I call the friends who gave me these beads at my mother blessing. They all light the candles they took home from the event, even Elizabeth, who is at a conference at a law school on the west coast. This little ritual leaves me feeling cared for and content. I putter around the house for an hour. As the contractions begin to intensify, I decide to do the labor project I had decided on months ago—something not too strenuous, fairly monotonous, not intellectually challenging, outside, and with no chance of finishing it too soon—weeding dandelions. Richard, up from his nap, brings me a weeding tool and a stool to sit on. As I lower myself awkwardly down, there is a sudden pop! Something bursts with a faint explosion, half sound, half sensation. It feels like the baby has punched downward toward my cervix. My waters have broken. A gush of pink fluid drenches my dress and underpants, flowing into my sandals. I am covered in bloody water, and I am thrilled. It is happening! We really are going to have this baby today.

Grinning and happy, I get undressed in the garden and make my way into the bathtub to rinse off. Richard hands me the phone in the tub, so I can call Maia and then Sarah. Maia reminds me not to use much hot water since we're going to need it all for the kiddie pool Richard is starting to inflate on our sun porch. I think to myself, that pool could take a while to fill and I'm going to need some relief now, since my water's already broken. So I go ahead and take a nice deep bath. I call Sarah, and she says to me, "My sister's coming at four o'clock to pick up her baby. That's six minutes from now. It takes another six minutes to drive from my house to yours. I can be there by ten minutes after four. Will that be okay?" I tell her that's fine, but she must detect some note of urgency in my voice, because later she tells me that when her sister hadn't arrived in five minutes, she suddenly decided not to wait for her, but to leave the children with her husband and take off for my house. When her husband said, "But your sister will be here in five minutes, Sarah replied, 'I'm not sure I have five minutes.'"

Meanwhile, my contractions have become very painful. Not agonizing yet, but close. I yell from the tub for Richard to find someone to take Max, and fill up that pool, now! I move to my bedroom, where I sit on a giant, red, physical therapy ball, the birth ball. It feels great, with excellent counterpressure and an easy, rocking, bouncing movement that forces my hips apart as I straddle it. The only problem is that it keeps rolling away with me on it, tossing me to the floor like a horse tossing an uncertain rider. Finally, I figure out how to wedge it against the side of the bed. Maia and Sarah arrive and ask how I'm doing. I grunt, "Okay. It hurts." Sarah unloads her equipment.

Richard says to me, "Let's try that ovarian breathing we learned in class." All I can think is "What are you talking about? My ovaries can't breathe." I snarl "No," and he backs off a bit. He tries again to help, saying, "The wave always hits the shore," our mantra from the first time. For no good reason, I get pissed off and say, "Try again." Richard goes to get his cheat sheet. He comes back and, reading from his notes, says, "You are so strong. Follow your next outward breath all the way out. Breathe the baby down. Let it all go." That's better. I find my breath and a tiny bit of calm.

Our friend, Elaine, has still not arrived to take Max, and I can feel that on some level, I'm not really letting myself go. I had thought I might want him at the birth, but now I know I want him out of there so I can yell. Finally, just after five o'clock, she arrives and then hangs out, chatting, for what feels like forever, but is actually about ten minutes. As this is going on, I'm laboring by myself in the bedroom. My contractions peak quickly and hold on hard, then suddenly taper off. They are about a minute apart, and I find I am able to use some of the pain-coping techniques I've learned. I say to myself, "Soften around the pain. Find the edges of the pain." On the next wave of agony, I tell myself, "Inhale. I am. Exhale. I surrender. Notice your breath." This feels good. Then, for several minutes, I am able to use nonfocused awareness. I say to myself, "Max is talking. I can hear the water pouring into the pool from the hose." But pretty soon it gets all speeded up from the way we practiced. Now it's more like, "Kids! Water! Uhhh!" I am acutely aware that I am just trying to hold it together until Max leaves. So the next time Richard checks in on me, I tell him, "Get them out of here, NOW!"

As Richard shoos Elaine and Max out the front door, I practically run from the bedroom to the pool, whipping off my clothes:

the short, loose, dark purple and red cotton dress I had so wanted to wear when I labored in the hospital with Max but the hospital made me trade for an ugly butt-revealing robe. Now, my doula, Maia says, "Oh, what a beautiful dress. How perfect for labor." I think I manage a smile.

I do take off the dress to clamber my big-bellied way into the pool. It isn't quite full, since, as Maia predicted, we did run out of hot water. Richard is in the kitchen boiling water in big pots on the stove, looking like a parody of the stereotypical birth scene. Nonetheless, the pool is sublime—for about three contractions. Then, all of a sudden, I am rising out of the water like a surfacing submarine. My moans escalate to wails. "They're not stopping in between," I cry. I feel a wave of pain and panic. Sarah nods and says, "Yeah, I know." I see my belly hardening like a boulder and have one or two contractions that are like being in a hideous storm. I remember Max's labor and tell myself I am not drowning, just being pulled by the current, this time with my head above water. I tell myself it's okay to surrender. I will survive. Then I start wailing. "Ohhhhhhh! Whoaahhhh!"

Maia, my doula, puts her hands firmly on my shoulders and rubs, saying, "Great noises." She gives me a sip of a sports drink, as she does after every other contraction, then says, "You are stronger than this pain." I hear this, and I repeat it to myself over and over. Maia is steadying me with her physical touch and telling me exactly what I need to hear. Internally, I hear my own voice saying, surrender, let go, surrender, let the baby go. I imagine my cervix opening.

After the next contraction, Sarah asks if she can check me. It is 5:25 P.M. She does and asks, "Do you want to know numbers?" I take a minute to have an actual thought—no easy task at this point—and figure if she's asking me, then I'm not fully dilated. So I hesitate, then answer, "I don't know. No." She says, "Well, you've made excellent progress. The baby is very low." Later she tells me I was at seven centimeters, with the baby at plus two station (very low).

Another wicked contraction. I'm thrashing a bit in the water, so Sarah suggests I gaze at the candle burning on a nearby table. I do and immediately feel more centered. It still hurts like hell, and I am alone inside the pain, but I am also aware of the help my attendants offer. On the next contraction, I feel incredible pressure. The infamous bowling ball sensation. I can feel the baby moving down. It is so different from the first time, when I pushed without really knowing where the baby was. Now I am not pushing; the baby is pushing itself out. This is definitely the expulsive phase. Expulsion is the perfect word for what I feel. It is incredible. I tell Sarah, who nods and disappears for minute; she's bringing her kit from the bedroom to the pool.

I feel sick and somebody thrusts a stainless-steel bowl under my face. Maia says, "Remember this birth." It seems an odd time for this suggestion. Here I am feeling yucky, weepy, and nauseated. But her comment wakes me up a bit, and I know I do want to remember this. I do want to be aware, even when it's hard. With the next contraction I say, "I need to push, but it can't be time." I know I wasn't fully dilated just three contractions ago. It could be hours before it's time to push. But Sarah says, "If you feel like you need to push, push. Listen to your body." No, I think to myself, I don't want to swell my cervix. I'm double-guessing, playing the textbook game. I tell myself I'm going to breathe through the next one. I'm *not* going to push. But after one more contraction, I know I can't hold back anymore. It feels like the baby is just going to rocket out of me, so I ask Sarah, "Are you ready?" She smiles, amused, and says, "Yes, I'm ready. We're ready to have this baby." And then she gives me a look I will never forget—benign, positive, supporting, connected—and says, "You are so strong." I can feel her strength, her calm, her confidence. And suddenly I feel grounded, solid, and confident. I feel strong.

From what seems like somewhere far behind me but is actually only a foot or so, Maia asks "Would you like to change positions?" I don't want to be sitting down to give birth, so I flip over like a rotating beach ball buoyed by the water and get on my knees. My body is upright and leaning against the side of the pool, my backside facing my midwife. With the next contraction,

I vomit into the bowl Maia is still holding. Sarah says, "This baby is coming. This baby is coming now." I feel myself let go, just totally release. One second later, Sarah says, "There's a little miracle about to happen here." It is excruciating. Pain like nothing else in the world. She asks if I want to touch the head, but I can't let go of Richard's hands, which I am clutching hard. Sarah says, forcefully, "Catherine. Your baby's head is crowning now." I get very conscious and think, no tearing, ease the baby out. Even in the moment, I feel absurdly proud that I am remembering how to make little blowing sounds and control the urge to just blast the baby out and have it be over. I pant and hold back a little, imagining my perineum stretching, stretching. And then, as Sarah gently cradles my baby's emerging head, I throw up again.

As the shoulders begin to push out, I pull away from the baby, up away from the pain. For a moment, I am fully surrounded by pain; nothing else exists. Then, suddenly, I am conscious again, thinking, the shoulders, sometimes they get stuck and they say a change of position helps. So in this second that feels like a minute, I lean forward and move my hips. Release. My body is released and so is my baby. It is behind me, up out of the water, in the hands of my midwife who says firmly in my ear, "Catherine, lift your left leg." She passes the baby under my raised leg, and I take it in my arms. I sit back with a huge wet purple baby on my chest, an actual being who didn't exist a moment ago. I laugh and say, "A baby! A baby!" I feel so surprised; it looks impossibly big and so unfamiliar. I don't know anything about it or who it is. I remind myself that getting to know each other will take time. Right now, it feels so animal. I stare into a pair of small, dark eyes, alert and yet dazed, so empty of meaning, so incredible. I am connected to something alive but not quite human. A quiet presence. I am suspended. In a minute it is covered by a blanket and is wearing a little cap.

It is 5:34 P.M. I went from seven centimeters dilated to ten centimeters, pushing, and having the baby, in nine minutes. I can't believe the baby is actually here. Everything is so calm. Sarah doesn't even do any suctioning; the baby is breathing fine on his own. After a minute, Richard, who looks happy and stunned, says, "Oh, it's done. I was just starting to pace myself, I thought we had hours to go. Oh, wow. Is it a boy or a girl?" I'm thinking, it's a girl, it's my girl, look at her. But then I notice something in the palm of my left hand, which is cradling the baby's bottom. A soft, rounded presence. I move my hand to reveal a set of enormous, rosy newborn testicles and everybody says, "It's a boy!" Sarah peers in his face and says, "Oh look, he's an old soul." He has tiny, pointed, elfin ears, and a sprinkling of red marks called stork bites across the bridge of his nose. His fingers are long and delicate, and his skinny legs and feet look vaguely frog-like. He is beautiful. He is perfect.

A wave of relief joins my ecstasy over his birth. After a few minutes, Sarah gets me to move to the bed, where she can see better if I am bleeding. I don't bleed much and certainly don't hemorrhage. More relief. The baby begins to nurse as soon as we are settled in the bed, his tiny mouth stretched in a wide kiss over my nipple. It hurts a bit, and I feel a sense of surprise to find this tiny stranger at my breast, but still I am thrilled. When the placenta arrives, maybe twelve minutes later, Sarah says, "This is something a little unusual," and shows us a place in the placenta that looks like a tiny, curved backbone. "It could just be a scar from where the placenta might have pulled away and then re-sealed itself, but it could be a twin who died early in the pregnancy. It seems like it was another baby." My euphoria over my wonderful birth ebbs a little as I wonder about this other baby. Was it a girl? Will my baby feel something missing in his life, the way twins who are separated at birth sometimes report they do? I feel the first hint of sadness for him. Then it's time to double-bag the placenta and put it into the freezer next to the ice cream so we can plant a tree with it later.

Sarah reports that I haven't torn at all. She seems pleased with herself. In fact, she has said in the past that she prides herself on her intact perineums. She tells me that when the baby is crowning, she's very careful not to let the head jerk up because that gives spider tears near the urethra and, although they heal nicely, they hurt like crazy. I feel *so* much better this time than with Max. It is night and day. After tearing the first time, I couldn't walk easily for days, and I hurt like crazy for weeks. I carried an embarrassing rubber donut to sit on everywhere I went for the first two months. This time, I am walking that evening and feel like myself within the week.

We decide to name our baby Emrys Gabriel. Emrys was the name Max picked, the birth name of Merlin when he was a boy in Wales. It is still a fairly common name in Wales. I call my parents to tell them the news, and my father, who is from England, says, "Well, Emrys Jones was one of the best rugby players ever to come out of Wales. Maybe he'll take after the athlete and not the wizard." Max gets back from his friend's house and says, "Oh goody, my Emrys! I love our baby. I love our baby more than all my toys." He'll live to retract that statement, but right now, it feels pretty sweet.

Maia cleans the house while Sarah does a newborn exam on Emrys. She gently weighs him in a little fleece sling hung from a handheld scale, like a grocer weighing soft peaches. Then she chats with me for a while. We look at the picture I drew in my childbirth class of the "landscape of labor," which I have taped to the wall by my bed. We marvel how closely my labor mirrored its short, rushing stream full of rapids, its sudden, easy opening of the canal into the wide lake of birth. After drawing it, I had fretted about the fact that it didn't have a proper depiction of the impedance of the pushing stage and had halfheartedly added a log jam. Now that I've experienced the inexorable pull of a baby who pushed himself out, my first draft looks exactly right. I think about the power of suggestion. I know the mind-body connection is strong at birth and wonder to what degree I might have influenced my labor by looking at this picture for weeks and weeks, telling myself this is the way it would be. After a few hours, Sarah leaves for the night, and we sleep, Emrys in a bassinet right next to the bed. Actually, Richard and Emrys sleep. I doze, nurse, and end up spending much of the night peering over the side of the bassinet at the amazing baby that lies there.

Sarah returns the next morning, looking beautiful in a long, dark-green dress that makes her eyes shine. I give her a final gift in exchange for all she has done. She is pleased but expresses her own gratitude for being part of Emrys' birth, and we both know that my gift is but a tiny token compared to all that she has given me and my family.

Her friendship throughout my pregnancy made me feel loved and special. Her skill, her fond attention, and her peaceful attitude during my labor and birth made me feel safe, supported, trusting, and, yes, empowered. She made me feel as if I were, briefly, the center of the universe, a woman engaged in a miracle, connected to all that is universal in birth. Being at home meant that everyone's priority was me and the baby. There were no other patients, no other people giving birth, no schedules, and no people going off shift. Everything revolved around what we needed, and that was absolutely wonderful.

How something so full of pain and vomit and bodily fluids can be so beautiful and so spiritual may be hard to grasp. Yet it was one of the most vital and powerful moments of my life. If I choose to, I can recall this birth any time I face a challenge, from the daily challenges of the often crushing boredom of motherhood, the mess of spit-up and leaky diapers, the endless flow of laundry, the ambivalent vacillations between parenting and other work, to other challenges, both emotional and physical. And while I am as prone to sulky bouts of insecurity as anyone else, I now know that I can find the strength I need within me and within those I call on for help. My midwife did not just attend the birth of my baby; she attended the birth of a new, powerful, confident, and loving part of my self. Although I know that it was I who brought forth both my baby and this stronger self, I will be forever grateful for my midwife's role in my unfurling and in the safe passage of my baby.

CONCLUSIONS

IT is spring again. The wind storms are here once more, kicking up towering dust devils in the empty lots and bending the budding irises in my garden. One year has passed since I began this journey with midwives, a year filled with long nights of waiting, tense moments resolved, physical challenges, and newborn infants—some already approaching toddlerhood—all attended by a group of women fiercely committed to supporting and enriching labor, birth, and motherhood. As I nurse my baby and feel the thick, disabling fog of sleep deprivation roll in, clear, then thicken again, I call Claire Hamilton, one of the midwives I observed. I tell her that I've become so immersed in the world of midwifery (as well as so brain-dead from sleeplessness) that I need her to remind me why a women who doesn't know anything about midwives might want one.

Claire chuckles at my spacey state and reassures me I'll sleep again some day. Then, since she and I have had some long talks over the past year about the transformative nature of birth, she begins by saying, "You know, even for women who aren't interested in empowerment or spirituality, midwives offer something different than waiting for hours in a waiting room for a nurse to weigh you, then waiting again for a doctor to slap a Doppler on you, tell you you're fine, and leave. I had that with my first baby, and I wouldn't actually classify myself as a very spiritual person, but I knew the second go-round that I didn't want to go through that again. Women don't have to do something hip and groovy, but they can be treated with more dignity and respect and still have the technology available if they want it. Women need to know that they can have a say in what is a relatively mundane but very important part of their life." She pauses, "Plus, you haven't already forgotten that we get better results when it comes to healthy moms and babies, right?"

No, I haven't forgotten. Respect for birthing women, treating pregnancy and birth as normal but significant life events, and shepherding women into motherhood by instilling confidence and competence were some of the constants that emerged in the diverse practices of the midwives I observed. True, good obstetricians also bring these qualities to their practices, but as midwifery scholar and historian Judith Pence Rooks points out, midwifery and medical obstetrics are "separate but complementary professions with different philosophies and overlapping but distinct purposes and bodies of knowledge." For both professions, healthy babies and mothers are the primary goal, but, Rooks adds, "they are not the midwife's *only* goals. Midwives value birth as an emotionally, socially, culturally, and often spiritually meaningful life experience—something to be experienced positively, with potential for making women feel stronger, and *be* stronger." For midwives, the baby is a central outcome of the pregnancy, but not the only outcome. "Pregnancy results in a *mother* as well as a baby," Rooks reminds us, thus, "breast-feeding and mothercraft are part of the focus of midwifery." Another way the medical model and the midwifery model differ noticeably is in how they approach potential health threats to mother and child. For midwifery, the outside possibility of a problem emerging does not justify interventions that might compromise the woman's experience of birth. Midwives are there to watch for possible problems and treat them appropriately if and when they emerge, while the medical model usually calls for a preventive approach where interventions like hep locks, IVs, and continuous fetal monitoring are used "just in case" a problem should arise.[1]

How these differences between the two professions arose is a long and fascinating history that a number of authors have thoroughly documented elsewhere.[2] Interestingly, when doctors first began attending births in place of midwives, they often did so at home. And although this began the displacement of midwives and the eons-long tradition of women attending other women at birth, it wasn't until doctors moved their practices into the hospital that women's traditional birth culture was truly dissolved. Scholars Judith Leavitt and Della Pollock have both written about how, as Pollock says, "medical control over birth literally corresponds to the change in birthplace."[3] When doctors attended women at home, they entered a domestic sphere dominated by the woman of the house and her female friends and relatives, who retained a certain authority over how to approach the birthing process. Pollock writes that although "hospital birthing was not a conspiracy wrought by men against women," inevitably, it "broke the connections between birth and social life that had imbued the act of giving birth with social power." Pollock finds:

> The ideal of a safe birth had its costs, among them the collapse of women's birthing culture and the power that culture secured for women as women. . . . Without the provisions of a woman's culture—social solidarity, empathy, traditional wisdom, shared values, manual skills, domestic help, and, above all, a common sense of the importance and difficulty of birthing and mothering—the birthing woman lost control over both her experience and the means of interpreting it. Deprived of its determinations within women's culture, birth became less a sign of women's power than a symbolic internment of female passivity.[4]

Contemporary midwifery revives women's birthing culture. There are a few male midwives, and I'm sure they are skilled practitioners who may even have tremendous empathy for their birthing clients. I don't think women have to be attended by other women to have a positive experience in childbirth, but for me there was something very comforting about being in the company of women. No doubt this has to do with culture and history—the history of power relations between men and women, especially the domination of men over women, the history of sexual politics, the way institutions and even spaces can become gendered, and the intertwining of these realms. This is a complicated realm, different for every woman. For a victim of abuse or rape, having a man present at birth may be particularly difficult. But even for women positively engaged in heterosexual desire, those whose pregnancies are the result of love, lust, or companionship, we, too, are part of a gendered history that may leave us feeling more secure and more supported when attended by women.

It strikes me as a sad truth that the demise of the female birth culture of the home and the rise of the male-dominated birth culture of the hospital has chipped away at birth as a symbol of female power and encouraged female passivity around birth. As Sheila Kitzinger says, "Every woman having a baby in the hospital is transformed into a patient."[5] Midwives at the hospital work to prevent this transformation and to allow women their power in birth. But it is an uphill battle; one that is limited by many of the assumptions of our culture.

I am reminded of the work of anthropologist Robbie Davis-Floyd, who has written extensively on the impact of medical culture on birth. Davis-Floyd's premise is that although we tend to think of rites of passage as primitive events in primitive settings, birthing is still a rite of passage even when it takes place in the technological sphere of the hospital. She points out how the standardization of the process of pregnancy and labor in doctors' offices and hospitals is "reminiscent of the standardized rituals that make up rites of passage in traditional societies," and she observes that "these rituals, also known as 'standard procedures for normal birth,' work to effectively convey the core values of American society to birthing women,"[6] core values that are often patriarchal and technological in nature. She writes:

Cumulatively, routine obstetrical procedures such as intravenous feeding, electronic monitoring, and episiotomy are
felt by those who perform them to transform the unpredictable and uncontrollable natural process of birth into a
relatively predictable and controllable technological phe-
nomenon that reinforces American society's most fundamen-
tal beliefs about the superiority of technology over nature. . . .
The pregnancy/childbirth process has been culturally transformed in the United States into a male-dominated initia-
tory rite of passage though which birthing women are taught
about the superiority, the necessity, and the "essential" nature of the relationship between science, technology, patri-
archy and institutions.[7]

Davis-Floyd points out that while most women's beliefs become fused with this dominant belief system, many resist it, either by resisting the rituals themselves or by perceiving the
doctors and hospitals as being their servants instead of the op-
posite.

For most women, having a baby places them in a high-tech
medical world in which the focus on the pathology of pregnancy,
the things that can go wrong, has shaped the way we define birth.
Birth historian and sociologist Barbara Katz Rothman says that in
defining birth as a medical event, we are "narrowing our scope of
perception. The other equally salient, humanly meaningful aspects of childbirth are lost to us, outside our narrow range of vision."[8] Sadly, this has often resulted in a polarizing of the way we
see our choices. We tell ourselves we can have either pain and
power or pain-relieving drugs and passivity. We tell ourselves we
can have either the comfort of home or the safety of the hospital.
Either a transformative experience or a healthy baby. But these
are false opposites. Although birth options in the United States
are currently quite narrow, a wide spectrum of choices could exist, as they do in most European countries.

In order for women to have both the safest form of birthing
and one that does not deny them their power, it seems to me that

we need to rethink the hospital as the main site for birth and doctors as the main attendants for normal pregnancies and births. Ninety-three percent of women have their babies with doctors, and 99 percent of births in America take place in the hospital. And yet the World Health Organization (WHO) states that the "preferred location for most births is outside the hospital, either at home or in a birthing center, and that out-of-hospital birth should be implemented and maintained as the basic standard for all midwifery education and training programs."[9]

When people find out that I had my baby at home, they often say, "How brave!" But I know it was not bravery and that I took no more risks than any mother in the hospital. I knew my midwife was competent to handle any problem that could arise. Yes, if I had had some rare problem emerge at home, I might have been slightly more at risk than I would have been in the hospital, but the risk is so small. It's like saying, I'm not going to walk by the river today because I might slip, fall, tumble into the water, and drown. Well, yes, there is that risk, but that minuscule chance doesn't stop me from taking that walk, because the experience I stand to gain is so much more sure than what I stand to lose.

A friend of mine recently told me, "Thank God for pain-free childbirth in the hospital. It's great. Having an epidural was a wonderful experience, and I am so glad I'm having my babies in the twenty-first century." Or as writer Anne Lamott says, "I think the epidural is right up there with the most important breakthroughs in the West, like the Salk polio vaccine and salad bars in supermarkets. It's an individual thing."[10] To them, I say "Great. More power to you. I'm glad you're getting the birth you want." But to all the women who have felt that their births left them disappointed, dissatisfied, or unprepared for motherhood, or that the importance of their experience was trivialized, and to all the women who have not had babies but want to do so in a safe, supportive, uplifting environment, I think we have a lot to learn from midwives, whether they are working to change the culture of the hospital or to raise the acceptability of birthing outside of the hospital.

What can we do to improve birthing in America and to ensure that women are not denied birthing choices? First and foremost, if we are having healthy pregnancies, we can see a midwife for our care. If there are no midwives in our town or city, we can request that our obstetricians or hospitals hire them, or we can help recruit home-birth midwives by requesting that our doctors provide medical backup. We can support midwives in their struggles to start birth centers or change inappropriate hospital protocols. We can suggest that large midwifery practices experiment with new models of "team midwifery," like those being tried in England, that assign prenatal clients three or four midwives who will share information among themselves, one of whom will attend the client's birth, thus ensuring some continuity of care. We can work to change the laws in states where direct-entry midwifery and home birth are unlawful, as home birth is always safest where it is legal and not forced underground. We can advocate that insurance companies cover out-of-hospital births and postpartum home visits. In Holland, all families can get postpartum support from home-aides who help with everything from breastfeeding advice to doing laundry to picking up older children, thus easing the transition into parenthood. We can support public health initiatives for birthing women like one in my town that provides doulas and translators to immigrant women for whom language barriers can make the experience of birthing in the hospital especially alienating. We can write to government representatives, asking them to include midwives in maternity care legislation. We can become doulas, or even midwives, ourselves and work directly to provide skillful, loving care to birthing women.

When I began work on this book, I wanted my journey with midwives to be about information and enlightenment. Inevitably, it turned out to be about politics as well. Access to midwifery is a political issue, and the health of mothers and babies as well as the disempowerment of women during the act of giving birth are feminist issues. Midwifery itself can be seen as a feminist practice, according to Barbara Katz Rothman, who writes that "midwifery works with the labor of women to transform, to create, the birth experience to meet the needs of women. It is a social, political activity, dialectically linking biology and society, the physical and the social experience of motherhood."[11] In her groundbreaking work, *Of Woman Born,* Adrienne Rich wrote, "to change the experience of childbirth means to change women's relationship to fear and powerlessness, to our bodies, to our children; it has far-reaching psychic and political implications."[12] My guess is that most midwives see their work as a form of activism but also look forward to the day when that will no longer be true, when they can simply be the skilled caregivers they already are. Right now, their work engages them in a mission that, if successful, will save billions of dollars currently spent on the superfluous use of expensive and often unnecessary technologies and procedures, and will radically improve birth for women and babies both emotionally and physically.

Women want and deserve these improvements. Although women's images of the ideal birth may be phenomenally diverse, they share core similarities. Women want healthy babies, a way to cope with pain, and respectful treatment. And yet, it is in the details that their experience will be formed. How will they feel about themselves in childbirth? How will they be shepherded into their role as mother? How will their family be guided? These are critical issues for women's physical and emotional health and the health of their babies and families. Women should be able to have whatever option they want, whether that is a doctor or a midwife, a hospital or a birth center or a home birth, anesthesia or its alternatives. Women deserve to be truthfully informed about the options, and, like their sisters in the rest of the industrialized world, they should be able to get excellent personal care along with excellent health outcomes. The United States spends more money on childbirth than any other country in the world, and still we rank a miserable, embarrassing, twenty-second from the top when it comes to healthy mothers and babies. Birthing women in the United States deserve better than what they're getting, and midwives can be central to that improvement.

I know for myself, if I ever have another baby (and right now, the demands of two seem overwhelming enough), I'm going to keep my dreams for childbirth big. So often we are afraid to dream, afraid to "think big" because it might jinx us, because thinking big might be the pride that leads to a fall. We think we should be more humble. And while humility is not a bad idea in the face of the awesome power and unpredictability of birth, big dreams and high standards are also appropriate. Am I romanticizing birth? Perhaps, but I am not closing my eyes to reality. I know that if I were to be in labor again, the pain might be worse, and despite my plans for a home birth with a midwife, I might need to go to the hospital for drugs, or unforeseen complications might make me an unsuitable client for a midwife. I might even end up with a caesarean with a doctor. If that happens, I'll be disappointed, but I know that there, too, emotional support and respect would be crucial to shaping my experience. Unless, and until, that happens, I can still shoot for what I want most. I'm thinking maybe next time I'll give birth under the stars, or in a shady garden, or in front of a crackling fire. Dreams matter; they are the way change begins. Midwives have a dream that one day all birthing women will get the highest level of care and respect, that birth technologies will be available to all who need them but used only when they truly need them, that the creation of a family, no matter what it looks like, will be honored, supported, and celebrated, and that birth will be both a sacrament and a safe passage.

NOTES

INTRODUCTION

1. Mary J. Renfrew, Walter Hannah, Leah Albers, and Elizabeth Floyd, "Practices That Minimize Trauma to the Genital Tract in Childbirth: A Systematic Review of the Literature," *Birth*, vol. 25 no. 3 (September 1998), 143–60; and Professor Leah Albers, interview with the author February 14, 2001.

2. Wenda Trevathan, *Human Birth: An Evolutionary Perspective* (New York: de Gruyter, 1987). Cited in Natalie Angier, *Woman: An Intimate Geography* (New York: Houghton Mifflin, 1999), 308.

3. *Williams Obstetrics, 21st ed.* (New York: McGraw-Hill, 2001), 430–31. Williams says second stage is usually limited by physicians to two to three hours for a first birth, one to two hours for subsequent births, but longer times may also have good outcomes.

4. Joyce Roberts, D. Woolley, "A Second Look at the Second Stage of Labor," *JOGNN*, vol. 25 no. 5 (1996), 415–23. Mary J. Renfrew, et al., "Practices that Minimize Trauma to the Genital Tract in Childbirth: A Systematic Review of the Literature," *Birth*, vol. 25 no. 3 (September 1998), 143–60.

5. Marshal H. Klaus, John H. Kennell, and Phyllis H. Klaus, *Mothering the Mother: How a Doula Can Help You Have a Shorter, Easier, and Healthier Birth* (Reading, MA: Perseus Books, 1993), 3, 37–41.

6. National Center for Health Statistics, 9.5.01, www.cdc.gov/nchs.

7. These figures are from "Trends in the Attendant, Place, and Timing Births, and in the Use of Obstetric Interventions: United States, 1989–97," *National Vital Statistics Reports*, vol. 47 no. 27, at www.cdc.gov/

nchs/releases/99facts/99sheets/attendant.htm as cited in "Bulletins," *Mothering Magazine* (March–April 2000), 30.

8. Sheila Kitzinger, *Rediscovering Birth* (New York: Pocket Books, 2000),163. Kitzinger says Britain has 25,000 midwives, 3,000 obstetricians, and the United States has 34,000 obstetricians, 6,000 nurse-midwives, and 3,000 direct-entry midwives. Marsden Wagner, a former officer of the World Health Organization, says Great Britain has approximately 35,000 midwives and less than 1,000 obstetricians, with more than 75 percent of births attended by midwives, while the United States has approximately 6,000 midwives and more than 32,000 obstetricians, according to his lecture handout of June 1998.

9. Suzanne Arms, *Immaculate Deception II; Myth, Magic, & Birth* (Berkeley, CA: Celestial Arts, 1996), 49–51; Marsden Wagner, *Pursuing the Birth Machine: The Search for Appropriate Birth Technology* (Camperdown, Australia: Ace Graphics, 1994); and Judith Pence Rooks, *Midwifery and Childbirth in America* (Philadelphia: Temple, 1997), 353, 410 ff.

10. National Center for Health Statistics, 1997 National Hospital Discharge Survey, quoted in *Mothering Magazine* (March–April 2000), 32.

11. S. J. Ventura , S. C. Curtin, F. Menacker, and B. E. Hamilton, "Births: Final Data for 1999," *National Vital Statistics Reports,* vol. 49 no. 1; National Center for Health Statistics, 2001, Hyatsville, MD.

12. M. F. MacDorman, and G. K. Singh, "Midwifery Care, Social and Medical Risk Factors, and Birth Outcomes in the USA," *Journal of Epidemiology and Community Health,* vol. 52 (1998), 310–17.

13. Rooks, *Midwifery and Childbirth in America,* 30.

14. Jan Tritten, "Who Are We?" in *Life of a Midwife: A Celebration of Midwife* (Eugene, OR: Midwifery Today, 1995), 10.

15. Laura Meckler, "The Doctor's Still in, but New Study Finds Midwives on the Increase," December 2, 1999, The Associated Press, ABCNEWS.com.

CHAPTER ONE

1. Barbara Harper, *Gentle Birth Choices* (Rochester, VT: Healing Arts Press, 1994),18; Suzanne Arms, *Immaculate Deception II,* 104; and Mary J. Renfrew, et al., "Practices That Minimize Trauma to the Genital Tract in Childbirth: A Systematic Review of the Literature," *Birth,* vol. 25 no. 3 (September 1998), 143–60.

2. Elizabeth Davis, *Heart and Hands: A Midwife's Guide to Pregnancy and Birth* (Berkeley: Celestial Arts, 1997), 102.

3. Barbara Harper, *Gentle Birth Choices,* 18, cites Judith Goldsmith, *Childbirth Wisdom* (Brookline, MA: East-West Health Books, 1990), 32.

4. Margaret Talbot, "Pay on Delivery," *New York Times Magazine,* October 31, 1999, 19.

5. Judith Rooks, "The Midwifery Model of Care," *Journal of Nurse-Midwifery,* vol. 44, no. 4 (July/August 1999), 373. She cites both S. Biasella, "Epidural Anesthesia," *Journal of Perinatal Ed,* vol. 3 no. 4 (1994), 67–9; and J. Lothian, "Why Do Women Choose Epidural?" *Journal of Perinatal Ed,* vol. 2 no. 2 (1993), ix–x.

6. George Ella Lyon, "Birth," in *Cries of the Spirit: A Celebration of Women's Spirituality,* ed. by Marilyn Sewell (Boston: Beacon Press, 1991), 67.

CHAPTER TWO

1. "ACR Standard for the Performance of Antepartum Obstetrical Ultrasound" (Res 37), Revised 1999, Effective 1/1/00, www.acr.org/cgi-bin/fr?tmpl:standards00,pdf:pdf/antepartum_obstetrical_ultrasound.pdf; and A. M. Gulmezoglu, P. Fajans, M. Q. Islam, M. K. Usher-Patel, and E. Ahman, "Planning and Programming for Reproductive Health," *WHO Annual Technical Report,* 1999 at www.who.int/hrp/atr/1999/pdf/planning%20and%20prog51–90.pdf.

2. Natalie Angier, *Woman: An Intimate Geography* (New York: Houghton Mifflin, 1999), 155.

3. "Breastfeeding and the Use of Human Milk," *Pediatrics,* vol. 100 no. 6 (December 1997), 1035–39 on the www.aap.org website. Also, Natalie Angier, *Woman: An Intimate Geography,* 144–155.

4. Ibid.,146,153,160.

5. Suzanne Arms, "Giving Birth: Challenges and Choices," a videotape created, produced, and directed by Suzanne Arms. A BirthingTheFuture Production, a division of Roots, Inc. Contact www.BirthingtheFuture.com.

6. Ellice Lieberman, J. M. Lang, F. Uletto, D. K. Richardson, S. Ringer, A. Cohen, "Epidural Analgesia, Intrapartum Fever, and Neonatal Sepsis Evaluation," *Pediatrics,* vol. 99 no. 3 (March 1997), 415–19.

CHAPTER THREE

1. "Letter to the Editor of *Newsweek,* Re: The Cesarean Birth Article," *Midwifery Today,* no. 57 (Spring 2001), 24.

2. Robbie Davis-Floyd, *Birth as an American Rite of Passage* (Berkeley, CA:

University of California Press, 1992),130–31. Another source that finds nearly 50 percent of caesareans unnecessary is M. Gabay and S. M. Wolfe, "Unnecessary Caesarean Sections: Curing a National Epidemic" (Washington DC: Public Citizen Health Research Group, 1994).

3. Natalie Angier, *Woman: An Intimate Geography,* 311, Klaus, M. H. and Kennel, J. H. "The doula: an essential ingredient of childbirth rediscovered." *Acta Paediatr* 1997; 86: 1034–6, and Goer, Henci, *The Thinking Woman's Guide to a Better Birth* (New York: Perigee Books, 1999).

CHAPTER FOUR

1. American College of Nurse-Midwives, "The Core Competencies for Basic Midwifery Practice," May 1997.

2. Peter Curtis, Jacqueline C. Resnick, Susan Evens, and Corleen J. Thompson, "A Comparison of Breast Stimulation and Intravenous Oxytocin for the Augmentation of Labor," *Birth,* vol. 26 no. 2 (June 1999), 115–122; and Peter Curtis, "Breast Stimulation to Augment Labor: History, Mystery, and Culture," *Birth,* vol. 26 no. 2 (June 1999), 123–26.

3. Susan McCuthcheon-Rosegg with Peter Rosegg, *Natural Childbirth the Bradley Way* (New York: Penguin, 1984); Suzanne Arms, *Immaculate Deception II,* 104.

4. Susan Moore Daniels, CNM, conversation with author, winter 1999.

5. Laura Meckler, "The Doctor's Still in, but New Study Finds Midwives on the Increase," The Associated Press, December 2, 1999, ABCNews.com.

6. Judith Rooks, *Midwifery and Childbirth in America,* 319.

7. Suzanne Arms, *Immaculate Deception II,* 103.

8. Judith Rooks, *Midwifery and Childbirth in America,* 319.

9. Ibid., 319.

10. Ibid., 320, cites S. F. Bottoms, V. J. Hirsch, R. J. Sokal, "Medical Management of Arrest Disorders of Labor: A Current Overview," *American Journal of Obstetrics and Gynecology,* vol. 156 (1987), 935–39.

11. Rooks, *Midwifery and Childbirth in America,* 316. For one view of the debate, see Stephen H. Halpern, Barbara L. Leighton, Arne Ohlsson, Jon F. R. Barrett, and Amy Rice, "Effect of Epidural vs. Parenteral Opioid Analgesia on the Progress of Labor: A Meta-Analysis," *Journal of the American Medical Association* (23/30 December 1998) vol. 280 no. 24, 2105–10, and a response to this article in *The Birth Gazette,* vol. 15 no. 3 (Summer 1999), 41.

12. Rooks, *Midwifery and Childbirth in America,* 316, cites J. A. Thorp, D. H. Hu, R. M. Albin, J. McNitt, B. A. Meyer, G. R. Cohen, and J. D. Yeast, "The Effect of Intrapartum Epidural Analgesia on Nulliparous

Labor: A Randomized, Controlled, Prospective Trial." *American Journal of Obstetrics and Gynecology,* vol. 169 (1993), 851–58, and S. C. Morton, M. S. Williams, E. B. Keeler, J. C. Gambone, and K. L. Kahn, "Effect of Epidural Analgesia for Labor on the Cesarean Delivery Rate," *American Journal of Obstetrics and Gynecology,* vol. 83 (1994), 1045–52.

13. Professor Leah Albers, conversation with author, February 14, 2001, New Mexico.

14. American College of Nurse-Midwives, "The Core Competencies for Basic Midwifery Practice," May 1997.

15. Alfirevic, Z. "Oral misoprostol for induction of labour (Cochrane Review). In: *The Cochrane Library,* 1, 2002. Oxford: Update Software, Goodman, David. "Forced Labor," Mother Jones (January/February 2001), http://www.motherjones.com/mother_jones/JF01/labor.html, Gaskin, Ina May, "Cytotec: Dangerous experiment or panacea?" Salon (http://www.salon.com/health/feature/2000/07/11/cytotec/print.html, Wagner, Marsden, "Misoprostol (Cytotec) for Labor Induction: A Cautionary Tale," *Midwifery Today* No. 49 (Spring 1999), http://www.midwiferytoday.com/articles/default.asp?t=cytotecwagner. For the full text of the drug manufacturer's (Searle) letter of warning, see "Important Drug Warning Concerning Unapproved Use of Intravaginal or Oral Misoprostol in Pregnant Women for Induction of Labor or Abortion," at the FDA website (www.fda.org) or the website of the Association for Improvements in Maternity Services (www.aims.org.uk/searle.htm). For a summary of labeling changes from April 2002 see also the FDA website.

16. W. Prendiville, J. Harding, D. Elbourne, and G. Stirrat, "The Bristol Third Stage Trial: Active Versus Physiological Management of the Third Stage of Labour," *British Medical Journal,* vol. 297 (1988), 1295–3000; J. Rogers, J. Wood, R. McCandlish, S. Ayers, A. Truesdale, and D. Elbourne, "Active Versus Expectant Management of Third Stage of Labour; the Hinchingbrooke Randomized Controlled Trial," *Lancet,* vol. 351 (1998), 693–99.

17. Rooks, *Midwifery and Childbirth in America,* 129, and Sheila Kitzinger, *Rediscovering Birth,* 145.

18. Barbara Harper, *Gentle Birth Choices,* 23.

19. Henci Goer, *Obstetric Myths Versus Research Realities: A Guide to the Medical Literature* (Westport, CT: Bergin & Garvey, 1995), 83–105.

20. Henci Goer, *Obstetric Myths Versus Research Realities,* 89 cites K. H. Sheehan, "Caesarean Section for Dystocia: A Comparison of Practices in Two Countries," *Lancet* vol. 1 no. 8532 (1987), 548–51.

21. Rooks, *Midwifery and Childbirth in America,* 320.

22. Ibid., 316.

23. Lois Wessell, "Electronic Fetal Monitoring," *Every Baby Magazine,* vol. 1 no. 1 (2001), 36–39. Leah Albers, "Monitoring the Fetus in Labor: Evidence to Support the Methods," *Journal of Midwifery and Women's Health* (November–December, 2001); S. B. Thacker and D. F. Stroup, "Continuous Electronic Heart Rate Monitoring for Fetal Assessment During Labour" (Cochrane Review) *The Cochrane Library,* Issue 2 (2000) Oxford: Update Software.

24. Rooks, *Midwifery and Childbirth in America,* 314.

25. Karin B. Nelson, James M. Dambrosia, Tricia Y. Ting, and Judith K. Grether, "Uncertain Value of Electronic Fetal Monitoring in Predicting Cerebral Palsy," *New England Journal of Medicine,* vol. 334 no. 10 (March 7, 1996), 613–618.

26. Rooks, *Midwifery and Childbirth in America,* 93, cites K. J. Ryan, "Giving Birth in America, 1988," *Family Planning Perspectives,* vol. 20 (1988), 298–301.

27. 1998 Data: S. J. Ventura, J. A. Martin, S. C. Curtin, T. J. Matthews, and M. M. Park, "Births: Final Data for 1998," *National Vital Statistics Reports,* vol. 48 no. 3, Hyatsville, Maryland, National Center for Health Statistics (2000). 1988 Data: L. L. Albers, and C. J. Krulewitch, "Electronic Fetal Monitoring in the United States in the 1980s," *Obstetrics and Gynecology,* vol. 82 (1993), 8–10. Also, Laura Meckler, Associated Press, "Midwives, Induced Labors on the Rise," from *AP Science* online, December 2, 1999, gives stats as 68 percent in 1989 and 83 percent in 1997.

28. Laura Meckler, op. cit.

29. Lois Wessel, "Electronic Fetal Monitoring," *Every Baby Magazine,* Issue One (2001), 37.

30. Hodnett, E. D. "Continuity of caregivers for care during pregnancy and childbirth (Cohrane Review). In: *The Cochrane Library,* 1, 2002. Oxford: Update Software. www.cochrane.org/cochrane/revabstr/ab000062.htm

31. Marshall H. Klaus, John H. Kennell, and Phyllis H. Klaus, *Mothering the Mother;* M. Enkin, M.N.J.C. Keirse, M. J. Renfrew, and J. P. Neilson, *A Guide to Effective Care in Pregnancy and Childbirth, 2d. ed.* (New York: Oxford University Press, 1995) cited in Rooks, 309.

32. Rooks, *Midwifery and Childbirth in America,* 310.

33. J. A. Martin, B. E. Hamilton, and S. J. Ventura, "Births: Preliminary Data for 2000," *National Vital Statistics Report,* 49, no. 5 (Hyatsville, MD: National Center for Health Statistics, 2001); S. M. Wolfe, *Unnecessary Caesarean Sections: Curing a National Epidemic* (Washington, DC: Public Citizen Health Research Group, 1994).

34. Margaret Talbot, "10.31.99, The Way We Live Now, Pay on Delivery," *The New York Times Magazine* (31 October 1999), 19–20.

CHAPTER SIX

1. Suzanne Arms, *Immaculate Deception II,* 161; Klaus, Kennell, and Klaus, *Mothering the Mother,* epigraph prior to table of contents.

2. Klaus, Kennell, and Klaus, *Mothering the Mother,* 4; Barbara Harper, *Gentle Birth Choices,* 209–210. Liddell and Scott, *An Intermediate Greek-English Lexicon* (Oxford: Clarendon Press), 210.

3. Kitzinger, *Rediscovering Birth,* 122; and Klaus, Kennell, and Klaus, *Mothering the Mother,* 4, attribute the term's use to anthropologist Dana Raphael.

4. Kitzinger, *Rediscovering Birth,* 122; Sosa study: R. Sosa, J. Kennel, M. Klaus, et al, "The effect of a supportive companion on perinatal problems, length of labor and mother-infant interaction," *New England Journal of Medicine,* vol. 305 no. 11 (1980), 585–7; J. Kennell, J. Klaus, M. McGrath, et al, "Continuous Emotional Support During Labor in a U.S. Hospital: A Randomized Controlled Trial," *Journal of American Medical Association,* vol. 265 no. 17 (1991), 2197–2201; E. D. Hodnett and R. W. Osborn, "A Randomized Trial of the Effects of Monitrice Support During Labor: Mothers' Views Two to Four Weeks Postpartum," *Birth,* vol. 16 no. 4 (1989), 177–83.

5. Klaus, Kennell, and Klaus, *Mothering the Mother,* 33

6. Ibid.,35–37.

7. Ibid.,43.

8. Adrienne Rich, *Of Woman Born; Motherhood as Experience and Institution* (New York: W.W. Norton,1986),158.

9. Emily Martin, *The Woman in the Body: A Cultural Analysis of Reproduction* (Boston: Beacon Press), 83.

10. Barbara Katz Rothman, *Recreating Motherhood; Ideology and Technology in a Patriarchal Society* (New York: W.W. Norton, 1989), 28, 155.

11. Kitzinger quoted in Rothman, *Recreating Motherhood,* 57, from Kitzinger, *Women as Mothers: How They See Themselves in Different Cultures* (New York: Vintage Books, 1978), 74.

12. Suzanne Arms, *Immaculate Deception II,* 50.

13. Ibid., 50.

CHAPTER SEVEN

1. Pattiann Rogers, *The Dream of the Marsh Wren: Writing as Reciprocal Creation* (Minneapolis, MN: Credo, 1999), 29.

2. Waterbirth International, "Survey of Waterbirth Practice," *Journal of Nurse-Midwifery,* vol. 34 no. 4 (1989), 86.

3. Mary J. Renfrew, et al., "Practices That Minimize Trauma to the Genital Tract in Childbirth: A Systematic Review of the Literature," *Birth,* vol. 25 no. 3 (September 1998), 143–60, 157.

CHAPTER EIGHT

1. Patricia Akins Murphy and Judith Fullerton, "Outcomes of Intended Home Births in Nurse-Midwifery Practice: A Prospective Descriptive Study," *Obstetrics and Gynecology,* vol. 92 no. 3 (September 1998), 461–70; O. Olsen, "Meta-Analysis of the Safety of Home Birth," *Birth,* vol. 24 (1997), 4–13; M. Tew and S.M.I. Damstra-Wijmenga, "The Safest Birth Attendants: Recent Dutch Evidence," *Midwifery,* vol. 7 (1991), 55–65. The website for Citizens for Midwifery lists twenty-four sources describing the safety of home birth from journals such as the *Journal of the American Medical Association* (JAMA), the *British Journal of Obstetrics and Gynaecology,* and the *Journal of Reproductive Medicine.* Henci Goer, *Obstetric Myths Versus Research Realities* is another source for information on home birth safety.

2. O. Olsen, "Meta-Analysis of the Safety of Home Birth," *Birth,* vol. 24 (1997), 4–13, cited in *The Birth Gazette,* vol. 15 no. 3 (Summer 1999).

3. "Breastfeeding and the Use of Human Milk," *Pediatrics,* vol. 100 no. 6 (December 1997), 1035–39 at www.aap.org.

4. *Williams Obstetrics, 21st ed.,* 983.

5. *Williams Obstetrics, 21st ed.,* 984.

CHAPTER NINE

1. See footnote #74.

2. James Lord, *Giacometti: A Biography* (London: Faber & Faber, 1986), 117.

3. Judith Leavitt, *Brought to Bed: Childbearing in America, 1750–1950* (New York: Oxford University Press, 1986) quoted in Della Pollock, *Telling Bodies, Performing Birth* (New York: Columbia University Press, 1999), 14.

CHAPTER ELEVEN

1. Judith Rooks, et al., "Outcomes of Care in Birth Centers: The National Birth Center Study," *New England Journal of Medicine,* vol. 321 (1989), 1806.

2. Marsden Wagner lecture handout, on file with the author; and for low birthweight as a predictor of infant mortality, see also "New Study

Shows Lower Mortality Rates for Infants Delivered by Certified Nurse Midwives," National Center for Health Statistics (May 19, 1998) at www.cdc.gov/nchs/releases/98news/midwife.htm.

3. Laura Meckler, "The Doctor's Still in, but New Study Finds Midwives on the Increase," The Associated Press, ABCNEWS.com, December 2, 1999.

4. Northern New Mexico Women's Health and Birth Center, GBS fact sheet.

5. Barbara Harper, *Gentle Birth Choices,* 27; Natalie Angier, *Woman: An Intimate Geography,* 148; and Professor Leah Albers, correspondence with the author January 22, 2002.

CHAPTER TWELVE

1. Pam England, *Birthing from Within: An Extra-Ordinary Guide to Childbirth Preparation* (Albuquerque, NM: Partera Press, 1998), 32–33.

2. Della Pollock, *Telling Bodies, Performing Birth,* 17.

3. Ibid., 15.

4. Beth Weinhouse, "Hard Labor," *Parents* (August 1999), 90–5.

CONCLUSIONS

1. Judith Pence Rooks, "The Midwifery Model of Care," *Journal of Nurse-Midwifery,* vol. 44 no. 4 (July/August 1999), 370, 373.

2. Mary Breckenridge, *Wide Neighborhoods: A Story of the Frontier Nursing Service* (Lexington, University Press of Kentucky, 1981); Barbara Ehrenreich and Deirdre English, *Witches, Midwives, and Nurses: A History of Women Healers* (New York, The Feminist Press, 1973); Sheila Kitzinger, ed., *The Midwife Challenge* (London: Pandora, 1988); Kitzinger, *Rediscovering Birth*; Judith Leavitt, *Brought to Bed: Childbearing in America*; J. B. Litoff, *The American Midwife Debate: A Sourcebook on Its Modern Origins* (New York: Greenwood Press, 1986); Jessica Mitford, *The American Way of Birth* (New York: Penguin Books, 1992); Ann Oakley, *The Captured Womb: A History of Medical Care of Pregnant Women* (New York: Basil Blackwell, 1984); Judith Rooks, *Midwifery and Childbirth in America*; Jean Towler and Joan Bramall, *Midwives in History and Society* (London and New York: Croom Helm, Ltd., 1986); Laurel Thatcher Ulrich, *A Midwife's Tale; The Life of Martha Ballard, Based on her Diary, 1785–1812* (New York: Vintage Books, 1991).

3. Della Pollock, *Telling Bodies, Performing Birth,* 11.

4. Ibid., 12–13.

5. Sheila Kitzinger, *Rediscovering Birth,* 9.

6. Robbie Davis-Floyd, *Birth as an American Rite of Passage,* 1–2.

7. Ibid., 2, 305.
8. Barbara Katz Rothman, *Recreating Motherhood,* 171.
9. www.cfmidwifery.org/resource/_fact3a.html.
10. Anne Lamott, *Bird by Bird: Some Instructions on Writing and Life* (New York: Pantheon Books, 1994), 164.
11. Barbara Katz Rothman, *Recreating Motherhood,* 170.
12. Adrienne Rich, *Of Woman Born,* 182.

RESOURCES

SUGGESTED READING

Angier, Natalie. *Woman: An Intimate Geography.* New York: Houghton Mifflin, 1999.

Arms, Suzanne. *Immaculate Deception II: Myth, Magic, & Birth.* Berkeley, CA: Celestrial Arts, 1996.

Armstrong, Penny and Sheryl Feldman. *A Midwife's Story.* New York: Ivy Books, 1986.

Balaskas, Janet. *Active Birth: The New Approach to Giving Birth Naturally.* Cambridge, MA: Harvard Common Press, 1992.

Buss, Fran Leeper. *La Partera: Story of a Midwife.* Ann Arbor, MI: The University of Michigan Press, 1980.

Chester, Penfield and Sarah Chester. *Sisters on a Journey: Portraits of American Midwives.* Rutgers, NJ: Rutgers University Press, 1997.

Dancy, Rahima Baldwin, *Special Delivery: A Guide To Creating the Birth You Want for You and Your Baby.* Berkeley, CA: Celestial Arts, 1986.

David-Floyd, Robbie. *Birth As An American Rite of Passage.* Berkeley, CA: University of California Press, 1992.

Davis, Elizabeth. *Heart & Hands: A Midwife's Guide to Pregnancy & Birth.* Berkeley, CA: Celestial Press, 1997.

Enrenreich, Barbara and Deirdre English. *Witches, Midwives, and Nurses: A History of Women Healers.* New York: The Feminist Press at The City University of New York, 1973.

England, Pam and Rob Horowitz. *Birthing From Within; An Extra-Ordinary Guide to Childbirth Preparation.* Albuquerque, NM: Partera Press, 1998.

Gaskin, Ina May. *Spiritual Midwifery.* Summertown, TN: The Book Publishing Company, 1990.

Goer, Henci. *The Thinking Woman's Guide to a Better Birth.* New York: Perigee, 1999.

Goer, Henci. *Obstetrical Myths Versus Research Realities: A Guide to the Medical Literature.* Westport, CT: Bergin & Garvey, 1995.

Harper, Barbara. *Gentle Birth Choices.* Rochester, VT: Healing Arts Press.

Kitzinger, Sheila. *Rediscovering Birth.* New York: Pocket Books, 2000.

Klaus, Marshall H., John H. Kennell, and Phyllis H. Klaus. *Mothering the Mother: How a Doula Can Help You Have a Shorter, Easier, and Healthier Birth.* Reading, MA: Perseus Books, 1993.

Leavitt, Judith Walzer. *Brought to Bed: Childbearing in America 1750–1950.* New York: Oxford University Press, 1986.

McCutcheon-Rosegg. *Natural Childbirth the Bradley Way.* New York: Plume, 1996.

Rooks, Judith Pence. *Midwifery and Childbirth in America.* Philadelphia: Temple University Press, 1997.

Rothman, Barbara Katz. *In Labor: Women and Power in the Birthplace.* New York: W.W. Norton, 1982, 1991.

Rothman, Barbara Katz, ed. *Encyclopedia of Childbearing: Critical Perspectives.* Phoenix, AZ: Oryx Press, 1993.

Van Olphen-Fehr, Juliana. *Diary of a Midwife.* Westport, CT: Bergin & Garvey, 1998.

PUBLICATIONS
Midwifery Today
P.O. Box 2672
Eugene, OR 97402
www.midwiferytoday.com

Mothering
PO Box 1690
Santa Fe, NM 87504
www.mothering.com

ORGANIZATIONS
Academy of Certified Birth Educators and Labor Support
    Professionals (ACBE)
2001 East Prairie Circle, Suite I
Olathe, KS 66062

(800) 444-8223
barb@acbe.com
www.acbe.com

American College of Nurse-Midwives (ACNM)
818 Connecticut Avenue NW, Suite 900
Washington, D.C. 20006
(202) 728-9860
info@acnm.org
www.midwife.org

Association of Labor Assistants & Childbirth Educators (ALACE)
P.O. Box 390436
Cambridge, MA 02139
(617) 441-2500
alacehq@aol.com
www.alace.org

Citizens for Midwifery
P.O. Box 82227
Athens, GA 30608-2227
(888) 236-4880
www.cfmidwifery.org

Doulas of North America (DONA)
13513 North Grove Drive
Apline, UT 84004
(888) 788-DONA (3662)
info@dona.org
www.dona.org

International Childbirth Education Association (ICEA)
P.O. Box 20048
Minneapolis, MN 55420
(952) 854-8660
www.icea.org

International Lactation Consultant Association (ILCA)
1500 Sunday Drive
Suite 102

Raleigh, NC 27607
(919) 787-5181
ilca@erols.com
www.ilca.org

La Leche League International
1400 North Meacham Rd.
Schaumburg, IL 60173
1-800-LALECHE
(847) 519-7730
lllihq@llli.org
www.lalecheleague.org

Lamaze International
2025 M Street NW, Suite 800
Washington, D.C. 20036-3309
(800) 368-4404
(202) 367-1128
www.lamaze.org

Midwives Alliance of North America (MANA)
4805 Lawrenceville Highway
Suite 116-279
Lilburn, GA 30047
(888) 923-MANA (6262)
info@mana.org
www.mana.org

INDEX

ACNM (American College of Nurse Midwives), 20, 96, 105
Active management of midwives, 110–11
AFP (alphafetoprotein) test, 42, 197–98
Albers, Leah, 90, 103, 197
Alphafetoprotein (AFP) test, 42, 197–98
Alternative medicines, 53, 54–55
American College of Nurse Midwives (ACNM), 20, 96, 105
Amniocentesis, 197, 198, 200, 201–2
Anderson, David, 165–66
Angier, Natalie, 45
Antibiotics, 101–2
Antibody screen, 61
Arms, Suzanne, 73, 162, 223
Aromatherapy, 55

Baby Friendly Hospitals (Unicef), 255
Background, midwives staying in, 27–28
Balancing midwifery, 129–42
    breaking of water, 134
    continuity of care, 120–22, 131–33
    decisions of patients, 105–8, 136
    doulas, 141–42
    epidurals, 135, 136
    family of patients and midwives, 132
    hospital boundaries, 130–31
    inducing labor, 140
    Joanne White, 129–37, 138–40, 141
    occiput posterior babies, 133
    pain reduction, 47, 58, 136, 140–41, 155
    parenting and midwifing, 129–31

Pitocin, 140
placenta birthing, 140
pushing, 138–39
umbilical cord, saving, 133, 134
Barrett, Nina, 164
B&B labor extract, 206–7
Beaded labor bracelet, 279–81, 283
Belly casting, 278–79
Belly dancing, 270–71
Birth art, 275–76, 290
Birth attendants. See Doulas
Birth ball, 284–85
Birth center, 239–69
    bleeding postpartum, 233, 235, 266, 267
    blood pressure, 245, 252, 261
    business aspects of, 252
    caesarean sections, 255
    calcium-magnesium, 247
    chart keeping by patient, 245
    chlorophyll, 253
    colostrum, 265–66
    competence, sense of, 251
    congestion, 250–51
    diet, 252–53
    digestive tightness, 253
    doctors at, 239, 242–43
    doulas, 244
    Elizabeth Gilmore, 239–40, 241–57, 268–69
    fetal kick counts, 250
    fetascope, 248
    Group B Strep (GBS) test, 262

Birth center (*cont.*)
  Heidi Rinehart, 243, 244
  hemorrhaging postpartum, 266, 267
  home birth, 243–44, 249, 261
  inducing labor, 256, 266
  IV for fluids, 267
  Joan Norris, 257–62, 264–68
  lochia, 261
  methergine, 266, 267
  obstetrician (local) and, 242–43
  patient participation, 245, 261, 262
  Pitocin, 266
  placenta previa, 242
  prenatal exams, 244–53, 260
  psychological side of labor, 250
  real birth-center birth, 268
  Rudy Fedrizzi, 243
  standards of care, 255–56
  temperature of newborn, 266–67, 268
  ultrasound (Doppler), 247
  umbilical cord problems, 261
  urine test, 245, 260–61
  value of mothers, 246
Birth control, 49–50, 61–62, 67
Birth Cottage, 241
Birthing
  choices, need for, 297–300
  safety, 13–14, 53, 86, 159–60, 256
  See also Childbirth
Birthing from Within (England), 144, 183, 275
Birthing in awareness, 150
Bleeding
  checking in clinic, 47–48, 64
  postpartum, 233, 235, 266, 267
Blood pressure
  position and, 116
  readings, taking, 245, 252, 261
Blue/black cohosh, 206–7, 209
Boundaries in hospitals, 130–31
Bowling ball sensation, 274, 287
Bracelet, beaded labor, 279–81, 283
Bradley, Hasan, 222, 223, 230–35
Bradshaw, Julie, 173–79, 180–83, 205–15
Brain damage to baby, 216–17
Breaking of water
  balancing midwifery, 134
  Earth Day birthday, 284
  medical midwives, 100–101
Breast exams, 60
Breast-feeding
  choosing a midwife and, 187

  clinics and midwives, 44–45, 53, 66–67
  Earth Day birthday, 289
  home birth, 182
  hospitals and midwives, 27, 30
  medical midwives, 100
Breath awareness technique, 148–49
Breeches, 50
Brought to Bed: Childbearing in America (Leavitt), 219
Brown, Doreen, 104
Business aspects of birth center, 252

Caesarean births
  birth center, 255
  clinics and midwives, 50–51, 54, 65
  doula school, 157
  managed care, 72–73
  medical midwives, 104–5, 123–25
Calcium-magnesium, 247
Calling to be midwife, 223–24
Canadian birthing safety rates, 14
Candles from mother blessing, 283–84
Canova, Isabella, 107, 108
Carter, Nora, 170–71
Cascade of interventions, 104–5, 126
Castor oil, 8, 153
Catching your own baby, 232
Cephalopelvic disproportion (CPD), 116–17, 212–13
Certification of doulas, 162
Certified nurse-midwife (CNM), 4–5, 187–93
Chart keeping by patient, 245
Childbirth, 270–81
  beaded labor bracelet, 279–81, 283
  belly casting, 278–79
  belly dancing, 270–71
  birth art, 275–76, 290
  classes, 48, 270–78
  community from classes, 278
  crowning phase, 274
  distractions, dealing with, 273
  episiotomy vs. tearing, 182, 274
  foot massages, 149, 276, 277, 278
  hospital classes, 277–78
  hospitals for, 19–20, 21–22, 23–27
  ice water dramatization, 271–73
  images for labor, 276
  mother blessing, 279–81
  need for classes, 48
  nonfocused awareness, 272–73
  pain-coping techniques, 271–73

Pam England, 270–75, 278
partners and, 156, 276–77, 284, 285, 286, 288
positions for birthing, 273
pushing, 273–74
Sarah Walker-Adams, 279–81
squatting birth position, 273
tearing vs. episiotomy, 182, 274
See also Balancing midwifery; Birth center; Choosing a midwife; Doula school; Home birth; Medical midwives; Prenatal/conception; With women
Chlorophyll, 253
Choosing a midwife, 185–202
alphafetoprotein (AFP) test, 42, 197–98
amniocentesis, 197, 198, 200, 201–2
breast-feeding, 187
certified nurse-midwives, 4–5, 187–93
chorionic villi sampling (CVS), 198
disabled babies, 199–200
Down's syndrome babies, 197–99, 202
ectopic (tubal) pregnancies, 201
false positive test rates, 42, 198
home birth, 185–86, 188–89, 193, 195
hospital midwives, 186–87
Jane Elliott, 187–88, 196
power of birth, 3, 27, 35, 78, 126–28, 192, 230, 291
prenatal tests, 197–99, 200, 201, 202
Sarah Walker-Adams, 189–93, 195, 219–20
Chorionic villi sampling (CVS), 198
Chromosomal abnormalities, 42
Classes, childbirth, 48, 270–78
Clinics and midwives, 39–68
alphafetoprotein (AFP) test, 42, 197–98
alternative medicines, 53, 54–55
antibody screen, 61
birth control, 49–50, 61–62, 67
bleeding, checking, 47–48, 64
breast exams, 60
breast-feeding, 44–45, 53, 66–67
breeches, 50
caesarean births, 50–51, 54, 65
childbirth classes, need for, 48
chromosomal abnormalities, 42
culture clash, 44, 45–46
emotional situation of mother, 61, 62, 63–64
epidural risks, 57–59
false positive test rates, 42, 198

fevers from epidurals, 57–58
headaches, 64
heartbeat (baby's), 41–42, 60–61
herbs, 53, 54–55
inducing labor, 65
journaling, 53
Liz Donahue, 43, 60–68
low birth weight, 42
managed care's impact, 59–60
medical administrations and, 44, 45–46, 68
multiple births, 42, 50
Nancy Elder, 51–59
Native American clients, 52
neural tube defects, 42
nurses' opinions on midwives, 65
obstetricians vs., 54
pain reduction, 47, 58, 136, 155
pap smears, 49
postpartum exams, 52–54, 66–67
prenatal exams, 46–48, 56–58, 60–65
preterm labor, 61, 62
risk factors and obstetricians, 50
Sarah Walker-Adams, 41–51
sexual history of client, 49
social situation of mother, 61, 62
stretch marks, 47
support groups, 53
teen pregnancies, 55–56, 62–63
ultrasound (Doppler), 41–42, 42–43, 48, 60
vaginal births after caesarean (VBACS), 51
well-woman exams, 48–50, 49–50
work situations, 64–65
CNM (certified nurse-midwife), 4–5, 187–93
Coalition for the Improvement of Maternity Services, 255
Colostrum, 265–66
Community from classes, 278
Congestion during pregnancy, 250–51
Connecting with individuals, 89, 90–91
Continuity of care, 120–22, 131–33
Contractions
doula school, 154–56
Earth Day birthday, 284–88
women helping with, 230–32
Cost-effectiveness of midwives, 15, 87–88
Couvade (sympathy pains), 122
CPD (cephalopelvic disproportion), 116–17, 212–13

318   *Index*

Crowning phase, 274
Cultural blocks to home birth, 44, 45–46, 218, 295–96
Culture clash in clinics, 44, 45–46
Culture of childbirth, 229–30
Cutbacks at managed care facilities, 75–76, 84–85, 86, 88–89
CVS (chorionic villi sampling), 198

Davies, Alison, 83–84, 85, 125
Davis-Floyd, Robbie, 73, 295–96
Decisions of patients, 105–8, 136
Delegating tasks to family, 176–77
Deproprovera, 49, 50
Desire for children, 1–4
Diet, prenatal, 252–53
Digestive tightness, 253
Dillard, Annie, 3
Direct-entry (lay) midwives, 5, 226–27
Disabled babies, 199–200
Disappointment in birthing, 11, 13
Distractions, dealing with, 273
Doctors
  birth center and, 239, 242–43
  co-managing cases, 107–8, 115, 116, 122–26
  midwives vs., 14–15
  refusing hospital backup, 219
Donahue, Liz
  clinic midwife, 43, 60–68
  hospital midwife, 29–37
  managed care midwife, 72, 73–74, 75, 85, 86–88
  medical midwife, 125
Doppler. *See* Ultrasound
Doulas (birth assistants)
  balancing midwifery, 141–42
  birth center and, 244
  Earth Day birthday, 283, 285, 286, 287, 290
  roles of, 13, 145, 159
Doula school, 143–71
  birthing in awareness, 150
  breath awareness technique, 148–49
  caesarean sections, 157
  castor oil, 153
  certification of doulas, 162
  contractions, 154–56
  doula bag contents, 147–48
  drinking during labor, 153, 156
  drugs and labor, 150, 154
  eating during labor, 153

effectiveness of doulas, 146–47
epidurals, 160–61
experiences with doulas, 165–71
father's roles vs. doulas, 149
foot massages, 149
"If You Give an Elk an Epidural" (England), 160–61
institutional barriers, 160
labor portion of class, 153–58
low-income communities, 163
massage techniques, 148, 161–62
medicalization of childbirth, 158–59
Mommy stories, 159
Netherlands birthing safety rates, 13, 14, 159–60
nipple stimulation, 153
noises (power), 152–53, 156
nurses and doulas, 153–54, 156
open to ideas for birthing, 143–44, 151
pain and labor, 150–51, 152
pain-reduction techniques, 155
Pam England, 143–45, 149–54, 156–57, 158, 159–60, 163, 183
partners, helping, 156
positions for birthing, 151–52
postpartum depression, 159
postpartum visits, 147, 159
prenatal visualizations, 151–52
private clients, 163–64
pushing, 156–57
relaxation techniques, 148
rite of passage from pain, 151
role-playing sessions, 149
roles of, 13, 145, 159
slow labor, 153
suffering vs. pain, 152
touch breathing, 148
transitions, 155–56
Down's syndrome babies, 197–99, 202
Doyle, Heike, 119, 235–36
Dr. Susan Love's Breast Book (Love), 2
Drinking during labor, 153, 156
Drug-free pain reduction, 21–22
Drug influence on decisions, 97
Drugs and labor, doulas, 150, 154

Earth Day birthday, 282–91
  beaded labor bracelet, 279–81, 283
  birth ball, 284–85
  bowling ball sensation, 274, 287
  breaking of water, 284
  breast-feeding, 289

candles (lighting) from mother blessing, 283–84
contractions, 284–88
doulas, 283, 285, 286, 287, 290
expulsion phase, 287
home birth, 283–91
labor project, 284
nonfocused awareness, 285
partner and, 284, 285, 286, 288
perineums, 289–90
placenta birthing, 289
positions for birthing, 287
pushing, 287, 288
Sarah Walker-Adams, 284, 285, 286–91
stork bites, 289
transformative nature of birth, 3, 27, 35, 78, 126–28, 192, 230, 291
visualizing contractions, 282–83
vomiting before delivery, 288
water birth, 286
See also Home birth; Home birth challenges
Eating during labor, 153
Economic blocks to home birth, 218–19
Economic discussions at managed care facilities, 73–75, 82–83, 87
Ectopic (tubal) pregnancies, 201
Edmond, Gloria, 108–10
EFM (electronic fetal monitoring), 117–19
Eisner, Nima, 221–23, 230–35
Elder, Nancy
  clinic midwife, 51–59
  home birth midwife, 215, 216–18
  managed care midwife, 78–83, 88–90, 91–92
Electronic fetal monitoring (EFM), 117–19
Eliason-Ward, Anne
  managed care midwife, 85
  medical midwife, 107, 108
Elliott, Jane, 187–88, 196
Emotional situation of mother, 61, 62, 63–64
Empathy belly, 206
Energetic experience of crisis, 217–18
England, Pam
  childbirth, 270–75, 278
  doula school, 143–45, 149–54, 156–57, 158, 159–60, 163, 183
Epidurals
  benefits of, 297
  caesarean sections and, 104
  disadvantages of, 96, 97, 160–61

doctor-assisted births and, 37
  electronic fetal monitoring (EFM), 117
  fevers from, 57–58
  hospitals and, 30–31, 79, 90
  labor-sitting, 110
  maternal demand for, 90, 136
  midwives' view of, 106–7
  risks of, 57–59
Episiotomy vs. tearing, 182, 274
European birthing safety rates, 13, 86
Expulsion phase, 287

Failure to progress, 153, 228
False positive test rates, 42, 198
Family of patients
  home birth role, 176–77, 177–78
  midwives and, 132
Father's roles vs. doulas, 149
Fedrizzi, Rudy, 243
Feminist practice of midwifery, 298–99
Fennel seed tea, 53, 54
Fetal kick counts, 250
Fetascope, 248
Fevers from epidurals, 57–58
First trimester. *See* Balancing midwifery; Choosing a midwife; Doula school; Home birth; Medical midwives
First trimester exhaustion, 77
First vs. second birth, 77–78, 208
Foot massages, 149, 276, 277, 278
Frank, Yvonne, 166–69
Friedman, Emmanuel, 102
Frigoletto, Fredric, 118, 256
Fundal massage, 100

Gaskin, Ina May, 223–24, 224–25, 239, 260
Gelsinium, 207
Gilmore, Elizabeth, 239–40, 241–57, 268–69
Goer, Henci, 117, 162
Great Britain birthing safety rates, 13
Group B Strep (GBS) test, 262
Guide to Effective Care in Pregnancy and Childbirth, 103

Hamilton, Claire, 223, 231–35
Hansen, Maren, 11
Headaches during pregnancy, 64
Healy-Karr, Anne, 223–29, 231–35
Heartbeat (baby's), 41–42, 60–61

Hemorrhaging postpartum
  birth center, 266, 267
  medical midwives, 110–11, 112
  women helping with, 233, 235
Hep lock, 8
Herbs, 53, 54–55
Hern, Robin, 95–101, 105, 107–12
Herrera, Mandy, 96–97, 101, 103–4, 105
Hoffman, Tracy, 115–17, 119–20, 122, 124
Home birth, 172–84
  birth center and, 243–44, 249, 261
  breast-feeding, 182
  choosing midwife for, 185–86, 188–89,
    193, 195
  cultural blocks, 44, 45–46, 218, 295–96
  delegating tasks to family, 176–77
  doctors refusing hospital backup, 219
  economic blocks, 218–19
  family's role in, 176–77, 177–78
  hospitals and, 106–7, 122, 182, 185–86,
    212–14
  Julie Bradshaw, 173–79, 180–83
  malpractice insurance, 218
  meconium, 181
  medical model vs., 229–30, 236,
    293–94, 295
  nux vomica, 179
  peri bottle, 182
  perineum tears and, 182
  placenta birthing, 181
  pushing, 180–81
  religious community support of, 179
  siblings attending, 177–78
  ultrasound (Doppler), 175, 177
  umbilical cord cutting, 182
  vomiting during labor, 178, 288
  water birth, 176–82, 206–9, 210–11
  See also Earth Day birthday; Home
    birth challenges
Home birth challenges, 205–20
  B&B labor extract, 206–7
  blue/black cohosh, 206–7, 209
  brain damage to baby, 216–17
  cephalopelvic disproportion (CPD),
    212–13
  cultural blocks, 44, 45–46, 218, 295–96
  doctors refusing hospital backup, 219
  economic blocks, 218–19
  empathy belly, 206
  energetic experience of crisis, 217–18
  gelsinium, 207

  hospital, need for, 106–7, 122, 182,
    185–86, 212–14
  IV for fluids, 209
  Julie Bradshaw, 205–15
  malpractice insurance, 218
  meconium, 208, 217
  Nancy Elder, 215, 216–18
  neonatal resuscitation, 217
  position for birthing, 208
  pushing, 211–13
  retained placenta, 214
  rigid os, 208
  second vs. first birth, 208
  ultrasound (Doppler), 206, 210
  water birth, 176–82, 206–9, 210–11
Hospitals and midwives, 19–38
  background, midwives in, 27–28
  birthing environment, 19–20, 21–22,
    23–27
  boundaries on midwives, 125–26, 128,
    130–31
  breast-feeding, 27, 30
  childbirth classes, 48, 277–78
  choosing a midwife, 186–87
  drug-free pain reduction, 21–22
  epidurals, 30–31, 37
  home birth and, 106–7, 122, 182,
    185–86, 212–14
  Joanne White, 29, 36–37
  labor-delivery-recovery (LDR), 22
  Liz Donahue, 29–37
  nurses' opinions on midwives, 32
  placenta birthing, 27, 35–36
  positions for birthing, 25, 30, 33
  power of birth, 3, 27, 35, 78, 126–28,
    192, 230, 291
  pushing, 24–26, 31–34
  Ring of Fire, 26
  Sarah Walker-Adams, 20–28
  separating baby from mother, 37–38
  squat bar, 24, 33
  umbilical cord cutting, 27, 35
  vacuum (Mighty Vac), 34–35, 37
  water drinking during labor, 24
  women helping with birthing, 227–28
  See also Medical midwives
Hysterical pregnancy, 70

Ice water dramatization, 271–73
"If You Give an Elk an Epidural"
  (England), 160–61

Images for labor, 276
Immaculate Deception (Arms), 223
Inducing labor
   balancing midwifery and, 140
   birth center, 256, 266
   clinics and midwives, 65
   managed care, 79–80, 81
   medical midwives, 96, 97, 99, 100,
      102–4, 108, 110, 114, 120, 123
   prenatal decision, 8
   women helping with, 235
Infant death rates and midwives, 14
"Informed consent," 90
Institutional barriers to doulas, 160
Insurance companies, 75, 82–83, 88
Internal monitors, 117, 119
Intravenous (IV) drip, 7–8, 209, 267

Journaling, 53, 79

Kaplan, Jeremy, 72, 75, 76
Kegel exercises, 233–34
Kennell, John, 35, 147, 171
Kitzinger, Sheila, 159, 295
Klaus, Marshall, 35, 147
Klaus, Phyllis, 147
Kolesky, Janelle, 115–16

Labor and midwives, 7–11. *See also*
      Childbirth
Labor-delivery-recovery (LDR) room, 22
Labor portion of doula class, 153–58
Labor project, Earth Day birthday, 284
Labor-sitting, 96, 110
Lamott, Anne, 297
Lay (direct-entry) midwives, 5, 226–27
Layoffs at managed care facilities, 75–76,
      84–85, 86, 88–89
Lazarre, Jane, 164
LDR (labor-delivery-recovery) room, 22
Leaving an active patient, 95–96
Leavitt, Judith, 219, 294
Leiris, Michel, 217–18
Levine, Sharon, 163–64
Licensing of midwives, 225–26
Lieberman, Ellice, 58
Lithotomy position, 25
Lochia, 261
Love, Susan, 2
Low birth weight, 14, 42
Lower back pain relief, 78–79

Low-income communities, 163
Lucero, Maria, 60–62, 67
Lyon, George Ella, 36

Malpractice insurance, 218
Managed care midwives, 69–92
   Alison Davies, 83–84, 85
   Anne Eliason-Ward, 85
   birthing safety rates, 86
   caesarean births, 72–73
   clinics and, 59–60
   connecting with individuals, 89, 90–91
   cost-effectiveness of midwives, 15, 87–88
   cutbacks, 75–76, 84–85, 86, 88–89
   economic discussions, 73–75, 82–83, 87
   Elaine Romero, 72, 74
   epidurals, 79, 90
   inducing labor, 79–80, 81
   "informed consent," 90
   insurance companies, 75, 82–83, 88
   Joanne White, 74, 75, 85
   journaling, 79
   layoffs, 75–76, 84–85, 86, 88–89
   Liz Donahue, 72, 73–74, 75, 85, 86–88
   lower back pain relief, 78–79
   Nancy Elder, 78–83, 88–90, 91–92
   nighttime staffing of midwives, 74
   nurses' opinions on midwives, 85–86
   oxytocin, 80
   Pitocin, 79–80
   prenatal exams, 78–80
   profitability impact, 72
   reimbursement to midwives, 75, 76, 82,
      88
   staffing of midwives, 73, 74, 84
   support expectations of patients, 91
   time protocols, hospitals, 79, 81–82
   unnecessary intervention protection for
      patient, 91–92
   volume emphasis of, 80–81, 83, 90–91
Martin, Emily, 158
Martinez, Vicky, 95, 97–101
Massage techniques, doulas, 148, 161–62
Meconium, 109, 181, 208, 217
Medical administrations and midwives,
      44, 45–46, 68. *See also* Hospitals and
      midwives; Managed care
Medicalization of childbirth, 158–59
Medical midwives, 95–128
   active management, 110–11
   Alison Davies, 125

Medical midwives (*cont.*)
   Anne Eliason-Ward, 107, 108
   antibiotics, 101–2
   blood pressure and position, 116
   breaking of water, 100–101
   breast-feeding, 100
   caesarean sections, 104–5, 123–25
   cascade of interventions, 104–5, 126
   cephalopelvic disproportion (CPD),
      116–17
   continuity of care, 120–22, 131–33
   couvade (sympathy pains), 122
   decisions of patients, 105–8, 136
   doctors co-managing cases, 107–8,
      115, 116, 122–26
   drug influence on decisions, 97
   electronic fetal monitoring (EFM),
      117–19
   epidurals, 96, 97, 104, 106–7, 110, 117
   fundal massage, 100
   hemorrhaging postpartum, 110–11, 112
   home birth, 106–7, 122
   hospital boundaries, 125–26, 128
   inducing labor, 96, 97, 99, 100, 102–4,
      108, 110, 114, 120, 123
   internal monitors, 117, 119
   Janelle Kolesky, 115–16
   labor-sitting, 96, 110
   leaving an active patient, 95–96
   Liz Donahue, 125
   meconium, 109
   natural vs. normal childbirth, 126–27
   nipple stimulation, 97
   nursing situation and, 111–12
   "on the clock," 101–2, 105
   passive management, 111
   patients, choosing care, 105–6, 107–8
   physical vs. spiritual aspects of child-
      birth, 126–28
   Pitocin, 96, 97, 99, 100, 102–4, 108,
      110, 114, 120, 123
   placenta birthing, 99, 110, 111, 113
   positions for birthing, 95, 97, 98–99, 116
   preclampsia, 120
   prolonged labor, 102–3
   Robin Hern, 95–101, 105, 107–12
   Sarah Walker-Adams, 111–17, 119–24
   spiritual vs. physical aspects of child-
      birth, 126–28
   technology and midwives, 119
   therapeutic relationship, 96, 120–21
   traction on umbilical cord, 110, 111, 113
   umbilical cord cutting, 113, 114
   See also Hospitals and midwives
Medical model vs. home birth, 229–30,
   236, 293–94, 295
Methergine, 235, 266, 267
Midwifery and Childbirth in America
   (Rooks), 117–18
Midwives, 292–300
   benefits of, 292–95
   birthing choices, 297–300
   cultural blocks to home birth, 44, 45–46,
      218, 295–96
   feminist practice of midwifery, 298–99
   medical model vs. home birth, 229–30,
      236, 293–94, 295
   out-of-hospital births, 297
   team midwifery, 298
   See also Balancing midwifery; Birth
      center; Choosing a midwife; Doula
      school; Home birth; Medical mid-
      wives; Prenatal/conception; With
      women
Mighty Vac, 34–35, 37
Mitford, Jessica, 162
Mommy stories, doula school, 159
Morning sickness, 77
Mother blessing, 279–81
*Mothering the Mother: How a Doula Can
   Help You Have a Shorter, Easier, and
   Healthier Birth* (Klaus and Kennell),
   147
Mother Knot, The (Lazarre), 164
Mother Mysteries (Hansen), 11
Mother's milk tea, 53, 54
Multiple births, 42, 50

Natural vs. normal childbirth, 126–27
Neonatal resuscitation, 217
Netherlands birthing safety rates, 13, 14,
   159–60
Neural tube defects, 42
Nighttime staffing of midwives at man-
   aged care facilities, 74
Nipple stimulation, 97, 153
Noises (power), 152–53, 156
Nonfocused awareness, 272–73, 285
Normal vs. natural childbirth, 126–27
Norris, Joan, 257–62, 264–68
Norris, Kathleen, 270
Nurse-midwives, 5, 226–27
Nurses
   doulas and, 153–54, 156

medical midwives and, 111–12
midwives and, 32, 65, 85–86
Nux vomica, 179

Obstetrician (local) and birth center,
    242–43
Obstetricians vs. midwives, 54
*Obstetric Myths Versus Research Realities:
    A Guide to the Medical Literature*
    (Goer), 117
Occiput posterior babies, 133
Odent, Michel, 273
Of Woman Born (Rich), 152, 299
"On the clock," 101–2, 105
Open to ideas for birthing, 143–44, 151
Out-of-hospital births, 297
Owens, Michelle, 60
Oxytocin, 80

Pain and labor, doulas, 150–51, 152
Pain-coping techniques, 271–73
Pain of labor, 7–9, 11, 15–16
Pain reduction, 47, 58, 136, 140–41, 155
Pap smears, 49
Parenting and midwifing, 129–31
Partners and birth, 156, 276–77, 284,
    285, 286, 288
Passive management of midwives, 111
Patients
    choosing care, 105–6, 107–8
    participation with own care, 245, 261,
        262
Pelvic tone, 233–34
Peri bottle, 182
Perineums, 182, 274, 289–90
Physical vs. spiritual aspects of childbirth,
    126–28
Pitocin usage, 8
    balancing midwifery and, 140
    birth center, 266
    managed care, 79–80
    medical midwives, 96, 97, 99, 100,
        102–4, 108, 110, 114, 120, 123
    women helping with, 235
Placenta birthing
    balancing midwifery and, 140
    Earth Day birthday, 289
    home birth, 181
    hospitals, 27, 35–36
    medical midwives, 99, 110, 111, 113
    women helping with, 233
Placenta previa, 242

Play Group, The (Barrett), 164
Pollock, Della, 276–78, 294
Positions for birthing
    doula school, 151–52
    Earth Day birthday, 287
    home birth, 208
    hospitals and midwives, 25, 30, 33
    medical midwives, 95, 97, 98–99, 116
    squatting birth position, 273
Postpartum depression, 159
Postpartum exams
    clinics and midwives, 52–54, 66–67
    doulas, 147, 159
Power noises, 152–53, 156
Power of birth, 3, 27, 35, 78, 126–28,
    192, 230, 291
Preclampsia, 120
Pregnancy confirmed, 71–72
Prenatal/conception, 1–16
    castor-oil cocktail, 8
    certified nurse-midwife (CNM), 4–5,
        187–93
    cost-effectiveness of midwives, 15,
        87–88
    desire for children, 1–4
    direct-entry (lay) midwives, 5, 226–27
    disappointment in birthing, 11, 13
    doctors vs. midwives, 14–15
    doulas (birth assistants), 13
    first trimester exhaustion, 77
    hep lock, 8
    history of midwives, 14–15
    increase of midwives, 15
    inducing labor, 8
    infant death rates and midwives, 14
    intravenous (IV) drip, 7–8
    labor, 7–11
    low birth weight, 14
    midwives, 4–5, 12–13, 14
    morning sickness, 77
    pain of labor, 7–9, 11, 15–16
    Pitocin, 8
    power of birth, 3, 27, 35, 78, 126–28,
        192, 230, 291
    pregnancy confirmed, 71–72
    pushing phase, 9–10
    rooming in, 10
    safety rates of birthing, 13–14, 53, 86,
        159–60, 256
    second vs. first pregnancy, 77–78,
        208
Valsalva pushing, 10

Prenatal/conception (*cont.*)
  See also Clinics and midwives; Hospi-
    tals and midwives; Managed care
    midwives
Prenatal exams
  birth center, 244–53, 260
  clinics and midwives, 46–48, 56–58,
    60–65
  managed care midwives, 78–80
Prenatal tests, 197–99, 200, 201, 202
Prenatal visualizations, 151–52
Preterm labor, 61, 62
Private clients, doulas, 163–64
Profitability, managed care, 72
Prolonged labor, 102–3
Psychological side of labor, 250
Pushing
  balancing midwifery and, 138–39
  doula school, 156–57
  Earth Day birthday, 287, 288
  home birth, 180–81, 211–13
  hospitals and midwives, 24–26,
    31–34
  phase, 9–10, 273–74
  Valsalva pushing, 10
  women helping with, 232

Raphael, Dana, 145
Rattey, Phyllis, 118
Real birth-center birth, 268
Red raspberry tea, 55
Registered nurse (RN), 20
Reimbursement from managed care, 75,
    76, 82, 88
Relaxation techniques, 148
Religious support of home birth, 179
Retained placenta, 214
Rich, Adrienne, 152, 299
Rigid os, 208
Riley, Maureen, 107, 108
Rinehart, Heidi, 243, 244
Ring of Fire, 26
Risk factors and obstetricians, 50
Rite of passage from pain, 151
Rogers, Pattiann, 174
Role-playing sessions, 149
Romero, Elaine, 72, 74
Rooks, Judith Pence, 15, 117–18, 293
Rooming in, 10
Rothman, Barbara Katz, 158, 296,
    298–99

Safer Motherhood Initiative (WHO), 255
Safety rates of birthing, 13–14, 53, 86,
    159–60, 256
Second trimester. *See* Home birth chal-
    lenges; With women
Second vs. first birth, 77–78, 208
Separating baby from mother, 37–38
Sexual history of client, 49
Shepherd's purse, 235
Siblings attending home birth, 177–78
Sidoli, Emmanuela, 97
Slow labor, 153, 228
Social situation of mother, 61, 62
Spirituality of childbirth, 3, 27, 35, 78,
    126–28, 192, 230, 291
Spiritual Midwifery (Gaskin), 223, 239, 260
Spouses and birth, 156, 276–77, 284,
    285, 286, 288
Squat bar, 24, 33
Squatting birth position, 273
Staffing of midwives at managed care
    facilities, 73, 74, 84
Standards of care for women, 255–56
Stork bites, 289
Stretch marks, 47
Suffering vs. pain, 152
Support expectations of patients, 91
Support groups, 53
Sympathy pains (couvade), 122

Team midwifery, 298
Tearing vs. episiotomy, 182, 274
Teas, 53, 54, 55
Technology and midwives, 119
Teen pregnancies, 55–56, 62–63
Telling Bodies, Performing Birth (Pollock),
    276
Temperature of newborn, 266–67, 268
Textbook of Medical Physiology, The, 68
Therapeutic relationship, 96, 120–21
Third trimester. *See* Birth center; Child-
    birth; Earth Day birthday
Time protocols of hospitals, 79, 81–82
Touch breathing, 148
Traction on umbilical cord, 110, 111, 113
Transformative nature of birth, 3, 27, 35,
    78, 126–28, 192, 230, 291
Transitions, 155–56
Transports to hospitals, 228–29
Tubal (ectopic) pregnancies, 201
Twilight sleep, 22

Ultrasound (Doppler)
  birth center, 247
  clinic midwives, 41–42, 42–43,
    48, 60
  home birth, 175, 177, 206, 210
Umbilical cord
  home birth cutting of, 182
  hospital cutting of, 27, 35
  medical midwives cutting of,
    113, 114
  saving, 133, 134
  wrapped around baby, 232–33, 261
UNICEF, 44, 255
United States birthing safety rates, 13, 14,
    15, 256
Unnecessary intervention protection for
    patient, 91–92
Urine test, 245, 260–61

Vacuum (Mighty Vac), 34–35, 37
Vaginal births after caesarean (VBACS), 51
Valsalva pushing, 10
Value of mothers, 246
Venus of Willendorf, 280
Visualizing contractions, 282–83
Volume emphasis of managed care, 80–
    81, 83, 90–91
Vomiting during labor, 178, 288

Wagner, Marsden, 229–30
Walker-Adams, Sarah
  choosing a midwife, 189–93, 195,
    219–20
  clinic midwife, 41–51
  Earth Day birthday, 284, 285, 286–91
  hospital midwife, 20–28
  medical midwife, 111–17, 119–24
  mother blessing, 279–81
Water birth
  Earth Day birthday, 286
  home birth, 176–82, 206–9, 210–11
  women helping with, 231–32
Water breaking. *See* Breaking of water
Water drinking during labor, 24
Weil, Simone, 152
Well-woman exams, 48–50, 49–50

White, Joanne
  balancing midwifery, 129–37, 138–40,
    141
  hospital midwife, 29, 36–37
  managed care midwife, 74, 75, 85
With women, 221–36
  Anne Healy-Karr, 223–29, 231–35
  bleeding postpartum, 233, 235, 266, 267
  calling to be midwife, 223–24
  catching your own baby, 232
  challenges of, 236
  Claire Hamilton, 223, 231–35
  contractions, 230–32
  culture of childbirth, 229–30
  direct-entry vs. nurse-midwives, 5,
    226–27
  failure to progress, 153, 228
  hemorrhaging postpartum, 233, 235
  hospital births, 227–28
  inducing labor, 235
  kegel exercises, 233–34
  licensing of midwives, 225–26
  medical model vs. home birth, 229–30,
    236, 293–94
  methergine, 235
  nurse-midwives vs. direct-entry mid-
    wives, 5, 226–27
  pelvic tone, 233–34
  Pitocin, 235
  placenta birthing, 233
  power to give birth, 3, 27, 35, 78,
    126–28, 192, 230, 291
  pushing, 232
  shepherd's purse, 235
  transports to hospitals, 228–29
  umbilical cord, unwrapping, 232–33
  water birth, 231–32
Wolfe, Naomi, 162
Woman: An Intimate Geography (Angier), 45
Women with infants and children (WIC),
    62
Work situations, 64–65
World Health Organization (WHO),
    42–43, 44, 73, 229, 255, 297

Yale University, 21, 114, 190, 191, 224

ABOUT THE AUTHOR

Catherine Taylor's articles have appeared in *Premiere, Rolling Stone, New York Woman,* and *The Oxford Companion to Women's Writing in the United States*. She co-founded the Human Rights Watch Film Festival in New York City and has served as a producer, writer, and researcher on a number of PBS projects. For the past ten years, she has taught writing to pregnant teens and at-risk populations. She is the founder and editor of *The Harwood Review,* a literary magazine based in New Mexico. Catherine has taught English at Duke University and at the University of New Mexico. She attended Cornell and Oxford universities and has a Ph.D. from Duke University. She lives with her family in New Mexico.